CARDIOVASCULAR DISEASE IN DIABETES

DEVELOPMENTS IN CARDIOVASCULAR MEDICINE

120. R. Vos: Drugs Looking for Diseases. Innovative Drug Research and the Development of the Beta Blockers and the Calcium Antagonists. 1991. ISBN 0-7923-0968-5.
121. S. Sideman, R. Beyar and A.G. Kleber (eds.): Cardiac Electrophysiology, Circulation, and Transport. Proceedings of the 7th Henry Goldberg Workshop (Berne, Switzerland, 1990). 1991. ISBN 0-7923-1145-0.
122. D.M. Bers: Excitation-Contraction Coupling and Cardiac Contractile Force. 1991. ISBN 0-7923-1186-8.
123. A.-M. Salmasi and A.N. Nicolaides (eds.): Occult Atherosclerotic Disease. Diagnosis, Assessment and Management. 1991. ISBN 0-7923-1188-4.
124. J.A.E. Spaan: Coronary Blood Flow. Mechanics, Distribution, and Control. 1991. ISBN 0-7923-1210-4.
125. R.W. Stout (ed.): Diabetes and Atherosclerosis. 1991. ISBN 0-7923-1310-0.
126. A.G. Herman (ed.): Antithrombotics. Pathophysiological Rationale for Pharmacological Interventions. 1991. ISBN 0-7923-1413-1.
127. N.H.J. Pijls: Maximal Myocardial Perfusion as a Measure of the Functional Significance of Coronary Arteriogram. From a Pathoanatomic to a Pathophysiologic Interpretation of the Coronary Arteriogram. 1991. ISBN 0-7923-1430-1.
128. J.H.C. Reiber and E.E. v.d. Wall (eds.): Cardiovascular Nuclear Medicine and MRI. Quantitation and Clinical Applications. 1992. ISBN 0-7923-1467-0.

CARDIOVASCULAR DISEASE IN DIABETES

Proceedings of the Symposium on the Diabetic Heart sponsored by the Council of Cardiac Metabolism of the International Society and Federation of Cardiology and held in Tokyo, Japan, October 1989.

edited by

Makoto Nagano
Seibu Mochizuki
Department of Internal Medicine
Jikei University School of Medicine
Tokyo, Japan

Naranjan S. Dhalla
Division of Cardiovascular Sciences
St. Boniface General Hospital Research Centre
University of Manitoba, Winnipeg, Canada

Springer Science+Business Media, LLC

Library of Congress Cataloging-in-Publication Data

International Symposium on the Diabetic Heart (1989: Tokyo, Japan)
    Cardiovascular disease in diabetes : proceedings of the Symposium on the Diabetic Heart / sponsored by the Council of Cardiac Metabolism of the International Society and Federation of Cardiology held in Tokyo, Japan, October 1989 ; edited by Makoto Nagano, Seibu Mochizuki, Naranjan S. Dhalla.
        p cm. — (Developments in cardiovascular medicine : 130)
    ISBN 978-1-4613-6558-7   ISBN 978-1-4615-3512-6 (eBook)
    DOI 10.1007/978-1-4615-3512-6
    1. Cardiovascular system—Diseases—Congresses. 2. Diabetes--Complications and sequelae—Congresses. I. Nagano, Makoto, 1928–
  II. Mochizuki, Seibu. III. Dhalla, Naranjan S. IV. Council on Cardiac Metabolism. V. Title. VI. Series: Developments in cardiovascular medicine ; v. 130.
    DNLM: 1. Diabetes Mellitus—complications—congresses. 2. Heart Diseases—diagnosis—congresses. 3. Heart Diseases—drug therapy--congresses. 4. Heart Diseases—physiopathology—congresses. W1 DE997VME v. 130 / / WK 835 I588c 1989]
RC669.I64 1989
616.1—dc20
DNLM/DLC
for Library of Congress   91-35388
                                                                                 CIP

Copyright © 1992 by Springer Science+Business Media New York
Originally published by Kluwer Academic Publishers in 1992
Softcover reprint of the hardcover 1st edition 1992

All rights reserved. No part of this publication may be reproduced, stored in a retrieval system or transmitted in any form or by any means, mechanical, photocopying, recording, or otherwise, without the prior written permission of the publisher, Springer Science+Business Media, LLC

This book is dedicated
with great admiration to our wives

Brigitte Nagano
Kimi Mochizuki
Ranjit Dhalla

for their inspiration, understanding and support.

Contents

Preface xiii

Acknowledgements xv

A. Evaluation of Cardiovascular Problems in Diabetes

1. Assessment of cardiac function in diabetic patients by impedance cardiography 3
   H. Sasaki, K. Yokota, T. Mizokami, M. Shimizu, H. Yamada and Y. Isogai
   Third Department of Internal Medicine, Jikei University School of Medicine, Tokyo, Japan; Fuji Medical Center, Shizuoka Pref., Japan

2. Early diastolic dysfunction of left ventricle and its relation to pathologic finding in patients with diabetes mellitus 9
   M. Shimizu, N. Sugihara, Y. Kita, K. Shimizu, M. Minamoto and R. Takeda
   Second Department of Internal Medicine, School of Medicine, Kanazawa University, Kanazawa, Japan

3. Radionuclide assessment of left ventricular function in middle-aged asymptomatic non-insulin-dependent diabetic patients 21
   I. Yasuda, K. Kawakami, T. Shimada, K. Tanigawa, R. Murakami, S. Izumi, S. Morioka, Y. Kato and K. Moriyama
   Fourth and First Departments of Internal Medicine, Shimane Medical University, Izumo, Japan

4. Usefulness of exercise Tl-201 myocardial scintigraphy to detect asymptomatic heart disease in diabetic patients 35
   K. Kawakami, I. Yasuda, T. Shimada, R. Murakami, S. Morioka, K. Tanigawa, Y. Kato and K. Moriyama
   Fourth Department of Internal Medicine, Shimane Medical University, Izumo-city, Shimane-prefecture, Japan

5. Autonomic function test assessed by ambulatory ECG in diabetes
   K. Aihara, I. Taniguchi, S. Kageyama and Y. Isogai 47
   Third Department of Internal Medicine, Jikei University School of Medicine, Tokyo, Japan

6. Diabetic albuminuria and ischemic heart disease
   J. Ishiguro, T. Tsuda, T. Izumi, S. Ito and A. Shibata 53
   First Department of Internal Medicine, Niigata University School of Medicine, Niigata, Japan

7. Prognostic significance of treadmill exercise stress test in diabetic patients without cardiovascular signs 61
   K. Kawakubo, J. Oku, T. Murakami and T. Sugimoto
   Department of Health Administration, School of Health Science and Second Department of Internal Medicine, Faculty of Medicine, University of Tokyo, Tokyo, Japan

8. Coronary artery bypass grafting in the diabetic heart: Myocardial
   tolerance during surgery and late result   69
   M. Sunamori, T. Maruyama, J. Amano, H. Tanaka, H. Fujiwara, T. Sakamoto
   and A. Suzuki
   *Department of Thoracic-Cardiovascular Surgery, Tokyo Medical and Dental
   University, School of Medicine, Yushima, Tokyo, Japan*

B. Interactions of Diabetes and Hypertension

9. The influence of diabetes on myocardial contractility and energetics in
   spontaneously hypertensive rats   77
   N. Takeda, I. Nakamura, T. Ohkubo, A. Tanamura, T. Iwai, M. Kato, K.
   Noma and M. Nagano
   *Department of Internal Medicine, Aoto Hospital, Jikei University School
   of Medicine, Tokyo, Japan*

10. Hypertensive-diabetic cardiomyopathy in rats   85
    A. Malhotra
    *Department of Medicine, Montefiore Medical Center and Albert Einstein
    College of Medicine, Bronx, USA*

11. Combined effects of hypertension and diabetes on myocardial contractile
    proteins and cardiac function in rats   95
    M. Kato, N. Takeda, E. Kazama, J. Yang, T. Asano, H.Q. Yin and M. Nagano
    *Department of Internal Medicine, Aoto Hospital, Jikei University School
    of Medicine, Tokyo, Japan*

12. Diabetes does not accelerate cardiac hypertrophy in spontaneously
    hypertensive rats (SHR)   109
    T. Sato, Y. Nara, Y. Kato and Y. Yamori
    *Departments of Internal Medicine and Pathology, Shimane Medical
    University, Izumo, Japan*

13. A close correlation of fasting insulin levels to blood pressure in obese
    children   115
    H. Kanai, Y. Matsuzawa, S. Fujioka, K. Tokunaga and S. Tarui
    *Second Department of Internal Medicine, Osaka University Medical School,
    Osaka, Japan*

C. Pathophysiological Aspects of Cardiovascular Dysfunction in Diabetes

14. Cardiovascular involvements in a new spontaneously diabetic (WBN/Kob)
    rat   127
    Y. Sakaguchi, S. Kato, A. Fujimoto, S. Tsuruta, M. Tsuchihashi, A.
    Kawamoto, S. Uemura, Y. Nishida, S. Fujimoto, T. Hashimoto, T.
    Kagoshima, H. Ishikawa and R. Okada
    *First Department of Internal Medicine, Nara Medical University, Nara,
    Japan; Labo. for Cardiovasc. Research of Internal Medicine, Juntendo
    University, Tokyo, Japan*

15. Biochemical and morphologic alterations in cardiac myocytes in
    streptozotocin-induced diabetic rats 139
    T. Katagiri, Y. Umezawa, Y. Suwa, E. Geshi, T. Yanagishita and M. Yaida
    *Third Department of Internal Medicine, Showa University School of
    Medicine, Tokyo, Japan*

16. Diabetes prolongs the action potential duration in rat ventricular
    muscle probably via enhanced calcium current 155
    S. Nobe, M. Aomine, M. Arita, S. Ito and R. Takaki
    *Departments of Physiology and Medicine, Medical College of Oita, Oita,
    Japan*

17. Increases in voltage-sensitive calcium channel of cardiac and skeletal
    muscle in streptozotocin-induced diabetic rats 173
    A. Kashiwagi, Y. Nishio, T. Ogawa, S. Tanaka, M. Kodama, T. Asahina, M.
    Ikebuchi and Y. Shigeta
    *Third Department of Medicine, Shiga University of Medical Science,
    Shiga, Japan*

18. Changes in cell morphology, $[Ca^{2+}]_i$ and pH_i during metabolic
    inhibition in isolated myocytes of diabetic rats using dual-loading of
    fura-2 and BCECF 183
    H. Hayashi, N. Noda, H. Miyata, S. Suzuki, A. Kobayashi, M. Hirano, T.
    Kawai, T. Hayashi and N. Yamazaki
    *Third Department of Internal Medicine and Medical Photonics, Hamamatsu
    University School of Medicine, Hamamatsu, Japan; Hamamatsu Photonics
    K.K., Hamamatsu, Japan*

19. Abnormal phosphorylation: Cause of reduced responsiveness to
    isoproterenol in diabetic heart 199
    S.W. Schaffer, S. Allo and G. Wilson
    *Departments of Pharmacology and Anatomy, University of South Alabama
    School of Medicine, Mobile, USA*

20. Electron microscopic cytochemical studies on ATPase and acid phosphatase
    activities of cardiac myocytes in streptozotocin induced diabetic rats
    Y. Suwa, Y. Umezawa, M. Yaida, Y. Takeyama and T. Katagiri 211
    *Third Department of Internal Medicine, Showa University School of
    Medicine, Tokyo, Japan*

21. Myocardial isoenzyme distribution in chronic diabetes: Comparison with
    isoproterenol-induced chronic myocardial damage 225
    H. Hashimoto, Y. Awaji, Y. Matsui, K. Kawaguchi, N. Akiyama, K. Okumura,
    T. Ito and T. Satake
    *Second Department of Internal Medicine, Nagoya University School of
    Medicine, Nagoya, Japan*

22. In vivo ^{31}-NMR spectroscopic investigation of myocardial energy
    metabolism in alloxan-induced diabetic rabbits 237
    T. Misawa, Y. Kutsumi, H. Tada, S. Hayashi, H. Kato, H. Nishio, K.
    Toyoda, S. Kim, R. Fujiwara, T. Hayashi, T. Nakai and S. Miyabo
    *Third Department of Internal Medicine, Fukui Medical School, Fukui,
    Japan*

23. Characterization of beta-adrenoceptors in sinoatrial node and left
    ventricular myocardium of diabetic rat hearts by quantitative   251
    autoradiography
    K. Saito, A. Kuroda and H. Tanaka
    Health Service Center of National Institute of Fitness and Sports,
    Kanoya, Japan; First Department of Internal Medicine, Faculty of
    Medicine, Kagoshima University, Kagoshima, Japan

24. Effects of zinc deficiency on heart catecholamine concentrations in
    normal and diabetic rats   261
    H. Fushimi, S. Ishihara, M. Kameyama, T. Minami and Y. Okazaki
    Department of Medicine and Laboratory of Sumitomo Hospital; Department
    of Pharmacology, Kinki University, Osaka, Japan

25. Atrial natriuretic peptide levels in plasma and atrial auricles of the
    non-obese diabetic (NOD) mouse   267
    S. Yano, Y. Kobayashi, K. Tanigawa, S. Suzuki, T. Shimada, S. Morioka,
    Y. Kato and K. Moriyama
    First and Fourth Departments of Internal Medicine, Department of
    Pharamcology, Institute of Experimental Animals, Shimane Medical
    University, Izumo, Japan

D. Pharmacological and Therapeutic Aspects of Diabetic Heart

26. Effects of beta-adrenoceptor blocking agents on myocardium isolated from
    experimentally diabetic rats   283
    F. Nagamine, R. Sunagawa, K. Murakami, M. Sakanashi and G. Mimura
    Second Department of Internal Medicine and Department of Pharmacology,
    School of Medicine, Faculty of Medicine, University of the Ryukyus,
    Okinawa, Japan

27. Effects of autonomic agents on isolated and perfused hearts of
    streptozotocin-induced diabetic rats   297
    R. Sunagawa, F. Nagamine, K. Murakami, G. Mimura and M. Sakanashi
    Second Department of Internal Medicine and Department of Pharmacology,
    School of Medicine, Faculty of Medicine, University of the Ryukyus,
    Okinawa, Japan

28. Insulin-like actions of vanadyl sulfate trihydrate in streptozotocin-
    diabetic rats   315
    M.C. Cam and J.H. McNeill
    Division of Pharmacology and Toxicology, Faculty of Pharmaceutical
    Sciences, University of British Columbia, Vancouver, Canada

29. Different cardiac effects of hypoglycaemic sulphonylurea compounds   333
    Z. Aranyi, G. Ballagi-Pordány, M.Z. Koltai and G. Pogátsa
    National Institute of Cardiology, Budapest, Hungary

30. Reversibility of diabetic cardiomyopathy by therapeutic interventions in
    mild diabetes   349
    D. Stroedter, M. Schmitt, T. Broetz, K. Federlin and W. Schaper
    Third Medical Clinic and Policlinic, University of Geissen, Germany;
    Max-Planck-Institute, Bad Nauheim, Germany

31. Improvement of myocardial function and metabolism in diabetic rats by the carnitine palmitoyltransferase inhibitor etomoxir 361
    P. Rösen, F.J. Schmitz and H. Reinauer
    Department of Clinical Biochemistry, Diabetes-Forschungsinstitut, Düsseldorf, Germany

32. Abnormal mitochondrial oxidative phosphorylation of ischaemic and reperfused myocardium reversed by L-propionyl-carnitine 373
    R. Ferrari, E. Pasini, A. Cargnoni, E. Condorelli, F. De Giuli and A. Albertini
    Chair of Cardiology and Chemistry, University of Brescia, Brescia, Italy

Preface

It is now well known that a wide variety of cardiovascular complications are associated with diabetes. Although it is commonly held that macroangiopathy and microangiopathy occurring during the development of diabetes are responsible for the genesis of cardiovascular complications, critical evidence in this regard is still lacking in both diabetic patients and animal models of diabetes. In fact, cardiomyopathy has been identified to occur in the absence of the above mentioned pathological conditions in diabetics as well as in experimental animals. Accordingly, it is conceivable that dramatic changes in cardiac, vascular, endothelial, nerve and renal cells may occur independently or in association depending upon the stage and severity of diabetes. In addition, insulin deficiency or reduced responsiveness of organs to insulin can be seen to produce dramatic changes in cellular metabolism. Such changes directly or indirectly may result in restructuring of components in all cells including cardiac and vascular myocytes and thus may alter their functional behaviour. Irrespective of the mechanisms for the pathophysiology of cardiovascular dysfunction in diabetes, it has become clear that diabetes is an important risk factor for the ischemic heart disease. Furthermore, the combination of hypertension with diabetes has been demonstrated to result in congestive heart failure. It is therefore necessary to pay more attention to cardiovascular problems if we are to prolong the life span of diabetic patients.

In an attempt to clarify the situation regarding the diagnosis, pathogenesis and therapeutics of cardiovascular dysfunction in diabetes, an International Symposium on Diabetic Heart was held in Tokyo, Japan during October, 1989. Thirty-two selected articles from the poster presentations, compiled in this book, have been grouped in four sections, namely (a) Evaluation of Cardiovascular Problems, (b) Interactions of Diabetes and Hypertension, (c) Pathophysiological Aspects of Cardiovascular Dysfunction in Diabetes, and (d) Pharmacological and Therapeutic Aspects of Diabetic Heart for the sake of convenience for our readers. We hope that the contents of these chapters will provide adequate information regarding the current status of cardiovascular abnormalities in diabetes and this book will be of great interest to both clinical and experimental cardiologists as well as endocrinologists interested in diabetes.

Acknowledgements

We express our sincere appreciation to the Japanese Heart Foundation and several Japanese pharmaceutical companies for their generous financial support for the organization of the International Symposium on Diabetic Heart and the publication of this volume. The cooperation of the Council of Cardiac Metabolism of the International Society and Federation of Cardiology helped us to obtain high quality scientific contributions by well established investigators. Untiring efforts of Drs. N. Takeda, M. Kato and other members of the Department of Internal Medicine, Aoto Hospital during the organization of this conference contributed greatly to the success of this project. The help of Mary Brown, Kari Ausland and Florence Willerton for the preparation of this book is highly appreciated. Special thanks are also due to the editorial staff of Kluwer Academic Publishers, Boston for their interest and patience in compiling this book.

A. EVALUATION OF CARDIOVASCULAR PROBLEMS IN DIABETES

Assessment of Cardiac Function in Diabetic Patients by Impedance Cardiography

H. Sasaki, K. Yokota, T. Mizokami, M. Shimizu, H. Yamada* and Y. Isogai

*Third Department of Internal Medicine, The Jikei University School of Medicine, Tokyo, 105 JAPAN. *Fuji Medical Center, Shizuoka Pref., 417 JAPAN.*

Introduction

Although it has been known that cardiac dysfunction occurs in diabetes mellitus, there are only a few detailed reports on cardiac performance. In diabetics, cardiac function at postural stress and treadmill exercise test was measured by impedance method. In this study, the relationships among cardiac performance in diabetics and the degree of diabetic retinopathy as well as the duration of diabetes were investigated.

Materials and Methods

The subjects consisted of 23 patients (NIDDM; 9 males and 14 females, mean age 43.6 ± 9.7 years). Patients were divided into 2 groups according to the duration of diabetes and the degree of diabetic retinopathy (Table 1). Twenty healthy volunteers (9 males and 11 females, mean age 40.0 ± 8.0 years) served as a control group. No case in these groups had any cardiovascular complications and any abnormal findings in ECG and Master's double stress test.

Measurement of cardiac function

Cardiac function was measured by impedance cardiography (Bomed Co. Ltd. Model NCCOM-3^R) at postural stress and exercise test. Postural stress is physiological volume load from standing position to supine position. In the exercise test, we used the treadmill and the load level was three times oxygen consumption (VO_2) at rest. SV (stroke volume) and EVI (ejection velocity index) were used as parameters of cardiac function. Those parameters were calculated by impedance cardiography. EVI is also one of the parameter of cardiac contractility.

Nagano, M., Mochizuki, S., Dhalla, N.S. (eds.), CARDIOVASCULAR DISEASE IN DIABETES. Copyright © 1992. Kluwer Academic Publishers, Boston. All rights reserved.

Table 1. Subjects   y.o.: years old

DM(NIDDM) Group

    23 cases (9 males, 14 females)
    Ages 43.6 ± 9.7 y.o. (mean ± S.D.)

    Duration of Diabetes
        short (group s), ~ 5 years   11 cases
        medium (group m), 5 ~ 10 years   7 cases
        long (group l), 10 years   5 cases

    Duration of Diabetic Retinopathy
        None (group N)   10 cases
        Simplex (group S)   8 cases
        Proliferative (group P)   4 cases

Control Group

    20 cases (9 males, 11 females)
    Age 40.0 ± 8.0 y.o. (mean ± S.D.)

SV (stroke volume) and EVI (ejection velocity index) were used as parameters of cardiac function. Those parameters were calculated by impedance cardiography. EVI is also one of the parameters of cardiac contractility.

Statistical analysis

Results were expressed as mean ± S.D. Statiscal signifance was established by Student's t-test.

Results

At postural stress, increased ratio of SV and EVI in diabetics were significantly lower than those of normal subjects (Fig. 1,2,3,4). These findings were seen in accordance with the degree of retinopathy and the duration of diabetes (Fig. 1,2,3,4).

At treadmill exercise, increased ratio of SV and EVI in diabetics were significantly lower than those of normal subjects (Fig.5,6,7,8). Remarkably, increased ratio of SV was seen in accordance with the degree of retinopathy, the duration of diabetics (Fig. 5,6,7,8).

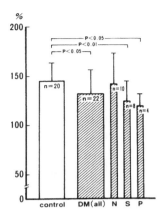

Fig. 1. The relationship between change in ratio of SV at postural stress and the of retinopathy.
SV: stroke volume, N: group N,
S: group S, P: group P.

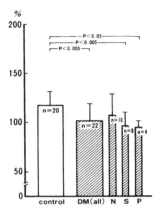

Fig. 2 The relationship between change in ratio of EVI at degree postural stress and the degree of retinopathy.
EVI: ejection velocity index,
N: group N, S: group S,
P: group P.

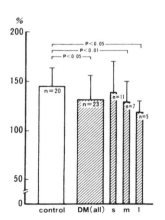

Fig. 3 The relationship between change in ratio of SV at postural stress and the duration of diabetes.

SV: stroke volume, s: group s,
m: group m, l: group l

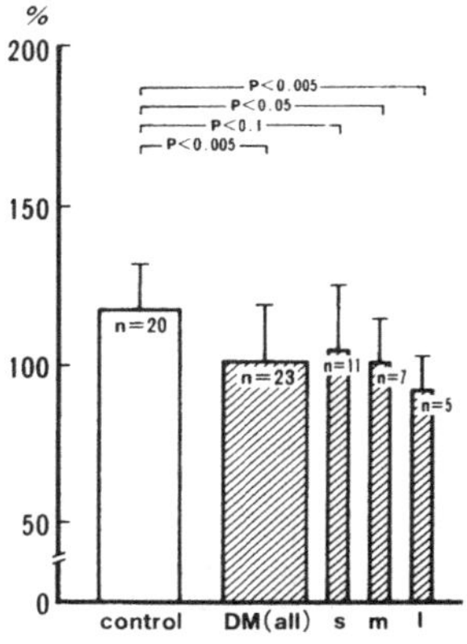

Fig. 4 The relationship between change in ratio of EVI at postural stress and the duration of diabetes.
EVI: ejection velocity index,
s: group s, m: group m,
l: group l.

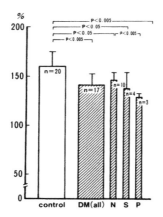

Fig. 5 The relationship between change in ratio of SV during exercise and the degree of retinopathy.
SV: stroke volume, N: group N,
S: group N, P: group P.

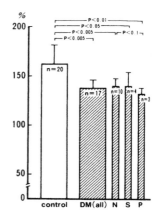

Fig. 6 The relationship between change in ratio of EVI during exercise and the degree of retinopathy.
EVI: ejection velocity index,
N: group N, S: group S,
P: group P.

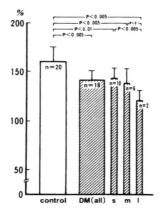

Fig. 7 The relationship between change in ratio of SV during exercise and the duration of diabetes.

SV: stroke volume,
s: group s, m: group m, l: group l

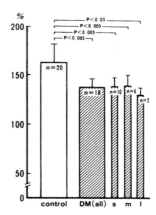

Fig. 8 The relationship between change in ratio of EVI during exercise and the duration of diabetes.
EVI: ejection velocity index,
s: group s, m: group m,
l: group l

Discussion

In this study, cardiac dysfunction was found in diabetics without clinical heart disease. It was suggested that cardiac dysfunction in diabetics was due to a decrease in cardiac reserve. This method is useful and safe for detection of cardiac dysfunction in diabetics and for the assessment of cardiac reserve.

It is considered that cardiac dysfunction in diabetics result from relaxation disturbance (1). SV is a parameter of cardiac function, and EVI is a parameter of cardiac contractility (2). In this study, SV decreased in parallel with EVI. So cardiac dysfunction in diabetics results from not only cardiac relaxation disturbance but also cardiac contractility disturbance. It was quite interesting that cardiac function decreased in accordance with the degree of retinopathy as well as the duration of diabetes.

These cardiac dysfunctions are considered to consist of multiple factors. For example, there are myocardial abnormality of contractile protein (3), metabolic disturbance (4,5), structural abnormality of capillaries (6) in diabetics.

Summary

Cardiac performance in diabetes at postural stress and treadmill exercise test was examined by the impedance method. The study group consisted of 23 diabetics (NIDDM) without clinical heart disease. Twenty healthy volunteers served as a control. Using impedance cardiography (NCCOM-30), stroke volume (SV) and ejection velocity index (EVI) were measured.

Results were as follows: 1) postural stress; increased ratio of SV in diabetics was lower than that in control. EVI of the control group was increased and that of diabetics was decreased. 2) treadmill exercise; increased ratio of SV, EVI in diabetics were lower than those in control. These phenomena were seen in accordance with the degree of diabetic retinopathy and the duration of diabetes. There were significant differences by statistical analysis.

It is suggested that cardiac dysfunction in diabetics was the reduction of cardiac reserve, which was due to decrease of contractility. And a good relationship among the reduction of cardiac reserve, the degree of retinopathy and the duration of diabetes was recognized.

References

1. Rubler S, Sajadi RM, Araoya MA, et al. Non-invasive estimation of myocardial performance in patients with diabetes. Diabetes 1978;27:127-135.
2. Bernstein DP. A new stroke volume equation for thoracic electrical bio-impedance: Theory and rationale. Crit Care Med 1986;14:904-909.
3. N. Takeda et al. Myocardial mechanical and myosin isoenzyme alterations in streptozotocin-diabetic rats. Jpn Heart J 1988;29:455-463.
4. Crall FA, Roberts WC. The extramural and intramural coronary arteries in juvenile diabetes mellitus, Analysis of nine necropsy patients aged 19 to 38 years with onset of diabetes before age 15 years. Am J Med 1978;64:221.
5. Penpargkul SS et al. The effect of diabetes on performance and metabolism of rat heart. Circ Res 1980;47:911-921.
6. Yokota K et al. A study of cardiac capillary casts in diabetics by means of scanninig electron microscope with correlation to morphometrical analysis. Jikei Med J 1984;31:211-228.

Early Diastolic Dysfunction of Left Ventricle and its Relation to Pathologic Finding in Patients with Diabetes Mellitus

M. Shimizu, N. Sugihara, Y. Kita, K. Shimizu, M. Minamoto and R. Takeda

*The Second Department of Internal Medicine, School of Medicine
Kanazawa University, Kanazawa, JAPAN.*

Introduction

In diabetes mellitus, the development of myocardial injury secondary to hypertension and coronary arteriosclerosis poses a major clinical problem. In addition, this issue has been the focus of great interest and it has been demonstrated that the existence of myocardial injury is not attributable to hypertension or coronary arteriosclerosis. It has also been reported in various pathological studies that even in the diabetic heart without hypertension and coronary artery lesions, various histological changes such as myocyte hypertrophy, perivascular fibrosis, and interstitial fibrosis are present (1-3). On the other hand, the existence of functional abnormalities such as left ventricular systolic and diastolic dysfunction has also been reported (4-12). It is, however, not yet clear which pathological changes account for these functional disturbances in the diabetic heart. To clarify this point we investigated the relation between systolic and diastolic function and the myocardial histological findings in diabetic patients.

Methods

1) Subjects:

The control group consisted of 6 non-diabetic patients in whom cardiac catheterization was undertaken because of complaints of chest oppression but in whom no organic abnormalities were found. Likewise, the diabetic group consisted of 8 patients who were suspected of having coronary arteriosclerosis because of chest oppression, but in whom coronary angiography revealed no significant stenosis. Patients with hypertension, renal failure, or any other condition influencing cardiac function were excluded from this study.

*Nagano, M., Mochizuki, S., Dhalla, N.S. (eds.), CARDIOVASCULAR
DISEASE IN DIABETES. Copyright © 1992. Kluwer Academic Publishers,
Boston. All rights reserved.*

Table 1. Clinical features of 8 diabetic patients

Case	Age(yr) & Sex	Duration (yr)	Treatment	FBS (mg/dl)	75gGTT 120 min	Scott	Creat (mg/dl)	Neuropathy ATR	Neuropathy VIB	Neuropathy OD
1	66 F	11	Diet	159	285	1	0.7	+	N	-
2	58 M	15	Diet	184	399	0	1.1	+	N	-
3	49 M	0.5	Diet	168	354	0	1.2	+	D	-
4	48 M	6	Diet	186	419	Ia	0.9	+	N	-
5	41 F	6	Diet	122	273	IIIb	0.9	-	D	-
6	39 M	8	Insulin	189	-	III	1.3	-	D	+
7	67 M	2	Drug	288	574	0	0.9	-	D	-
8	26 M	8	Insulin	233	-	0	0.8	+	N	-

M=male; F=female; FBS=fasting blood sugar; GTT=glucose tolerance test; Creat=creatinine; ATR=achilles tendon reflex; OD=orthostatic disturbance; N=normal; D=disturbed.

Clinical features of diabetic patients are shown in Table 1.

11) Echocardiography:

An echocardiogram was recorded within the week preceding cardiac catheterization. With the subjects at rest, the direction of the beam was confirmed with a B-mode echocardiographic long axis view, and the M-mode echocardiogram was recorded at the level of the tips of the mitral valve. A Toshiba SSH-11A, a Honeywell Model 1219 strip chart recorder, and a Toshiba LSR-20B line scan recorder were used and recordings were made at a paper speed of 100 mm/sec. Using a picture analyzer -5 (Medical System Research Company), the endocardial surface of the ventricular septum and posterior left ventricular wall were traced. Then, as shown in Fig 1, the left ventricular end-systole, end-rapid filling phase, end-slow filling phase, and atrial end-systole (left ventricular end-diastole) were identified from the electrocardiogram, phonocardiogram, and motion of the posterior left ventricular wall. Using a Teichholz equation, the volume at the end of each phase was calculated and from these differences the filling volumes of each phase were determined. The time from the aortic component of the second sound to the point of opening of the mitral valve was considered to be the left ventricular isovolumic relaxation time (IRT). Also, fractional shortening was sought as an index of systolic function.

III) Histopathological Investigations:

Cardiac catheterization was performed within 1 week after recording of the echocardiogram. Angiography confirmed that none of the patients had significant stenosis of the right or left coronary arteries. At the same time, using the Konno-Sakakibara bioptome, endomyocardial biopsies were obtained from the right ventricle side of the interventricular septum. The specimens were immediately submerged in a 10% neutral formalin buffer solution, and embedded in paraffin. The longitudinally sliced specimens were then cut into 4 um sections and stained with hematoxylin-eosin and Mallory-Azan. Myocyte diameter, percentage of fibrosis of the myocardial interstitium (% fibrosis), and eccentricity $\underline{e}$, which indicates the degree of myocardial dysarrangement, were quantified. Measurement of the myocyte diameter was performed on hematoxylin-eosin stained specimens, according to the method of Baandrup et al. (13). In longitudinally cut myocytes the distance across the cell at the narrowest plane across the nucleus was measured in at least 50 cells from each specimen under 400x magnification. The mean value and 1 standard deviation were sought.To determine the % fibrosis, Mallory-Azan stained specimens were used. Using the point-counting method (14,15), over 2000 points were recognized, and the proportion of interstitial fibrosis was expressed as a percentage. The degree of myocyte dysarrangement was quantified by seeking eccentricity $\underline{e}$, following the method of Tezuka (16). Nearly 300 um long straight lines were drawn at 15 degree intervals, and the number of myocytes crossed by each segment counted. The ratio of this number to the average number of intersecting points of all the directions was plotted on coordinates and an ellipse calculated. The eccentricity $\underline{e}$ of this ellipse was sought. When there is an increase in dysarrangement, the ellipse becomes more circular with $\underline{e}$ approaching 0. Conversely, when there is little dysarrangement, $\underline{e}$ approaches 1; $\underline{e}$ was sought in 3 places per specimen with the average value taken as the $\underline{e}$ of the specimen.

IV) Statistical Methods:

All data are expressed as mean ± one standard deviation. Differences

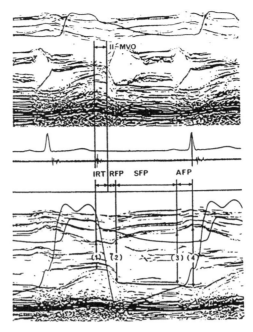

Figure 1. Echocardiographic measurements of each parameter. IRT=isovolumic relaxation time; II-MVO=the time from the aortic component of the second sound to the point of opening of the mitral valve; RFP=rapid filling phase; SFP=slow filling phase; AFP=filling phase during atrial systole; (1)=left ventricular internal dimension(LVD) at end-systole; (2)=LVD at end-rapid filling phase; (3)=LVD at end-slow filling phase; (4)=LVD at end-diastole. Each filling volume is calculated as the increment of ventricular volume during each filling phase.

between 2 groups were analyzed using Student's t-test and Wilcoxon signed rank test. The correlations between myocyte diameter, % fibrosis, $\underline{e}$, and various cardiac functional indices were investigated using Pearson's correlation formula and multiple regression analysis. The P value was considered statistically significant when it was less than 0.05.

Results
1) Cardiac Function:

The mean blood pressure, heart rate, and left ventricular wall thickness did not differ between the control and diabetic groups (Table 2). Systolic and diastolic indices determined by echocardiography are shown in Table 3.

Table 2. Hemodynamic data and wall thickness in the 2 groups.

	Case (M/F)	Age (yr)	MBP (mmHg)	HR (beats/min)	IVST (mm)	PWT (mm)
Control	(4/2)	46.8±6.3	100.0±4.8	63.8±8.7	9.5±0.8	9.2±1.2
D M	(6/2)	49.3±14.1	88.9±15.1	62.5±12.5	8.9±1.2	9.1±0.6

DM=diabetes mellitus; M=male; F=female; MBP=mean blood pressure; HR=heart rate; IVST=interventricular septal thickness; PWT=posterior wall thickness.

Table 3. Echocardiographic findings in control and diabetes mellitus groups

	LVEDVI (ml/m^2)	LVESVI (ml/m^2)	SI (ml/b/m^2)	FS (%)	IRT (msec)	RFVI (ml/m^2)
Control	67.1±11.6	23.7±5.7	43.4±8.3	40.2±5.0	50.0±16.7	15.4±4.6
D M	60.0±13.2	23.4±11.7	36.6±8.8	33.0±7.8	86.3±30.7#	11.8±3.1*

	SFVI (ml/m^2)	AFVI (ml/m^2)	RFV/SV (%)	SFV/SV (%)	AFV/SV (%)
Control	16.4±4.3	11.6±3.6	35.0±5.2	38.0±9.1	27.1±8.0
D M	14.6±5.7	14.1±6.8	29.9±6.5*	35.7±9.6	34.4±9.1

DM=diabetes mellitus; LVEDVI=left ventricular end-diastolic volume index; LVESVI=left ventricular end-systolic volume index; SV=stroke volume; SI=stroke volume index; FS=fractional shortening; IRT=isovolumic relaxation time; RFV=rapid filling volume; RFVI=rapid filling volume index; SFV=slow filling volume; SFVI=slow filling volume index; AFV=filling volume during atrial systole; AFVI=filling volume index during atrial systole; *p<0.05; #p<0.01.

Although there were no differences in the left ventricular end-diastolic volume index (LVEDVI) and end-systolic volume index between the 2 groups, the diabetic group LVEDVI and stoke volume (SV) index tended to be smaller. There was no difference in fractional shortening between the 2 groups. IRT was significantly prolonged in the diabetic group while rapid filling volume (RFV) index was significantly reduced. The 2 groups did not differ with respect to filling volume indices during the slow filling and atrial systolic periods.

Table 4. Multiple regression analysis.

	R	p	standard regression coefficient X_1	X_2	X_3
1) Y=IRT					
Y=389+1.93X_2-363X_3	0.686	<0.05	-	0.557	-0.292
2) Y=RFV/SV					
Y=83.3-0.386X_2-58.7X_3	0.736	<0.05	-	-0.742	-0.314

X_1=myocyte diameter; X_2=percentage of fibrosis; X_3=eccentricity $\underline{e}$.

When each filling volume was divided by the SV similar results were obtained.

II) Histopathological Findings:

Examination of the endomyocardial biopsy specimens revealed a mean myocyte diameter of 11.7 ± 0.4 and 13.1 ± 0.5 um in the control and diabetic groups (p<0.001), respectively, while the % fibrosis was 10.9 ± 1.9 and 20.9 ± 9.9% in the control and diabetic groups (p<0.01), respectively, with significantly higher values found in both cases in the diabetic group. $\underline{e}$ was 0.98 ± 0.01 in the control group and significantly smaller at 0.96 ± 0.03 in the diabetic group (p<0.05).

III) Comparative Study of Cardiac Function and Histological Findings:

We examined the correlations between the left ventricular early diastolic indices and the myocardial histological findings. No correlations were found between the myocyte diameter and IRT or RFV/SV (Fig 2). A significant positive correlation was found between % fibrosis and IRT (r=0.62, p<0.01), while a significant negative correlation was found between % fibrosis and RFV/SV (r=-0.63, p<0.01), as shown in Fig 3. No correlations were found between $\underline{e}$ and IRT or RFV/SV (Fig 4). Multiple regression analysis demonstrated that % fibrosis was more more closely associated with IRT and RFV/SV than myocyte diameter or $\underline{e}$ (Table 4).

Discussion

In diabetes mellitus, the high incidence of myocardial injury secondary to hypertension and coronary arteriosclerosis is well known. The findings that myocardial injury is present in diabetic patients who are without hypertension and coronary arteriosclerosis has also been reported and has received a great deal of attention. In 1972, Rubler et al. (1) studied the

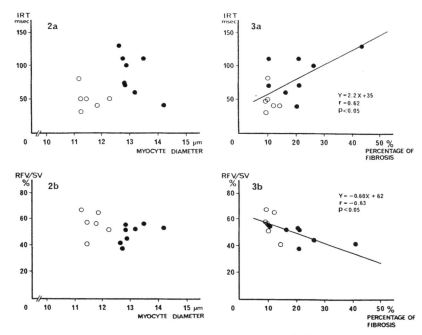

Fig. 2a and 2 b. Correlations between IRT and RFV/SV, and myocyte diameter. There are no significant correlations between IRT and RFV/SV, and myocyte diameter in the 2 groups.

Fig. 3a and 3b. Correlations between IRT and RFV/SV, and percentage of fibrosis. Significant correlations are seen between IRT and RFV/SV, and percentage of myocardial fibrosis in the 2 groups.

hearts of patients with diabetic glomerulosclerosis post-mortem. In 4 patients, in whom neither hypertension nor major coronary artery disease had been present, diffuse fibrosis of the myocardial interstitium, myofibrillar hypertrophy, and small intramural coronary arteriole wall thickening with narrowing of the lumen due to the deposition of acid mucopolysaccharide were found. The authors postulated that these findings represented a new type of cardiomyopathy. In 1974, Hamby et al. (2) in a study of the post-mortem diabetic heart found perivascular and interstitial fibrosis, proliferation of the endothelial lining cells with bridging across the lumens, and myocardial hypertrophy in hearts free from main coronary artery lesions. Accordingly, it was concluded that in diabetes mellitus a specific lesion of the small vessels

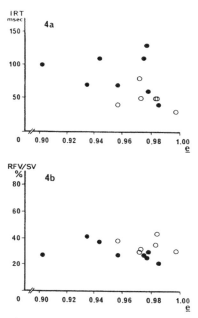

Fig. 4a and 4b. Correlations between IRT and RFV/SV, and eccentricity e. There are no significant correlations between IRT and RFV/SV, and e in the 2 groups. DM=diabetes mellitus; IRT=isovolumic relaxation time; RFV=rapid filling volume; SV=stroke volume; O=controls; ●=diabetics.

arises, which the authors named "diabetic cardiomyopathy". Ledet (3) reported similar histological findings, while Factor et al (17) reported the existence of capillary microaneurysms within the myocardium and suggested the possibility that microangiopathy itself may lead to myocardial injury. However, little is yet known about the origin and pathophysiology of diabetic myocardial injury which develops independently of hypertension and coronary arteriosclerosis. With this in mind, we investigated the correlations between the cardiac function and histopathological findings in a group of diabetic patients in whom hypertension and coronary arteriosclerosis were carefully excluded.

Various studies have been undertaken to evaluate cardiac function in diabetic patients using mechanocardiography (4-6), echocardiography (7-9), and nuclear medicine methods (10-12). Rynkiewicz (6), Sanderson (7), Shapiro (8) and their respective colleagues have reported prolongation of IRT in diabetic patients, and Kahn et al (11) in a study using radionuclide ventriculography pointed out abnormalities in the early diastolic phase indicated by a decrease in the peak filling rate in 21% of diabetic patients as well as a prolongation of the time to peak filling rate. We obtained similar results with prolongation of IRT and a decrease in the rapid filling volume index found in the diabetic group. Fractional shortening which is an index of systolic function did not differ between the control and diabetic groups. The diabetic patients investigated in the present study had relatively mild disease and it was surmised that in the early stage of diabetic myocardial dysfunction, disturbances of the early diastolic phase extended from the isovolumic relaxation period to the rapid filling period develop first.

Regan et al. (18) performed studies in the diabetic canine heart as well as in human diabetic subjects (19) and reported an elevation of the left ventricular end-diastolic pressure and a reduction in the left ventricular end-diastolic volume as well as changes in the left ventricular pressure-volume relation at the time of volume expansion, indicating increased left ventricular chamber stiffness. Although it is commonly accepted that chamber stiffness is largely due to left ventricular muscle itself (20), there was no difference in left ventricular wall thickness between the 2 groups studied in the present work. It is, therefore, surmised that myocardial injury itself is largely responsible for the early diastolic dysfunction.

With regard to the histopathological changes found in the diabetic myocardium, a number of studies have been undertaken, beginning with those of the above-mentioned Rubler et al. (1) and Hamby et al. (2), with myocyte hypertrophy and degeneration, interstitial fibrosis, and perivascular fibrosis (3,21,22). However, the relation between these histological changes and cardiac function has not been sufficiently investigated. Accordingly, using myocardial biopsy specimens, we attempted in the present study to quantitatively evaluate 3 items, namely, the degree of myocyte hypertrophy, the percentage of interstitial fibrosis, and the degree of myocyte dysarrangement, and investigated their relation to cardiac function. In the diabetic group compared to the control group, the mean myocyte diameter was significantly greater, and in addition there was a significant increase in interstitial fibrosis, and pronounced myocyte dysarrangement. Comparative study of these histological findings and cardiac function showed that only the % fibrosis was significantly correlated with early diastolic indices, whereas there were no significant correlations between myocyte diameter or degree of myocyte dysarrangement and early diastolic indices. Collagen fibers make up the majority of intramyocardial fibrosis. Borg et al (23), in their study using a scanning electron microscopy stated that the property of the diastole is determined by the existence of collagen fibers surrounding groups of myocytes. Also, Regan et al (18) in a study in the alloxan-induced diabetic dog proposed an increase of glycoprotein in the interstitium as the cause of the left ventricular diastolic dysfunction found in diabetes mellitus. From the above it is surmised that in the diabetic heart, left ventricular early diastolic dysfunction appears first and that the major histopathological change involved in its pathogenesis is interstitial fibrosis.

Summary

In order to study left ventricular function and its relation to pathologic findings in patients with diabetes mellitus, an echocardiographic study and endomyocardial biopsy were carried out on diabetic patients and non-diabetic control subjects without hypertension and coronary arteriosclerosis. Left ventricular systolic and diastolic indices were calculated from M-mode echocardiography. Right ventricular endomyocardial biopsies were performed to calculate the myocyte diameter, the percentage of fibrosis, and the eccentricity $\underline{e}$, which means the degree of myocardial dysarrangement. The results were as follows: isovolumic relaxation time (IRT) in the diabetic group was significantly longer than that of the control group. Ratio of rapid filling volume to stroke volume (RFV/SV) in the diabetic group was significantly smaller than that of the control group. In the diabetic patients, the myocyte diameter and the percentage of fibrosis were significantly larger, and the $\underline{e}$ was smaller, than those of control subjects.

Although there were no significant correlations between IRT, RFV/SV and the myocyte diameter, $\underline{e}$, there were significant correlations between IRT, RFV/SV and the percentage of fibrosis (r=0.62, r=-0.63). These studies show that early diastolic dysfunction occurs in patients with diabetes mellitus, and is correlated to the percentage of fibrosis.

References
1. Rubler S, Dlugash J, Yuceoglu YZ, Kumral T, Branwood AW and Grishman A. New type of cardiomyopathy associated with diabetic glomerulosclerosis. Am J Cardiol 1972;30:595-602.

2. Hamby RI, Zoneraich S, and Sherman L. Diabetic cardiomyopathy. JAMA 1974;229:1749-1754.
3. Ledet T. Diabetic cardiomyopathy. Quantitative histological studies of the heart from young juvenile diabetics. Acta Path Microbiol Scand Sect A 1976;84:421-428.
4. Ahmed SS, Jaferi GA, Narang RM and Regan TJ. Preclinical abnormality of left ventricular function in diabetes mellitus. Am Heart J 1975;89:153-158.
5. Zoneraich S, Zoneraich O and Rhee JJ. Left ventricular performance in diabetic patients without clinical heart disease. Evaluation by systolic time intervals and echocardiography. Chest 1977;72:748-751.
6. Rynkiewicz A, Semetkowska-Jurkiewicz E, and Wyrzykowski B. Systolic and diastolic time intervals in young diabetics. Br Heart J 1980;44:280-283.
7. Sanderson JE, Brown DJ, Rivellese A and Kohner E. Diabetic cardiomyopathy? An echocardiographic study of young diabetics. Br Med J 1978;1:404-407.
8. Shapiro LM. Echocardiographic features of impaired ventricular function in diabetes mellitus. Br Heart J 1982;47:439-444.
9. Bouchard A, Sanz N, Botvinick EH, Phillips N, Heilbron D, Byrd III BF, Karam JH and Schiller NB. Non-invasive assessment of cardiomyopathy in normotensive diabetic patients between 20 and 50 years old. Am J Med 1989;87:160-166.
10. Mildenberger RR, Bar-Shlomo B, Druck MN, Jablonsky G, Morch JE, Hilton JD, Kenshole AB, Forbath N and McLaughlin PR. Clinically unrecognized ventricular dysfunction in young diabetic patients. J Am Coll Cardiol 1984;4:234-238.
11. Kahn JK, Zola B, Juni JE and Vinik AI. Radionuclide assessment of left ventricular diastolic filling in diabetes mellitus with and without cardiac autonomic neuropathy. J Am Coll Cardiol 1986;7:1303-1309.
12. Ruddy TD, Shumak SL, Liu PP, Barnie A, Seawright SJ, McLaughlin PR and Zinman B. The relationship of cardiac diastolic dysfunction to concurrent hormonal and metabolic status in Type I diabetes mellitus. J Clin Endocrinol Metab 1988;66:113-118.
13. Baandrup U and Olsen EGJ. Critical analysis of endomyocardial biopsies from patients suspected of having cardiomyopathy. I:Morphological and morphometric aspects. Br Heart J 1981;45:475-486.

14. Nunoda S, Genda A, Sugihara N, Nakayama A, Mizuno S and Takeda R. Quantitative approach to the histopathology of the biopsied right ventricular myocardium in patients with diabetes mellitus. Heart Vessels 1985;1:43-47.
15. Sugihara N, Genda A, Shimizu M, Suematsu T, Kita Y, Horita Y and Takeda R. Quantitation of myocardial fibrosis and its relation to function in essential hypertension and hypertrophic cardiomyopathy. Clin Cardiol 1988;11:771-778.
16. Tezuka F. Muscle fiber orientation in normal and hypertrophied hearts. Tohoku J Exp Med 1975;117:289-297.
17. Factor SM, Okun EM and Minase T. Capillary microaneurysms in the human diabetic heart. N Engl J Med 1980;302:384-388.
18. Regan TJ, Ettinger PO, Kahn MI, Jesrani MU, Lyons MM, Oldewurtel HA and Weber M. Altered myocardial function and metabolism in chronic diabetes mellitus without ischemia in dogs. Circ Res 1974;35:222-237.
19. Regan TJ, Lyons MM, Ahmed SS, Levinson GE, Oldewurtel HA, Ahmad MR and Haider B. Evidence for cardiomyopathy in familial diabetes mellitus. J Clin Invest 1977;60:885-899.
20. Lewis BS and Gotsman MS. Current concepts of left ventricular relaxation and compliance. Am Heart J 1980;99:101-112.
21. Das AK, Das JP and Chandrasekar S. Specific heart muscle disease in diabetes mellitus-a functional structural correlation. Int J Cardiol 1987;17:299-302.
22. Genda A, Mizuno S, Nunoda S, Nakayama A, Igarashi Y, Sugihara N, Namura M, Takeda R, Bunko H and Hisada K. Clinical studies on diabetic myocardial disease using exercise testing with myocardial scintigraphy and endomyocardial biopsy. Clin Cardiol 1986;9:375-382.
23. Borg TK, Ranson WF, Moslehy FA and Caulfield JB. Structural basis of ventricular stiffness. Lab Invest 1981;44:49-54.

Radionuclide Assessment of Left Ventricular Function in Middle-Aged Asymptomatic Non-Insulin-Dependent Diabetic Patients

I. Yasuda, K. Kawakami, T. Shimada, K. Tanigawa*,
R. Murakami, S. Izumi, S. Morioka, Y. Kato* and K. Moriyama

The Fourth and First Departments of Internal Medicine,
Shimane Medical University, Izumo, JAPAN*

Introduction

The incidence of congestive heart failure is increased in patients with diabetes mellitus (1,2,3) and there is evidence that cardiac dysfunction occurs in diabetic patients with normal coronary arteries (4,5), but the causes of these abnormalities are still unclarified. Some authors (6,7) have suggested the existence of a specific diabetic cardiomyopathy. Rubler et al. (6) reported four adult-onset diabetic patients who had cardiomegaly and congestive heart failure in the absence of major coronary artery disease or hypertension. Hamby et al. (7) observed a high incidence of diabetes mellitus in their series of patients with idiopathic cardiomyopathy. On the other hand, it has been proposed that metabolic derangements of diabetes may impair the left ventricular function (4,8). Several investigators have shown that abnormalities of left ventricular systolic (9-14) or diastolic (4,8,15-17) function or both (18,19) are common in diabetics even without coronary artery disease and clinical manifestations of congestive heart failure. Abnormalities of the left ventricular function have been shown in diabetic patients at rest (4,9,20,21) and also during exercise (10-14). Whether these abnormalities result either from microangiopathy in the heart or from metabolic derangements inherent to diabetes mellitus remains unclear.

Previous studies have been made to detect subclinical left ventricular dysfunction in mainly young asymptomatic insulin-dependent diabetic (IDD) patients. There are few papers with respect to left ventricular systolic and diastolic functions in middle-aged asymptomatic non-insulin-dependent diabetic (NIDD) patients (14,16). In our study, we used exercise radionuclide ventriculography to investigate left ventricular systolic and diastolic function in middle-aged asymptomatic NIDD patients, with no signs of ischemic heart disease and any other cardiovascular diseases.

Methods

Study Subjects

Fifteen middle-aged asymptomatic NIDD patients (8 males and 7 females, aged 41 to 74 years, mean age 58.7 ± 10.5 years), selected among diabetic patients attending at the first Department of Internal Medicine, Shimane Medical University, were investigated. All patients were free of hypertension and any evidence of heart disease based on history, physical examination, electrocardiogram at rest and chest x-ray. They had no obvious perfusion defects in exercise thallium-201 myocardial scintigram and neither had angina nor showed abnormal exercise electrocardiogram. The duration of diabetes mellitus for the group ranged from 1 to 22 years, mean duration 9.1 ± 7.5 years. Five patients were treated with insulin injections. Six patients received oral antidiabetic treatment and 4 patients were treated by diet only. Glycosylated hemoglobin concentration (normal values < 8.0%) ranged from 8.5% to 15.6%, mean value 10.4 ± 2.0%. Two of 15 patients had proliferative retinopathy and three of them had proteinuria (Table 1).

Ten age- and sex-matched healthy control subjects were also studied for comparison. None of the control subjects had evidence of heart disease based on history, physical examination, electrocardiogram at rest and chest x-ray. They also had no obvious perfusion defects in exercise thallium-201 myocardial scintigram and showed no angina or significant ST shifts of 12-lead electrocardiogram upon exercise. Five asymptomatic NIDD patients who were suspected of coronary artery disease by exercise thallium-201 myocardial scintigraphy and/or exercise electrocardiography were excluded from this study. Three of them showed both perfusion defects in myocardial scintigrams and abnormal electrocardiograms on exercise. One of them showed only perfusion defect on myocardial scintigram and one showed only abnormal electrocardiogram on exercise.

Informed consent was obtained from all patients and control subjects before the study.

Myocardial Scintigraphy

The subjects were investigated in the postabsorptive state. A standard

Table 1. Clinical Features of 15 Diabetic Patients.

Case	Age (yr) & Sex	Duration of Diabetes (yr)	Treatment	Hgb A1 (g/100 ml)	Retinopathy	Urinary Protein
1	57 F	1	diet	8.5	(-)	(-)
2	41 F	22	I	12.5	(-)	(-)
3	71 F	1	diet	9.4	(-)	(-)
4	59 F	3	diet	11.7	(-)	(-)
5	55 M	4	OA	11.4	(-)	(-)
6	74 M	20	I	10.2	(+)	(-)
7	66 M	20	I	15.6	(+)	(+)
8	60 F	9	OA	12.0	(-)	(-)
9	51 F	7	OA	10.4	(-)	(+)
10	56 M	7	OA	9.2	(-)	(-)
11	66 M	9	I	9.0	(-)	(+)
12	53 M	2	OA	8.8	(-)	(-)
13	41 M	11	OA	8.8	(-)	(-)
14	73 F	18	I	9.9	(-)	(-)
15	51 M	3	diet	8.9	(-)	(-)

F = female; M = male; I = insulin; OA = oral agent
Hgb A1 = glycosylated hemoglobin A1

multistage exercise was performed on a motorized ergometer with simultaneous recording of a 12-lead electrocardiogram. The exercise load was begun at 20W for one minute and then increased by 20W step every one minute until symptoms such as leg fatigue appeared. One minute before termination of exercise, one bolus of 111 MBq of thallium-201 was injected intravenously. Blood pressure and 12-lead electrocardiogram were recorded at every one minute. Images were obtained twice within 5 minutes after exercise (early imaging) and 4 hours later (delayed imaging).

Radionuclide Ventriculography

All the patients underwent multigated radionuclide ventriculography with simultaneous electrocardiographic tracing. Twenty minutes after intravenous administration of 148 MBq stannous pyrophosphate, 925 MBq technetium pertechnetate were injected intravenously for in vivo labeling of the red blood cells. Imaging was performed in the subject lying on his back, using a mobile gamma camera equipped with a multipurpose collimator, built in a computer system (General Electric, Starcam, 400 AC/T). Imaging was carried on in the left anterior oblique projection. Eighty percent of total workload was used on exercise thallium-201 testing as the appropriate load. Each cardiac cycle was divided into 24 frames on a 64 x 64 matrix. Four hundred cardiac cycles at rest and at least 200 cardiac cycles during supine bicycle exercise were collected and stored by ECG gating. Ectopic beats were excluded from the data. During exercise, stabilization of the heart rate was allowed during the first one minute before data acquisition was begun. High temporal resolution left ventricular time-activity curves representing a measure of relative left ventricular volume changes with time throughout the average cardiac cycle, were generated from the cardiac image sequence with use of variable left ventricular and background region of interest. The left ventricular time-activity curves were reconstructed from the first four Fourier harmonics. First derivative curves (dv/dt) of these time-activity curves were computed and obtained over the entire circle.

Statistical Analysis

All data were analyized by F-test and followed by unpaired t-test. All data were shown as mean ± standard deviation.

Results

Exercise Capacity

There was no difference between the diabetic and control groups with respect to heart rate and blood pressure at rest. Termination of exercise was limited by exhaustion such as leg fatigue in all subjects. None showed chest pain, myocardial scintigraphic defects or electrocardiographic changes. Both groups attained similar total workload, peak heart rates, peak blood pressures and pressure-rate products. There was no significant difference between the diabetic and control groups with regard to exercise capacity. (Figure 1).

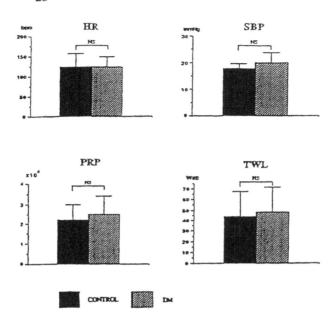

Figure 1. Indexes at Peak Exercise. No statistically significant difference in heart rate, systolic blood pressure, pressure-rate-product and total workload was recognized between the controls and the diabetic patients at peak exercise.

Ejection Fraction

No regional wall motion abnormalities in phase and amplitude analysis of the radionuclide ventriculography were observed in any subjects in either group at rest or during exercise. Left ventricular ejection fraction (LVEF) was 60% or more in all NIDD patients. The average LVEF at rest was 69.1 ± 5.3% (mean ± SD) in the NIDD patients and 65.6 ± 4.2% in the control subjects. The value of LVEF at rest was higher in the diabetic group than in the control group, but there was no significant difference. On exercise, the average LVEF changed to 68.3 ± 6.9% and 72.1 ± 5.0%, respectively. There was also no significant difference. While LVEF of the control group increased significantly on exercise ($p < 0.01$), the diabetic group did not change much (Figure 2). The average change of LVEF to exercise was -0.7 ± 7.6% in the diabetic group and +6.5 ± 2.6% in the control group. It was significantly different between these two groups.

If a normal response of LVEF to exercise was defined as an increase of

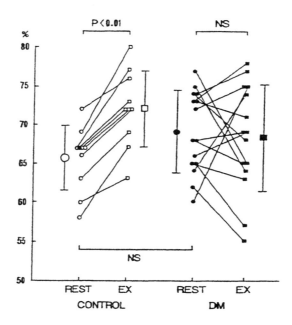

Figure 2. The response of LVEF to exercise. The average LVEF at rest was 69.1 ± 5.3% in the NIDD patients and 65.6 ± 4.2% in the control subjects. On exercise, the average LVEF changed to 68.3 ± 6.9% and 72.1 ± 5.0%, respectively. LVEF of the control group increased significantly (p < 0.01), but that of the diabetic group did not.

more than 4% during exercise, then 12 of 15 NIDD patients (80%) and 2 of 10 control subjects (20%) would be considered abnormal (Figure 3).

No statistical correlation was found between abnormal response of LVEF to exercise in the NIDD patients and various clinical variables, such as age, sex, duration of diabetes, glycosylated hemoglobin concentration, presence of retinopathy or nephropathy, heart rate or blood pressure at rest or on exercise, pressure-rate product, total workload or ejection fraction at rest.

Diastolic Filling

Left ventricular diastolic filling at rest was also impaired in the NIDD patients. Filling fraction the first third of diastole (1/3FF) at rest was significantly low in the diabetic group compared with the control group (p <

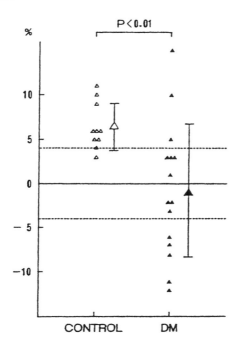

Figure 3. Average change of LVEF on exercise. The average change of LVEF on exercise was -0.7 ± 7.6% in the diabetic group and +6.5 ± 2.6% in the control group. There was a significant difference between these two groups. If a normal response of LVEF to exercise was defined as an increase of more than 4% during exercise, then 12 of 15 NIDD patients (80%) and 2 of 10 control subjects (20%) would be considered abnormal.

0.05). Filling rate at the first third of diastole (1/3FR) in the diabetic group was lower than in the control group. On the contrary, the peak filling rate (PFR) in the former was higher than in the latter. In addition, the time from end systole to peak filling rate (TPF) at rest was longer in the NIDD patients than in the control subjects. This remained true even when the TPF was normalized by the R-R interval and expressed as a percentage (TPF/R-R). Filling fraction of the first third of diastole was significantly different between the two groups and the other indexes were not significantly different (Figure 4).

Statistical correlation was not found between 1/3FF, TPF or TPF/R-R in the NIDD patients and various clinical variables such as age, sex, duration of diabetes, glycosylated hemoglobin concentration, presence of retinopathy or nephropathy, heart rate or blood pressure at rest or on exercise, pressure-rate product, total work load or ejection fraction at rest.

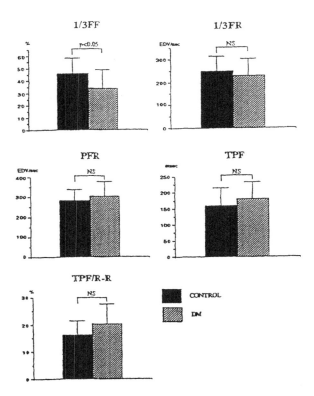

Figure 4. Indexes of LV Diastolic Function at Rest. Filling fraction during the first third of diastole (1/3FF) at rest was significantly lower in the diabetic group than in the control group (P < 0.05). In addition, the TPF at rest was longer in the NIDD patients than in the control subjects. This remained true even when the TPF was normalized by the R-R interval and expressed as a percentage (TPF/R-R).

Discussion

Coronary artery disease is one of the well-known diabetic complications (22,23). Coronary angiography is an accurate practical tool, but it is an invasive procedure which cannot be used indiscriminately. We carefully selected our patients to obtain an asymptomatic diabetic population on cardiovascular disease and having no factors likely to alter left ventricular function other than diabetes. Exercise thallium-201 myocardial scintigraphy was used to exclude coronary artery disease from the study. Five patients were excluded and three of them showed both perfusion defects in exercise thallium-201 myocardial scintigrams and abnormal exercise electrocardiograms. One of them showed only perfusion defect in exercise thallium-201 myocardial scintigram and the other one showed only abnormal exercise electrocardiogram. The former three patients had significant coronary lesions. The latter two patients had no significant coronary lesion, but they were also excluded from the study because the possibility of coronary artery spasm on exercise cannot be denied completely. However, it is sometimes difficult that three-vessel coronary artery disease with global myocardial ischemia might be detected even by exercise thallium-201 myocardial scintigraphy or exercise electrocardiography. Subclinical impairment of left ventricular function in asymptomatic diabetic patients has been suggested by evidence from echocardiography (9,16-20), systolic time intervals (4,9,16) and radionuclide ventriculography (10-14,16).

In the present study, there was no significant difference between the NIDD patients and the control subjects with regard to exercise capacity. In accordance with previous studies, our results indicated that LVEF remained preserved at rest but decreased or failed to increase during exercise in 80% of the NIDD patients in contrast to 20% of the control subjects. The causes of the higher incidence of abnormal LVEF response to exercise in our patients compared to some previous studies (42-72%) (10-14) may be due to another subset of diabetes mellitus. Our patient group consists of middle-aged asymptomatic NIDD patients. The value of the average change of LVEF to exercise of our control group (6.5 ± 2.6%) is also lower than that of the control group of the previous studies (10-15%) (10-14).

The causes of these abnormalities remain unclarified. In fact, different factors which have been considered capable of producing impairment of the left ventricular function in asymptomatic diabetic patients include metabolic factors (4), microangiopathy (6,7,18-21), neuropathy (15) and latent coronary artery disease (23). However, these factors are often present simultaneously in diabetic patients, making it difficult to assess their contribution.

A decrease in LVEF to exercise is a sensitive index of coronary artery disease (24,25). Diffuse global microvascular circulation disturbance is present in various organs of diabetes due to microangiopathy or hyperviscocity of the blood serum. The shift to the left of oxygen hemoglobin dissociation curve by glycosylated hemoglobin is partly concerned with reduction of oxygen supply to the myocardial cells in accordance with other organ cells in diabetes (26). One cause of abnormal response of LVEF to exercise can be latent global myocardial ischemia. Because it is very difficult for global myocardial ischemia, as well as three-vessel coronary artery disease, to be detected by exercise thallium-201 myocardial scintigraphy or exercise electrocardiography.

No statistical correlation was found between abnormal response of LVEF to exercise in the NIDD patients and various clinical variables, such as age, sex, duration of diabetes, glycosylated hemoglobin concentration, presence of retinopathy or nephropathy, heart rate or blood pressure at rest or on exercise, pressure-rate product, total workload or ejection fraction at rest. Reasons for this result could be considered as follows: (1) equivocal onset of non-insulin-dependent diabetes mellitus, (2) relatively wide range of age, (3) few severely complicated diabetic patients; only two patients with retinopathy and three with proteinuria.

We also detected impairment of left ventricular diastolic function at rest in the NIDD patients. Filling fraction during the first third of diastole (1/3FF) at rest was significantly low in the diabetic group compared with the control group. This fact suggests that early diastolic blood filling in diabetic patients decreases due to impairment of relaxation or distensibility of the left ventricle and the deteriorated early distolic filling can result in prolongation of the TPF. In the present study, the TPF at rest was longer and TPF/R-R, normalized by the R-R interval and expressed as a percentage was larger in the NIDD patients than in the control subjects. But the PFR in the NIDD patients was not low compared with that in the control subjects and this point is different from the previous studies (15-17). This conflicting result may be attributed to differences in the study population. Accumulation of glycoprotein and collagen and increased fibrosis of myocardial interstitium in the diabetic patients (8,13,27,28) may impair relaxation or distensibility of the left ventricle at early diastole.

Despite the normal ejection fraction at rest in the NIDD patients, left ventricular diastolic filling was already impaired in the diabetic patients in our study as well as in the previous studies (16,17). This shows that abnormalities in left ventricular diastolic function can be an earlier sign of diabetic myocardial disease than impaired systolic function at rest.

Summary

Radionuclide ventriculographic studies were performed at rest and during exercise on 15 middle-aged asymptomatic NIDD patients (mean age 58.7 ± 10.5 years) and 10 age- and sex-matched normal control subjects. They had no clinical evidence of cardiovascular diseases and no obvious perfusion defects in exercise thallium-201 myocardial scintigraphy. The average LVEF at rest was 69.1 ± 5.3% (mean ± SD) in the diabetic patients and 65.6 ± 4.2% in the control subjects. On exercise, the average LVEF changed to 68.3 ± 6.9% and 72.1 ± 5.0%, respectively. Average change of LVEF to exercise was -0.7 ± 7.6% in the diabetic group and +6.5 ± 2.6% in the control group. On the other hand, 1/3FF at rest was significantly low in the diabetic group compared with the control group. We conclude that not only the response of LVEF to exercise but also early left ventricular diastolic filling at rest is impaired in middle-aged asymptomatic NIDD patients as well as young asymptomatic IDD patients.

References
1. McKee PA, Castelli WP, McNamara PM, Kannel WB. The natural history of congestive heart failure. The Framingham study. New Engl J Med 1971;285:1441-1445,.
2. Kannel WB, Hjortland M, Castelli WP. The role of diabetes in congestive heart failure. The Framingham study. Am J Cardiol 1974;34:29-34.
3. Kannel WB, McGee DL. Diabetes and cardiovascular disease. The Framingham study. JAMA 1979;241:2035.
4. Regan TJ, Ettinger PO, Khan MI, Jesrani MU, Lyons MM, Oldewurfel HA, Weber M. Altered myocardial function and metabolism in chronic diabetes mellitus without ischemia in dogs. Circ Res 1974;35:222-227.
5. Ahmed SS, Jaferi GA, Narang RM, Regan TJ. Preclinical abnormality of left ventricular function in diabetes mellitus. Am Heart J 1975;89:153-158.
6. Rubler SR, Dluglash J, Yuceoglu YZ, Kumral T, Branwood AW, Grishman A. New type of cardiomyopathy associated with diabetic glomerulosclerosis. Am J Cardiol 1972;30:595-602.
7. Hamby RI, Zoneraich S, Sherman L. Diabetic cardiomyopathy. JAMA 1974;229:1749-1754.
8. Regan TJ, Lyons MM, Ahmad SS, Levinson GE, Oldewurtel HA, Ahmed MR, Halder B. Evidence for cardiomyopathy in familial diabetes mellitus. J Clin Invest 1977;60:884-899.
9. Zoneraich S, Zoneraich O, and Rhee JJ. Left ventricular performance in diabetic patients without clinical heart disease. Evaluation by

systolic time intervals and echocardiography. Chest 1977;72:748-751.
10. Vered Z, Batler A, Segal P, Liberman D, Yerushalmi Y, Berezsin M, Neufeld HN. Exercise induced left venetricular dysfunction in young men with asymptomatic diabetes mellitus (Diabetic cardiomyopathy). Am J Cardiol 1984;54:633-637.
11. Mildenberger RR, Bar-Shlomo B, Druch M, Jablonsky G, Morch JE, Hilton D, Keushole AB, Forbath N, McLaughlin PR. Clinically unrecognized ventricular dysfunction in young diabetic patients. J Am Coll Cardiol 1984;4:234-238.
12. Margonato A, Gerundini P, Vicedomini G, Gilardi MC, Pozza G, Fazio F. Abnormal cardiovascular response to exercise in young asymptomatic diabetic patients with retinopathy. Am Heart J 1986; Am Heart J 1986;112:554-560.
13. Fisher BM, Gillen G, Lindop GBM, Dargie HJ, Frier BM. Cardiac function and coronary arteriography in asymptomatic type I (insulin-dependent) diabetic patients: evidence for a specific diabetic heart disease. Diabetologia 1986;29:706-712.
14. Mustonen JN, Uusitupa MIJ, Tahvaninen K, Tarwar S, Laakso M, Lansimies E, KuiKKa JT, Pyorala K. Impaired left ventricular systolic function during exercise in middle-aged insulin-dependent and noninsulin-dependent diabetic subjects without clinically evident cardiovascular disease. Am J Cardiol 1988;62:1273-1279.
15. Kahn JK, Zola B, Juni JE, Vinik AI. Radionnuclide assessment of left ventricular diastolic filling in diabetes mellitus with and without cardiac autonomic neuropthy. J Am Coll Cardiol 1986;7:1303-1309.
16. Uusitupa M, Mustonen J, Laako M, Vainio P, Lansimies E, Talwar S, Pyorala K. Impairment of diastolic function in middle-aged type 1 (insulin-dependent) and type 2 (non-insulin-dependent) diabetic patients free of cardiovascular disease. Diabetologia 1988;31:783-791.
17. Ruddy TD, Shumak SL, Liu PP, Barnie A, Seawright SJ, McLaughlin PR, Zinman B. The relationship of cardiac diastolic dysfunction to conccurrent hormonal and metabolic status in type 1 diabetes mellitus. J Clin Endocrinol metab 1988;66:113-118.
18. Shapiro LM, Leatherdale BA, MacKinnon J, Fletcher RF. Left ventricular function in diabetics. Relation between clinical features and left ventricular function. Br. Heart J. 1981;45:129-132.

19. Shapiro LM, Echocardiographic features of impaired ventricular function in diabetes mellitus. Br Heart J 1982;47:439-444.
20. Seneviratne BIB. Diabetic cardiomyopathy: the preclinical phase. Br Med J 1977;1:1444-1446.
21. Sanderson JE, Brown DDJ, Rivellese A, Kohner E. Diabetic cardiomyopathy? An echocardiographic study of young diabetics. Br Med J 1978;1:404-407.
22. Gorcia MJ, McNamara PM, Gordon T, Kannel WB. Morbiditiy and mortality in diabetics in the Framingham population. Diabetes 1974;23:105-111.
23. Abenavoli T, Rubler S, Fisher VJ, Axelrod HI, Zuckerman KP. Exercise testing with myocardial scintigraphy in asymptomatic diabetic patients. Circulation 1981;63:54-64.
24. Caldwell, JH, Hamilton, GW, Jorensen SG, Richtie JL, Williams PL, Kennedy YW. The detection of coronary artery disease with radionuclide techniques: A comparison of rest-exercise thallium imaging and ejection fraction response. Circulation 1980;61:610.
25. Okada RD, Boucher CA, Strauss HW, Pohost GM. Exercise radionuclide approaches to coronary artery disease. Am J Cardiol 1980;46:1188-1204.
26. Ditzel J. Oxygen transport impairment in diabetes. Diabetes 1976;25(Suppl. 2):832.
27. Ledet T. Diabetic cardiopathy: quantitative histologic studies of the heart from young juvenile diabetes. Acta Pathol Microbiol Scand (A) 1976;84:421-428.
28. Genda A, Mizuno S, Nunoda S, Nakayama A, Igarashi Y, Sugihara N, Namura M, Takeda R, Bunko H, Hisada K. Clinical studies on diabetic myocardial disease using exercise testing with myocardial scintigraphy and endomyocardial biopsy. Clin Cardiol 1986;9:375-382.

Usefulness of Exercise T1-201 Myocardial Scintigraphy to Detect Asymptomatic Heart Disease in Diabetic Patients

K. Kawakami, I. Yasuda, T. Shimada, R. Murakami, S. Morioka, K. Tanigawa, Y. Kato, K. Moriyama.

The Fourth Department of Internal Medicine, Shimane Medical University, 89-1 Enya-cho, Izumo-city, Shimane-prefecture, JAPAN

Introduction

Diabetes mellitus is thought to be one of the risk factors of coronary heart disease (1,2). It is hard to detect ischemic heart disease in diabetic patients because many of them are asymptomatic. It is also considered that cardiomyopathy more often occurs in diabetic patients than in normal population (3,4,5). Exercise T1-201 scintigraphy are commonly used to detect myocardial viability in coronary heart disease (6,7,8) and cardiomyopathy (9). We evaluate how often the patients of diabetes mellitus without symptoms suffer from heart disease, using the scintigraphic method.

Methods

This investigation consists of forty-seven patients at our university hospital, 28 men and 19 women from 24 to 74 years of age (mean 58±12). They were selected if they passed the following criteria: (a) diagnosed as diabetic mellitus by the oral glucose tolerance test, (b) without any symptoms like angina pectoris in their past history, (c) stable clinical condition allowing exercise studies before choice, (d) without any handicaps interrupting the exercise study. The mean duration of the disease in these patients was 9±7 years. We compared the patient data on exercise to those of 27 healthy volunteers (control group). Control group consisted of 17 men and 10 women, and their mean age was 61±11 years. There was no significant difference between these two groups on sex and age. The medication such as ß-adrenergic receptor-blocking agents, calcium-channel blocker or other drugs which might effect the cardiac performance was stopped 3 days before the study.

Standard equipments and techniques were used to perform both exercise and myocardial perfusion imaging. All exercise studies were performed in the morning period on a motorized ergometer machine with supine position by the standard multistage method. Exercise load was started from 20 watts and then increased by 20 watts step every one minute. One minute before the maximal load 111 MBq of Tl-201 was injected intravenously. The end-point of the load was either ischemic change of the ECG or fatigue. A 12-lead electrocardiogram was continously monitored and recorded every one minute, at peak exercise, and at one, two and three minutes after exercise. The ST segment displacement was quantitated as the vertical distance from the base line (TP segment) at 80 millisecond after the J point. The first measurements was computed from the average of the value of consecutive 5 beats in the electrocardiogram lead showing maximal displacement; the second measurement was calculated in the same manner. At peak exercise 111 MBq of Tl-201 was injected into a peripheral arm vein, and then the patients exercised on for one more minute. Stress imaging began 4 minutes after stopping exercise. Single photon emission computed tomography (SPECT) imaging was taken first and planar imaging followed. To make the SPECT images, the gantry was rotated 180 degrees from left posterior oblique 45 degree to right anterior oblique 45 degree around the long axis of the patient. Data were collected from 60 views (25 second/view). Each planar image contained 500,000 counts that were recorded successively in the anterior, 45 degree left anterior oblique (LAO), and left lateral projections. Redistribution images were recorded 240 minutes after stopping exercise with exactly the same manner, in each view, as the initial images. Starcam 400-ACT scintillation camera (General Electric) equipped with a low energy all-purpose and parallel-hole collimator was interfaced to Starcam computer system (GE). Data were collected in 128 x 128 matrix.

Images were reconstructed into 10-mm-thick multiple slices in the transaxial planes by a filtered back-projection method with a Butterworth spatial filter (power factor: 10. cut-off frequency: 0.4 cycles/cm) as a pre-filter and a Ramp filter to reconstruct. Each reconstructed image contained 200,000 to 800,000 counts. The vertical short-axial (frontal), the long-axial (sagittal) and trans-axial (horizontal) sections of the heart were reconstructed by conventional method. In comparison with myocardial region of the most intense uptake on the images, myocardial segment was judged abnormal if the Tl-201 uptake reduced to 50% or more relatively. The myocardial scintigraphic findings were interpreted on the basis of segmental analysis predicting the responsible coronary arteries.

Table 1. Clinical data on exercise

	Diabetic	Control	p value
Number (male/female)	47(28/19)	27(17/10)	NS
Age (years)	58 ± 12	61 ± 11	NS
Duration of the disease (years)	9.7 ± 7	--	
Heart rate (bpm)			
at rest	67 ± 10	67 ± 11	NS
at the maximal exercise	123 ± 23	132 ± 16	p<0.01
increment	56 ± 22	67 ± 16	p<0.05
Systolic blood pressure (mmHg)			
at rest	145 ± 23	140 ± 23	NS
at the maximal exercise	199 ± 29	197 ± 24	NS
Exercise capacity (watts)			
maximal	103 ± 35	110 ± 30	NS
total	438 ± 210	473 ± 197	NS

Values are mean±SD   NS=not significant

Results

1) Heart rate at rest of diabetic group was 67±10 (bpm) and that of control group 67±11(bpm). There were no significant differences between these two groups, though the heart rate at the maximal exercise of diabetic group was 123±23 (bpm) and that of control group 134±16 (bpm) (p<0.01). The increment of the heart rate was 56±23 (bpm) in diabetic group and was 67±16 (bpm) in control group (p<0.05). We could not find any differences between these two groups about the blood pressure at rest and at maximal exercise, maximal work load and total work load.

Figure 1. Results of the scintigraphy

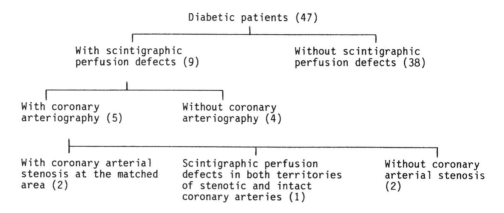

2) We revealed perfusion defects in 9 cases. Coronary arteriography was done 5 out of 9. Coronary arterial stenosis was detected in coincidence with the defective area in 3 of them. One of them also had perfusion defects in normal arterial territory. There were two cases with intact coronary arteries in which perfusion defect was detected. These results indicate that at least 6% (3/47) of asymptomatic patients suffer from microangiography, and 6% (3/47) of them have unexplainable scintigraphic perfusion defects which may indicate microangiopathy or metabolic disorder in the heart.

3) There was a case with ketoacidosis in which perfusion defect was detected and disappeared after the recovery from ketoacidosis (Fig. 2).

4) There was a case clinically diagnosed as dilated cardiomyopathy with intact coronary arteries (Fig. 3).

5) Scintigraphic asymmetrical hypertrophy was found in one case and was clinically diagnosed as hypertrophic cardiomyopathy (Fig. 4).

Discussion

Although there was no significant differences between the heart rate at rest in the two groups, heart rate at the maximal exercise was significantly lower in the diabetic group than in healthy volunteers. The lower maximal heart rate and work load in these subjects are consistent with previous reports (10,11,12). This change may be partly due to autonomic neuropathy

With ketoacidosis

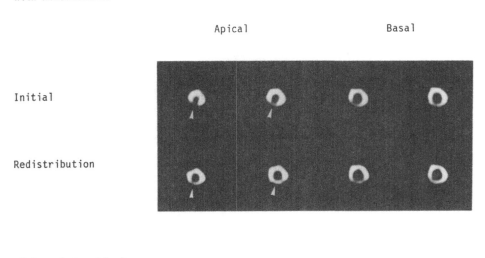

Without ketoacidosis

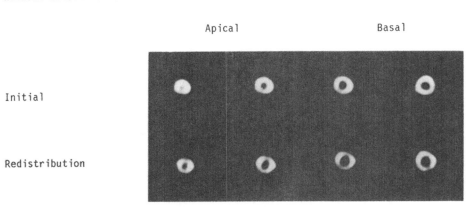

Figure 2. Stress myocardial scintigraphy of 32 year old male patient. Exercise induced perfusion defect in the inferior wall was detected in ketoacidosis (white triangle). However it disappeared one month after the recovery from ketoacidosis with insulin treatment.

Left ventriculogram

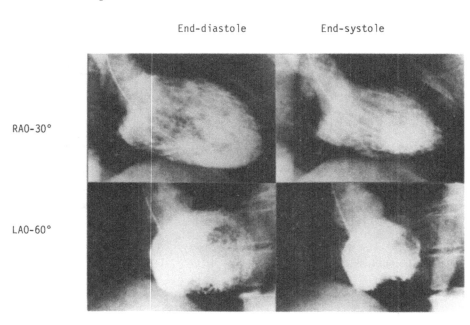

Myocardial scintigram

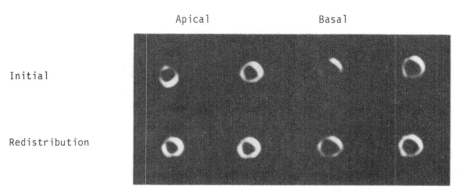

Figure 3. Stress myocardial scintigraphy and left ventriculography of 56 year old male patient. Left ventricular enlargement and small and multiple scintigraphic perfusion defects were noted.

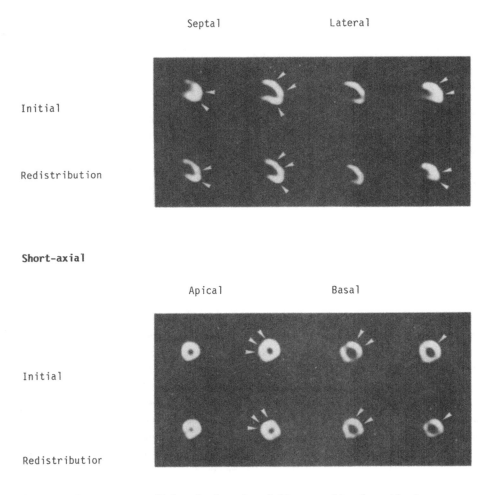

Figure 4. Stress myocardial scintigraphy of 66 year old male patient. Asymmetrical anterior and apical hypertrophy (white triangle) were noted.

which is known to reduce maximal heart rate and exercise capacity. We could not find any difference between the two groups concerning the exercise capacity in our study. This phenomenon might occur because of the difference of the severity of the diseases between our and their patients.

In previous studies, scintigraphic perfusion defects had been demonstrated in 30-50% in asymptomatic diabetic patients (9,10,11). In our study scintigraphic perfusion defects were found in only 19% (9/47). Coronary arteriography was performed in 5 out of 9 patients. At the matched area, coronary arterial stenosis was detected in 60% (3/5) of them. No significant coronary arterial stenosis was found in 60% (3/5) of them. Thus, approximately 11 (19x0.6)% of the asymptomatic patient has a chance to suffer from coronary arterial stenosis, and about 11 (19x0.6)% of them have the possibility of unexplainable perfusion defect. Our data on the scintigraphic perfusion defect were lower than the previous reports. We judged the perfusion defects as the count of 50% or less than the most intense uptake of the images. In this manner, we detected the exercise induced perfusion defects which occurred with the sensitivity 94.1% and the specificity 89.9% (6) because of the coronary arterial stenosis. However, the previous workers had rarely confirmed their own data with sensitivity and specificity of their institute. We observe less frequently the patient with diabetes mellitus who suffers from congestive heart failure with no coronary arterial stenosis. Therefore, we cannot believe so many patients are in diabetic cardiomyopathy. In a part of the Framingham study, Kannel et al. (16) reported that diabetic patients developed congestive heart failure more often than non-diabetic population. They reported that diabetic patients often developed cardiomyopathy and also speculated that the possibility of pathological changes in small coronary vessels was present in diabetic cardiomyopathy (4,5,17). The 56 year old male patient described in Fig. 4 was clinically diagnosed as dilated cardiomyopathy. In this case, small multiple perfusion defects with enlarged left ventricular cavity were found, so microangiopathy may play some role at the defective area. For this reason, this case might be so called diabetic cardiomyopathy. In the 32 year old male patient described in Fig. 3, the perfusion defect disappeared after the ketoacidosis had recovered. Some metabolic disturbance may affect this phenomenon rather than microangiopathy. It is hard to believe that microangiopathy disappeared within a month only. Tl-201 can play almost the same role as K^+ at the microcirculatory system of the myocardium. At the ketoacidotic state, the plasma concentration of H^+ rise up and may modify K^+ or Tl-201 in the cellular level. So the myocardial uptake of Tl-201 may decrease. There are some possibilities that the scintigraphic perfusion defect reflects both microangiopathy and metabolic disturbance of myocardium.

Scintigraphic myocardial perfusion defects are observed in both angiopathy and some metabolic disorders. Angiopathy consists of two possibilities. Some people have reported that silent myocardial ischemia was frequently seen in diabetic patients. Exercise myocardial scintigraphy can be a very useful method to detect silent myocardial ischemia in this disease. One is coronary microangiopathy which can be confirmed by coronary arteriography. The other is the microangiopathy of the heart which is frequently seen in other organs such as eyes and kidneys. Myocardial perfusion defects in normal coronary arterial territory might represent microangiopathy of the heart. However, some metabolic disorder might cause these perfusion defects just like the case in Fig. 3. Therefore, when we observe the perfusion defect in normal arterial territory in diabetic patients, we have to consider at least two possibilities that perfusion defect is affected from microangiopathy and some metabolic disturbance or both.

We could conclude that exercise Tl-201 myocardial scintigraphy is a useful non-invasive method to detect cardiac disease including ischemic heart disease, cardiomyopathy and some metabolic disorders in the asymptomatic patient of diabetic mellitus.

Summary

To evaluate cardiac involvements in diabetic patients without symptoms, exercise Tl-201 myocardial imaging was carried out in 47 patients (average age: 58.1±12.1 years, average duration of disease: 9.4±7.1 years). The heart rate at maximal exercise of the diabetic patient was 123±23 (bpm) and that of the control group was 134±16 (bpm); there was a significant difference between these two groups ($p<0.01$). Poor response of the heart rate increment to the exercise in diabetic patient may indicate autonomic nerve dysfunction. Scintigraphic perfusion defects were found in 9 out of 47 asymptomatic diabetic patients (19%). Coronary arteriography was performed in 5 out of 9 patients. Coronary arterial stenosis was recognized at the matched area in 3 patients, but one of them had another perfusion defect in the normal arterial territory. No arterial stenosis was found in the other two patients. Scintigraphic asymmetrical hypertrophy was found in one case.

Judging from the above described findings non-invasive Tl-201 myocardial scintigraphy can detect heart diseases of different types. Exercise myocardial scintigraphy was useful to detect not only coronary stenosis in asymptomatic patient but also coronary microangiopathy or some metabolic disturbances. Scintigraphic perfusion defect in normal coronary arterial territory may indicate both microangiopathy and some metabolic disorders of the heart.

References
1. Marks HH, Krall LP. Onset, course prognosis in diabetes mellitus. In: Diabetes Mellitus (eds.) Marble A, White P, Bradley RF, Krall LP. Philadelphia, Lea & Febiger; 1971:226.
2. Bradley RF. Cardiovascular disease. In: Joslin's Diabetes Mellitus (eds.) Marble A, White P, Bradley RF, IKrall L. Philadelphia, Lea & Febiger;1971:419.
3. Blumenthal HT, Alex M, Goldenberg S. A study of lesions of the intramural coronary artery branches in diabetic mellitus. Arch Pathol 1960;70:13.
4. Rubler S, Dlugash J, Yuceoglu YZ, Kumal T, Branwood AM, Grishman A. New type of cardiomyopathy associated with diabetic glomerulosclerosis. Am J Cardiol 1972;30:595.
5. Hamby RI, Zoneraich S, Sherman L. Diabetic cardiomyopathy. JAMA 1974;229:1749.
6. Kawakami K, Yasuda I, Shimada T, Murakami M, Morioka S, Moriyama K. Re-evaluation of Bullseye map in the patient with coronary heart disease. Jpn J Nuc Med 1989;26:921.
7. Richie JL, Zaret BJ, Strauss HW, Pitt B, Berma DS, Sherbert HW, Ashburn WN, Berger HJ, Hamiltom GW. Myocardial imaging with thallium-201: A multicenter study in patients with angina pectoris or acute myocardial infarction. Am J Cardiol 1978;42:345.
8. De Pasquale ED, Nody AC, De Puey EG, Garcia EV, Pilcher G, Bledlau C, Roubin G, Gober A, Gluentzig A, D'Amato P, Berger HJ. Quantitative rotational thallium-201 tomography for identifying and localizing coronary artery disease. Circulation 1988;77(2):316.
9. O'Gara PT, Bonow RO, Marson BJ, Damske BA, Lingen AV, Bacharash SL, Larson SM, Epstein SE. Myocardial perfusion abnormalities in patients with hypertrophic cardiomyopathy assessment with thallium-201 emission tomography. Circ 1987;76:6.

10. Hilsted J, Galvo H, Christensen NJ. Impaired cardiovascular responses to graded exercise in diabetic autonomic neuropathy. Diabetes 1979;28:313.
11. Storstein L, Jervell J. Response to the bicycle exercise testing in long-standing juvenile diabetes. Acta Med Scand 1979;205:227.
12. Airaksinen JKE, Kaila JM, Linnaluoto MK, Ikaheimo MJ, Takkunen JT. Cardiovascular response to exercise in young woman with insulin-dependent diabetes mellitus. Acta diabetol lat 1985;22:1.
13. Abenaboli TJ, Ruber S, Fisher VJ, Axelrod HI, Zucherman KP. Exercise testing with myocardial scintigraphy in asymptomatic diabetic males. Circulation 1981;63:54.
14. Mizuno S, Genda A, Nakayama A, Igarashi Y, Takeda R. Myocardial involvement in diabetic patients evaluated by exercise thallium-201 scintigraphy and cardiac catheterization. J Cardiography 1985;15:427.
15. Amano K, Sakamoto T, Oku J, Fujinami J, Sugimoto T. Diabetic cardiomyopathy: the relationship between 201-thallium myocardial scintigraphic perfusion defect and left ventricular function in symptomatic diabetes. Acta Cardiologica 1988;18(2):75.
16. Kannel WB, Hjortland M, Castelli WP. Role of diabetes in congestive heart failure: The Framingham Study. Am J Cardiol 1974;34:29.
17. Regan TJ, Lyons MM, Ahmed SS, Levinson GE, Oldewurtel HA, Ahmed MR, Haider B. Evidence for cardiomyopathy in familial diabetes mellitus. J Clin Inv 1977;60:885.

Autonomic Function Test Assessed by Ambulatory ECG in Diabetics

K. Aihara, I. Taniguchi, S. Kageyama and Y. Isogai

3rd Department of Internal Medicine, Jikei University School of Medicine,
Tokyo 105, JAPAN

Introduction

R-R interval variation of ECG has been used as an autonomic function test in diabetic autonomic neuropathy and various neurological disorders (1). Although R-R interval variation has been determined at various times of the day, it has not yet been clarified whether or not there are significant circadian variations and changes caused by sleep stages.

Therefore, we investigated the circadian variation and reproducibility of R-R interval variation using an ambulatory ECG.

Subjects and Methods

Subjects were 5 healthy males (23-32 years), 11 diabetics without autonomic neuropathy (31-53 years, 10 males and 1 female), and 5 diabetics with autonomic neuropathy (29-53 years, 5 males). Subjects were not taking either psychotropic, anti hypertensive drugs or any drug affecting the central nervous system. Diabetics with autonomic neuropathy denote those with orthostatic hypotension, diabetic diarrhea, impotence or sweating abnormalities. Blood glucose levels on the study day were within the range between 100 and 250 mg/dl, and hypoglycemia was not observed.

ECGs were recorded for 24 hours in each subject. They lay on a bed quietly for 20 min every 2 hours and 100 consecutive R-R intervals in ECG during the last 5 min of each 20 min resting period were analyzed. Coefficient of variation (CV_{R-R}) was calculated. Data show mean ± SD.

Results

Histogram and trendgram of R-R intervals of a case are shown (Fig. 1). Health subjects and diabetics without autonomic neuropathy showed a similar

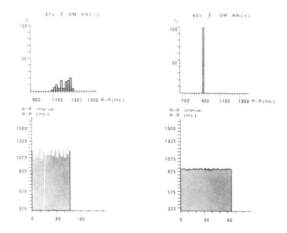

Figure 1. Analysis of heart rate variation using Holter ECG. AN: Autonomic neuropathy.

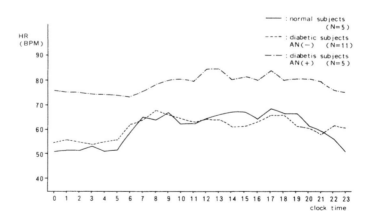

Figure 2. Daily profiles of mean heart rate in normal and diabetic subjects. AN: Autonomic neuropathy.

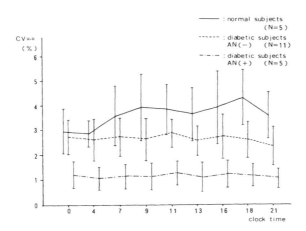

Figure 3. Daily profiles of CV_{R-R} in normal and diabetic subjects. AN: Autonomic neuropathy.

heart rate change, i.e. heart rate is increased during the day time and decreased during the night (Fig. 2, Table 1).

Coefficient of variation of R-R intervals (CV_{R-R}) (1) were over 1.5% in each case of the healthy subjects and the diabetics without neuropathy at any time of the day, while they were less than 2% in each case of the diabetics with autonomic neuropathy at any time point (Fig. 3, Table 1).

The difference between maximum and minimum of CV_{R-R} within a day were 2.2 ± 0.7% in healthy subjects, 1.7 ± 0.4% in diabetics without autonomic neuropathy, less than 3.3% in each case of two groups. It was within 0.7 ± 0.1% in those with neuropathy.

Discussion

Holter ECG has already been available for years in the diagnosis of cardiac diseases. There have also been reports on diabetic autonomic neuropathy using a Holter ECG, showing smaller diurnal variation of heart rate in diabetic neuropaths than healthy subjects (2,3). However, it has not yet been shown whether healthy subjects with greater daily activities also show such a small diurnal variation as diabetic neuropaths whose daily activities are limited. Therefore, we have examined heart rate variation using a Holter

Table 1. Mean R-R intervals and CV_{R-R} in normal and diabetic subjects. AN: Autonomic neuropathy.

mean ± SD

clock time	0	4	7	9	11	13	16	18	21
Normal (N=5)									
Mean R-R interval (msec)	1126±211	1097±203	964±163	900±981	938±146	869±118	940±94	868±92	958±142
CV_{R-R} (%)	2.98±0.84	2.85±0.54	3.59±1.2	3.91±1.34	3.83±0.99	3.62±1.08	3.91±1.64	4.29±1.07	3.57±0.92
Diabetics without AN (N=11)									
Mean R-R interval (msec)	1058±164	1050±202	933±176	861±101	915±175	938±147	998±198	901±138	1013±197
CV_{R-R} (%)	2.71±0.74	2.61±0.81	2.75±0.47	2.67±0.81	2.88±0.58	2.57±0.60	2.76±0.86	2.62±0.70	2.33±0.77
Diabetics with AN (N=5)									
Mean R-R interval (msec)	821±103	827±100	814±127	736+49	732±31	757±123	744±54	747±78	810±136
CV_{R-R} (%)	1.20±0.54	1.10±0.41	1.16±0.47	1.12±0.56	1.26±0.52	1.15±0.51	1.24±0.53	1.17±0.48	1.04±0.35

ECG apparatus in healthy subjects, diabetics without autonomic neuropathy and diabetics with advanced autonomic neuropathy.

Although a greater variation of CV_{R-R} was observed in healthy subjects and diabetics without autonomic neuropathy than those with advanced autonomic neuropathy, CV_{R-R} of those without autonomic neuropathy was never smaller than 1.5% which is assumed a critical level whether various autonomic symptoms appear (4). The difference between maximum and minimum of CV_{R-R} within a day was within 2%, and a significance of the results was not different regardless of time when ECG was recorded. On the other hand, those with advanced autonomic neuropathy showed a smaller diurnal variation of CV_{R-R} with the difference between maximum and minimum being less than 1%. Here, again, a clinical significance of the results did not differ regardless of the time of the day.

Therefore, it could be concluded that an autonomic function test using heart rate variation can be applied at any time of the day to subjects whether or not they have autonomic neuropathy. A method of using a Holter ECG described here is a useful way to assess autonomic function in diabetics.

Summary

Ambulatory ECGs were recorded in 5 normal subjects (group I), 11 diabetics without autonomic neuropathy (group II), and 5 diabetics with autonomic neuropathy (group III). Coefficient of variation of R-R intervals was calculated by processing 100 consecutive intervals at 0, 4, 7, 9, 11, 13,

16, 18 and 21 hours. CVs were over 1.5% at all time points in groups I and II, the latter being lower than the former during the night. The fluctuations of CV (max-min) were 2.2% (mean) in group I, 1.7% in group II, and less than 2% in each case of the 2 groups. CVs in groups III were less than 2% in each case at all time points, and fluctuation was 0.5% (mean) and less than 1% in each case. From the data obtained, it was concluded that it is possible to measure CV of R-R intervals at any time of the day as an index of diabetic autonomic neuropathy. The method described here using ambulatory ECG could be useful for determination of autonomic function in various disorders.

References
1. Kageyama S, Mochio S, Taniguchi I and Abe M. A proposal of quantitative autonomic function test. Jikeikai Med J 1981;28:81-85.
2. Bennet T, Riggot PA, Hosking DJ and Hampton JR. Twenty-four hour monitoring of heart rate and activity in patients with diabetes mellitus: A comparison with clinic investigations. Br Med J 1976;1:1250-1251.
3. Ewing DJ, Borsey DQ, Travis P, Bellavere F, Nielson JMM and Clarke BF. Abnormalities of ambulatory 24-hour heart rate in diabetes mellitus. Diabetes 1983;32:101-105.
4. Kageyama S, Taniguchi I, Tanaka S, Tajima N, Saito N, Ikeda Y and Abe M. A clinical level of diabetic autonomic neuropathy. Tohoku J Exp Med 1983;141(Suppl):479-483.

Diabetic Albuminuria and Ischemic Heart Disease

J. Ishiguro, T. Tsuda, T. Izumi, S. Ito and A. Shibata

First Department of Internal Medicine, Niigata University School of Medicine, Niigata, 951 JAPAN.

Introduction

It is well known that ischemic heart disease is a major cause of death in patients with diabetes mellitus (DM) and they have poor prognosis after myocardial infarction (1-4). However, even patients with serious ischemic lesions are apt to be asymptomatic. Some of the best diagnostic determinants of ischemic lesions in DM heart are yet to be identified (5-7). In this study, patients with non-insulin dependent diabetes mellitus (NIDDM) were examined using dipyridamole loading thallium-201 myocardial scintigraphy (Tl-201) to investigate how frequently they are associated with ischemic lesions in DM heart and to assess whether their occurrence is closely related to the presence of chest pain and the severity of diabetic nephropathy.

Methods

Fifty eight patients with NIDDM were examined. Thirty seven were male and 21 were female. The average age reached up 62.5 years old. Tl-201 scintigraphy was performed (Fig. 1) as previously reported by Albro et al. (8-11). An ischemic lesion in DM heart was justified with the scintigraphic documentation of myocardial ischemia and/or infarction.

The chest pain was inquired at the time of consultation. The albumin in the urine, albuminuria, was measured with the radioimmunoassay. The severity of the diabetic nephropathy was divided into three categories, namely, normoalbuminuria: below 20 microgram/min; micro-albuminuria: from 20 to 200 microgram/min; and macro-albuminuria: more than 200 microgram/min (12-13).
In this study, hypertension, hyperlipidemia, hyperuricemia, obesity and habitual smoking resorted to the coronary risk factors.

$X2$-test was employed for statistics.

Nagano, M., Mochizuki, S., Dhalla, N.S. (eds.), CARDIOVASCULAR DISEASE IN DIABETES. Copyright © 1992. Kluwer Academic Publishers, Boston. All rights reserved.

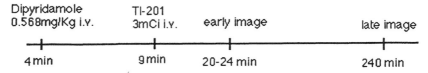

Figure 1. The method of dipyridamole loading thallium-201 myocardial scintigraphy: A dose of 0.568 mg/kg of dipyridamole was injected for four minutes. The early image used 3 mCi of Tl-201 and was taken five minutes after dipyridamole administration. The late image was taken after four hours.

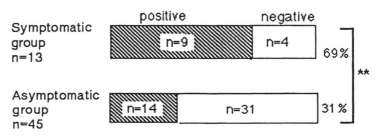

Figure 2. Positive documentation of dipyridamole loading thallium-201 myocardial scintigraphy in NIDDM patient;**:p<0.025.

Results

Twenty-three out of 58 NIDDM patients (40%) demonstrated a positive indication of the ischemic lesion in the scintigram. Among them, 11 males and 2 females complained of chest pain. As shown in Fig. 2, these symptomatic patients were documented. The ischemic lesions in the scintigram were frequent (69%) than in the other asymptomatic patients (31%). The symptomatic group did not differ in age, sex, hypertension and hyperlipemia from the asymptomatic. However, in smoking, hyperuricemia and obesity, the former had a higher ratio than the latter (Table 1).

Among symptomatic patients, the diabetic nephropathy was distributed as shown in Table 2. That is to say, 6 cases of macro-albuminuria (6 males only), 2 of macro-albuminuria (one to one) and 5 of normo-albuminuria (4 to one). By contrast, in asymptomatic, it consisted of 10 cases with macro-albuminuria (6 males and 4 females), 15 micro-albuminuria (11 to 4) and 20 normo-albuminuria (9 to 11). Concerning the coronary risk factors, only hypertension closely referred to the severity of albuminuria.

Table 1. Profile of NIDDM's patients ;M :male, F :female, y.o. :years old, * :p<0.05.

	symptomatic group	asymptomatic group
number	13	45
sex	M 11, F 2	M 26, F 19
age(y.o.)	62.3 ± 6.0	62.3 ± 9.3
hypertension	54%	42%
hyperlipemia	33%	38%
smoking *	54%	20%
hyperuricemia*	31%	11%
obesity*	38%	11%

Table 2. Clinical features and the albuminuria ;M :male, F :female, y.o. :years old, * :p<0.05

Symptomatic group

	Macroalbuminuria	Microalbminuria	Normoalbuminuria
number	6	2	4
sex	M=6, F=0	M=1, F=1	M=4, F=1
age(y.o.)	65.4 ± 6.2	73.5	67.4 ± 5.1
hypertension	50%	0%	80%
hyperlipemia	50%	50%	20%
smoking	67%	0%	60%
hyperuricemia	67%	0%	0%
obesity	33%	0%	40%

Asymptomatic group

	Macroalbuminuria	Microalbuminuria	Normoalbuminuria
number	10	15	20
sex	M=6, F=4	M=11, F=4	M=9, F=11
age(y.o.)	61.1 ± 9.2	63.4 ± 9.1	59.2 ± 9.1
hypertension*	80%	40%	25%
hyperlipemia	60%	33%	20%
smoking	0%	40%	15%
hyperuricemia	40%	0%	15%
obesity	10%	7%	15%

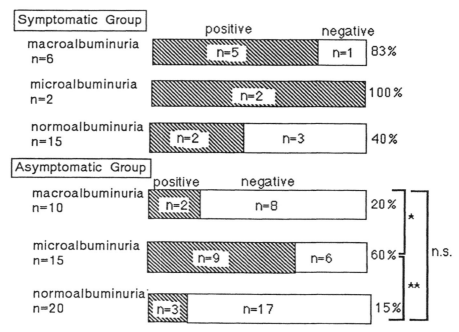

Figure 3. Differences of scintigraphic documentation depend on the severity albuminuria *: P<0.05, ***: p<0.01 n.s. :no significance.

As shown in Fig. 3, scintigraphic demonstration of the ischemic DM heart was affected by the severity of nephropathy. Among the symptomatic, on the one hand, the positive rate was exaggerated in patient with proteinuria despite of the small number of cases examined in this study, 83% (5/6) in the macro-albuminuria and 100% (2/2) in the micro-albuminuria. On the other hand, among asymptomatic, the micro-albuminuria was marked by a significant high frequency of the positive rate up to 60% in comparison with the two others, 20% in the macro-albuminuria and 15% in the normo-albuminuria.

It should be pointed out that a 54 year-old Japanese salesman had no history of chest pain, at any time. He was followed as NIDDM for five years. He developed micro-albuminuria during this time. His risk factor was limited to only hypertension. Fig. 4 illustrated his Tl-201 dipyridamole scintigram, where the ischemic lesion was detected in the posteroseptal wall. The right coronary artery documented severe atherosclerosis as shown in Fig. 5.

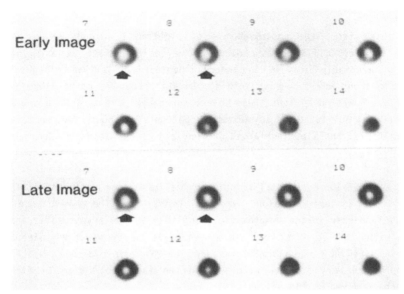

Figure 4. Eight representative short axial slices of early image and late image in Tl-201 SPECT of patient with posteroseptal wall ischemia. Improvement of distribution in posteroseptal wall is noted on late image.

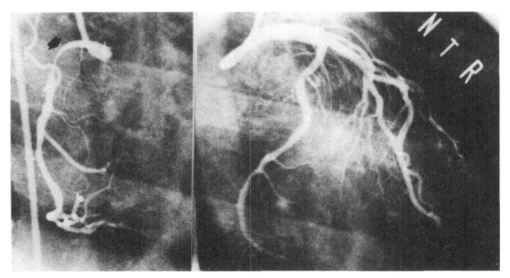

Figure 5. Right coronary artery documented severe atherosclerosis. Left coronary artery had no significant atherosclerosis.

Discussion

In this study, the positive rate of symptomatic group was very high (5/6:83%) in macro-albuminuria. However, the positive rate of asymptomatic group was invariably low in the macro-albuminuria. It was thought that asymptomatic group would develop into symptomatic group in macro-albuminuria. Eventually, it was noted that these severe coronary lesions of DM heart could not be recognized in such asymptomatic patients without two cooperative diagnostic tools: the albuminuria measurement and T1-201 scintigraphy.

Summary

1. With T1-201 myocardial scintigraphically, 40% of patients with NIDDM revealed the ischemic lesion in the heart. 2. The prevalence was significantly higher in the symptomatic group than in the asymptomatic and was affected with the severity of albuminuria. 3. A cooperative diagnostic probes, measurement of albuminuria and T1-201 dipyridamole myocardial scintigraphy are very helpful in detecting the ischemic lesion in diabetic heart, even in asymptomatic patients.

References

1. Kannel WB, McGee DL. Diabetes and cardiovascular disease: The Framingham Study. JAMA 1979;241:2035.
2. Yoshino H, Matuoka K, Horiuchi A et al. Painless myocardial infarction in diabetics. Tohoku J. Exp Med 1983;141 (Suppl.):547.
3. Garcia MJ, McNamara PM, Gordon T and Kannel WB. Morbidity and mortality in diabetics in Framingham Population: Sixteen year follow-up study. Diabetes 1974;23:105.
4. Smith JW et al. Prognosis of patients with diabetes mellitus after acute myocardial infarction. Am J Cardiol 1984;54:718.
5. Rubuler S et al. Predictive value of clinical and exercise variables for detection of coronary artery disease in men with diabetes mellitus. Am J Cardiol 1987;59:1310.
6. Chipkin SR et al. Frequency of painless myocardial ischemia during exercise tolerance testing in patients with and without diabetes mellitus. Am J Cardiol 1987;59:61.
7. Abenavoli T et al. Exercise testing with myocardial scintigraphy in asymptomatic diabetic males. Circulation 1981;63 (1):54.

8. Albro PC, Gould KL et al. Non-invasive assessment of coronary artery stenosis by myocardial imaging during pharmacologic coronary vasodilation. Am J Cardiol 1978;42:751.
9. Ruddy TD et al. Myocardial uptake and clearance of thallium-201 in normal subjects: Comparison of dipyridamole hyperemia with exercise stress. J Am Col Cardiol 1987;10:547.
10. Lam JYT et al. Safety and diagnostic accuracy of dipyridamole-thallium imaging in the elderly. J Am Col Cardiol 1988;11:585.
11. Francisco DA et al. Tomographic thallium-201 myocardial perfusion scintigrams after maximal coronary artery vasodilation with intravenous dipyridamole: Comparison of qualitative and quantitative approaches. Circulation 1982;66(2):370.
12. Jarrett RJ, Viberti GC, Argyropoulos A et al. Micro-albuminuria predicts mortality in non-insulin-dependent diabetes. Diabetic Med 1984;1:17.
13. Mogensen CD. Micro-albuminuria predicts clinical proteinuria and early mortality in maturity-onset diabetes. N Engl J Med 1984;310:356.

Prognostic Significance of Treadmill Exercise Stress Test in Diabetic Patients Without Cardiovascular Signs

K. Kawakubo, J. Oku, T. Murakami, and T. Sugimoto

Department of Health Administration, School of Health Science and Second Department of Internal Medicine, Faculty of Medicine, University of Tokyo, Tokyo, JAPAN 113.

Introduction

As in the Western countries, the incidence of coronary artery disease in diabetic patients is increasing in Japan. Early detection of coronary artery disease is important in the management of diabetic patients. However, because painless myocardial infarction is frequent in diabetics(1), silent ischemia might be also frequent in asymptomatic diabetic patients. Exercise electrocardiography is useful in the early detection of coronary artery disease, but no data was available concerning the incidence and prognostic significance of exercise electrocardiographic abnormalities in asymptomatic diabetic patients in Japan. To identify incidence and prognostic significance of exercise-induced abnormalities in asymptomatic Type 2 diabetic patients, we performed treadmill exercise stress tests in 176 consecutive patients with no symptoms and signs suggestive of cardiac disease and they were followed prospectively.

Methods

Patient population: The 176 study patients were from a population of patients with Type 2 diabetes followed at the Second Department of Internal Medicine, University of Tokyo Hospital. They were consecutively entered into the study, provided the patient was over 40 years old, had no history of chest pain suggestive of angina pectoris, and had no resting electrocardiographic abnormalities such as abnormal Q-waves and ST-T changes. The patients who were unable to walk on the treadmill were not included. The study patients included 113 men and 63 women with a mean age of 59 years (range 40 to 81 years).

Nagano, M., Mochizuki, S., Dhalla, N.S. (eds.), CARDIOVASCULAR DISEASE IN DIABETES. Copyright © 1992. Kluwer Academic Publishers, Boston. All rights reserved.

Treadmill exercise stress test: The patients exercised to limiting symptoms according to a standard Bruce protocol. Twelve lead electrocardiograms (ECG) and cuff blood pressure were recorded every 1 minute during exercise and the first 6 minutes of recovery. A positive exercise response was defined as more than 1 mm ST segment depression at 80 msec after the J point in the immediate post exercise ECG tracings (exercise-positive).

Non-exercise variables: The duration of diabetes, diabetic therapeutic regimen (diet, oral hypoglycemic agents, or insulin), incidence of complications (nephropathy, retinopathy, or hypertension), serum lipid values, and body mass index were compared between exercise-positive and exercise-negative patients.

Exercise Tl-201 scintigraphy using bicycle ergometer was performed in 13 patients and coronary arteriography was performed in 5 patients among exercise-positive patients.

Follow-up: Among 176 study patients, 172 patients (98%) could be followed more than 6 months. The mean follow-up interval was 23 months with a range of 6 to 36 months. The end-point of follow-up was occurrence of cardiac events (acute myocardial infarction or sudden cardiac death). Calcium antagonists were prescribed in patients with positive exercise test.

Statistical analysis was performed using a Student-t test and chi square method.

Results

Clinical characteristics and follow-up data of exercise-positive and exercise-negative patients (Table 1,2): Among 176 study patients, 29 patients (16.5%) had significant ST depression during treadmill exercise test (Table 1). Exercise-positive patients were significantly older than exercise-negative patients. The duration of diabetes, exercise tolerance time, and peak heart rate did not differ between the two groups. During the follow-up periods, 4 patients had acute myocardial infarction, 2 of which were fatal, and 1 patient died suddenly after complaining of chest discomfort. All of these 5 patients with cardiac events belonged to the exercise-positive group. The other clinical features such as diabetic therapy, frequencies of complications, serum lipid values, and body mass index did not differ between the two groups (Table 2).

Exercise Tl-201 scintigraphy (Ex Tl) and coronary arteriography (CAG) (Table 3): Among 13 patients who performed EX Tl, 3 patients had no exercise

Table 1. Characteristics of exercise-positive and exercise-negative patients.

	Exercise-positive	Exercise-negative	
No. of cases	29	147	
Male (%)	20(69%)	93(63%)	N.S.
Age	43 - 81y(63 ± 10)	40 - 81y(58 ± 9)	p < 0.01
Duration of diabetes	1 - 36y(13 ± 11)	1 - 40y(10 ± 8)	N.S.
Follow-up cases	29(100%)	143(97%)	N.S.
Cardiac events	5/29(17%)	0/143(0%)	p < 0.005

N.S.: not significant

induced perfusion defects. In other 10 patients, perfusion defects were mainly observed at the postero-inferior region (8 cases). Among 5 patients who performed CAG, 1 patient showed no significant stenosis. The other 4 patients had stenosis of left circumflex or right coronary artery.

Characteristics of 5 patients who had cardiac events during the follow-up periods (Table 4): During the follow-up periods, 3 patients had acute inferior myocardial infarction and 1 patient had acute anterior infarction, and 1 patient died suddenly after 6 to 29 months' follow-up. These five patients were relatively older male diabetic patients with a long history of diabetes (5 to 36).

Exercise electrocardiographic findings of exercise-positive patients with or without cardiac events (Table 5): Among exercise-positive patients, exercise duration and magnitude of maximum ST depression did not differ between those with and without cardiac events. However, the recovery time of ST depression after exercise was significantly longer in patients with cardiac events than those without cardiac events. Patients whose recovery time of ST depression was within 1 minute were more frequent among those without cardiac events.

Discussion

We performed treadmill exercise stress tests in 176 diabetic patients

Table 2. Clinical features of exercise-positive and exercise-negative patients.

		Exercise-positive (29)	Exercise-negative (147)
Diabetic therapy	Diet	15(52%)	54(37%)
	Oral agents	14(48%)	83(56%)
	Insulin	0	10(7%)
Complications	Nephropathy	5(17%)	26(18%)
	Retinopathy	10(35%)	51(35%)
	Hypertension	8(28%)	33(22%)
Serum lipids (mg/dl)	T-cho	211 ± 60	215 ± 46
	LDL-chol	111 ± 33	118 ± 36
	HDL-chol	52 ± 22	59 ± 24
Body mass Index (kg/m^2)		22.1 ± 2.8	22.2 ± 2.8

Values of serum lipids and body mass index are expressed as means ± SD

Table 3. Results of exercise ^{201}Tl scintigraphy (Ex Tl) and coronary angiography (CAG) in patients with positive-exercise tests.

Case	Ex Tl Ant	Post-inf	Lat	CAG LAD	LCX	RCA	Prognosis
1. 43M	○	○			normal		ok
2. 72M		●		⑨ 75%		③ 75%	Ant MI
3. 45M		○			⑫ 75%		ok
4. 56M		○	○	⑨ 90%	⑫ 90%		Inf MI
					⑬ 100%		
5. 67M	normal					② 75%	ok
6. 71M		△	△				Inf MI
7. 65M		●					Inf MI
8. 68M	○			not done			ok
9. 56M		○					ok
10. 55F	normal						ok
11. 67M		△					ok
12. 63F	normal						ok
13. 62M		●					ok

Ant: Anterior segment, Post-inf: Postero-inferior segment, Lat: Lateral aegment, ○: Transient defect, ●: Persistent defect, △: Defect with partial redistribution,
LAD: Left anterior descending coronary artery, LCX: Left circumflex coronary artery, RCA: Right coronary artery,
Ant MI: Anterior myocardial infarction, Inf MI: Inferior myocardial infarction, ok: without cardiac events

Table 4. Characteristics of 5 patients who had cardiac events during the follow-up periods.

No.	Age Sex	Exercise test		Follow-up		
		Exercise duration	End-point	Duration of follow-up	Cardiac events	Symptom
1.	72y male	10 min	leg fatigue	16 mo.	Ant MI dead	Chest pain
2.	71y male	3 min	leg fatigue	8 mo.	Inf MI alive	Dyspnea
3.	65y male	6 min	chest pain	10 mo.	Inf MI dead	Chest pain
4.	56y male	10 min	leg fatigue	6 mo.	Inf MI alive	Chest pain
5.	54y male	9 min	leg fatigue	29 mo.	Sudden death	Chest pain

Ant MI: Anterior myocardial infarction, Inf MI: Interior myocardial infarction.

without chest pain and ECG abnormalities, and significant ST depression was observed in 29 patients (16.5%). Screening of coronary artery disease using exercise stress test in asymptomatic population is of limited value because post-test likelihood depends on pre-test likelihood of coronary artery disease (2). In our study, we selected patients over 40 years old. Uhl et al. (3) reported in their review article that the incidence of exercise-induced ST depression in asymptomatic, apparently healthy, men was about 13%. The incidence of exercise-induced ST depression in our study (16.5%) was higher than this figure.

Lemp et al. (4) reported from their angiographic study that the risk of coronary artery disease increased with the severity of diabetes defined on the type of treatment received. In our study, exercise-positive patients were older than exercise-negative patients and the other clinical characteristics including the type of treatment did not differ between the two groups. These different results could be due to the method for defining coronary artery disease.

Table 5. Exercise electrocardiographic characteristics in exercise-positive patients with or without cardiac events.

	Cardiac events (+)	Cardiac events (-)	
No. of cases	5	24	
male (%)	5(100%)	15(63%)	N.S.
Age	54 - 72y	43 - 81y	
	(64 ± 8)	(63 ± 10)	N.S.
Exercise duration	3 - 10.2 min	2 - 14 min	
	(7.6 ± 3.1)	(7.4 ± 3.0)	N.S.
Magnitude of max ST depression	1.2 - 2.4 mm	1.0 - 3.8 mm	
	(1.7 ± 0.5)	(2.1 ± 0.7)	N.S.
Recovery time of ST depression	3 - 7 min	1 - 6 min	
	(5.0 ± 2.0)	(2.5 ± 1.8)	$p<0.05$
Recovery time of ST depression within 1 min	0/5	13/24	$p<0.05$
Exercise-induced VPC	1/5	6/24	N.S.

VPC: Ventricular premature contraction, N.S.: not significant

In our study, only a limited number of patients have undergone coronary arteriography. From the present study, however, we might recommend that the relatively older diabetic patients should perform exercise stress test for screening of coronary artery disease.

From the scintigraphic and angiographic studies of the exercise-positive patients, association between asymptomatic ST depression and infero-posterior ischemia was found in diabetic patients. The number of patients was too small to draw a conclusion from this study. However, Opasich et al. (5) reported from their study of post-infarction patients that the incidence of exercise-induced asymptomatic ischemia was more frequent in patients with inferior infarction than anterior infarction. Asymptomatic ischemia per se might be frequent in patients with inferior ischemia.

No data was available concerning the prognostic significance of exercise stress test in Japanese diabetic patients. Persson (6) reported the 9 years' follow-up study of 84 male diabetic patients who performed bicycle ergometer exercise test. The incidence of coronary artery disease was significantly higher in those who showed pathological ST depression, that is, ischemic and slowly ascending ST depression (31% vs 7%). More recently, Rubler et al. (7) and Gerson et al. (8) also reported the prognostic significance of exercise test parameters in diabetic patients. In Rubler's study, diabetic men who can exercise for 440 seconds on a treadmill using a Bruce protocol were at low risk of coronary event during 41 months' follow-up. In Gerson's study, 110 insulin-requiring diabetic patients were followed for 100 months and the peak treadmill heart rate was the most single important predictor of subsequent development of clinical coronary artery disease. In our present study of Type 2 diabetic patients over 40 years old, 5 cardiac events occurred from 172 patients during the follow-up for 23 months and they all belonged to exercise-positive group. These conflicting results could be due to type of diabetes and age of the study patients and the duration of follow-up.

Our data showed that exercise duration and the magnitude of maximum ST depression did not differ between those with cardiac events and without cardiac events during the follow-up periods. However, ST depression occurred during exercise and recovered quickly in patients with cardiac events and in more than half of patients without cardiac events, ST segment recovered within 1 minute. Lozner et al. (9) reported that ST segment resolved by one minute after exercise in all subjects who had more than 2 mm ST segment depression during exercise but did not have coronary artery disease. From these data, it is suggested that those patients whose exercise-induced ST depression persist more than 1 minute into the recovery should be followed carefully.

Limitation of our present study is the shortness of the follow-up periods and the small number of the patients who had cardiac events. We could not perform statistical analysis of the relation between the occurrence of cardiac events and other clinical variables. More prolonged follow-up studies should be performed.

Summary

We performed treadmill exercise stress test in 176 Type 2 diabetic patients over 40 years old without cardiovascular signs and symptoms. Twenty-nine patients (16.5%) exhibited ST depression and they were older than exercise-negative patients. During the mean follow-up duration of 23 months, 4 patients had acute myocardial infarction and 1 patient died suddenly. All of these 5 patients with cardiac events belonged to exercise-positive group.

In conclusion, exercise stress test was useful in the detection of latent coronary artery disease in patients with asymptomatic diabetes and those with positive results should be followed carefully.

References
1. Bradley RF, Schonfeld A. Diminished pain in diabetic patients with acute myocardial infarction. Geriatrics 1962;17:322-326.
2. Rifkin RD, Hood Jr WB. Bayesian analysis of electrocardiographic exercise stress testing. N Engl J Med 1977;297:681-686.
3. Uhl GS, Froelicher V. Screening for asymptomatic coronary artery disease. J Am Coll Cardiol 1983;1:946-955.
4. Lemp GF, Zwaag RV, Hughes JP, Maddock V, Kroetz F, Ramanathan KB, Mirvis DM, Sullivan JM. Association between the severity of diabetes mellitus and coronary arterial atherosclerosis. Am J Cardiol 1987;60:1015-1019.
5. Opasich C, Cobelli F, Assandri J, Calsamiglia G, Febo O, Larovere MT, Pozzoli M, Traversi E, Ardissino D, Specchia G. Incidence and prognostic significance of symptomatic and asymptomatic exercise-induced ischemia in patients with recent myocardial infarction. Cardiology 1984;71:284-291.
6. Persson G. Exercise tests in male diabetics. A nine-years' follow-up study with special reference to ECG changes and cardiovascular morbidity. Acta Med Scand 1977; 605(suppl):7-23.
7. Rubler S, Gerber D, Reitano J, Chokshi V, Fisher VJ. Predictive value of clinical and exercise variables for detection of coronary artery disease in men with diabetes mellitus. Am J Cardiol 1987;59:1310-1313.
8. Gerson MC, Khoury JC, Hertzberg VS, Fischer EE, Scott RC. Prediction of coronary artery disease in a population of insulin-requiring diabetic patients: Results of an 8-year follow-up study. Am Heart J 1988;116:820-826.
9. Lozner EC, Morganroth J. New critieria to enhance predictability of coronary artery disease by exercise testing in asymptomatic subjects. Circ 1977;56:799-802.

Coronary Artery Bypass Grafting in the Diabetic Heart: Myocardial Tolerance During Surgery and Late Result

M. Sunamori, T. Maruyama, J. Amano, H. Tanaka, H. Fujiwara, T. Sakamoto, A. Suzuki

Department of Thoracic-Cardiovascular Surgery, Tokyo Medical and Dental University, School of Medicine, Yushima, Bunkyo-ku, Tokyo, 113, JAPAN.

Introduction

It has been known that diabetic mellitus (DM) is listed as one of the risk factors in coronary artery bypass grafting (CABG). DM affects the coronary artery and arterioles to aggravate atherosclerotic lesions and result in impairment of cardiac function. In this regard, DM is responsible for late bypass graft patency and intra-operative surgical problems with respect to graftability of the coronary artery, completeness of coronary artery revascularization or myocardial tolerance to intra-operative ischemic insult. Further clinical characteristics on CABG for DM is aggravation of DM stimulated by surgical stress and increase in post-operative complication. Thus, we reviewed our clinical experience on CABG for the patients with DM with respect to perioperative ischemic tolerance and late surgical result.

Methods

Patients who underwent isolated CABG performed during the last five years were selected in this study, and they were divided into two groups; group 1 is non-diabetic patients (n=181, N-D) and group 2 is diabetic patients (n=39, D). In both groups, CABG was done using saphenous vein graft under cardiopulmonary bypass and K^+-Mg^{2+}-cardioplegia associated with moderate systemic hypothermia. Pre- and intra-operative clinical factors are listed in Table 1 and they were well matched among two groups. Post-operative enzyme release was measured and these include serum GOT, CPK, MB-CK and mitochondrial aspartate aminotransferase (m-AAT). Changes in ECG and hemodynamics, early

Nagano, M., Mochizuki, S., Dhalla, N.S. (eds.), CARDIOVASCULAR DISEASE IN DIABETES. Copyright © 1992. Kluwer Academic Publishers, Boston. All rights reserved.

Table 1. Clinical Profile

	Diabetic (n=39)	Diabetic (n=181)	P
Pre-op Factors			
Ejection Fraction (%)	59.0 ± 2.3	59.9 ± 1.2	NS
Left Vent. End-Diastolic Pressure (mmHg)	14.1 ± 1.5	13.3 ± 0.6	NS
Incidence of old myocardial infarction	20/39	69/181	p=0.22
Intra-operative Factors			
Cardiopulmonary bypass (min)	191.5 ± 9.4	191.2 ± 4.6	NS
Cardiac Arrest (min)	95.3 ± 5.8	98.4 ± 3.7	NS
Cardioplegic solution (ml)	1702 ± 98	1734 ± 70	NS
Level of hypothermia, Rectal °C	23.3 ± 0.3	23.4 ± 0.1	NS
Number of graft implanted	2.13 ± 0.11	2.16 ± 0.12	NS

Table 2. Bypass Graft Flow (ml/min, mean ± S.E.M.)

	DM		N-D	
Left Anterior Descending	73.1	6.6	74.9	4.0
Left Circumflex	61.6	7.5	58.4	4.6
Right Coronary	82.3	8.6	94.7	6.3

and late mortality and post-operative complication were studied and compared among two groups.

Statistical analysis was made using Student's t-test and chi-square test and p <0.05 was thought to be significant.

Results

Bypass graft flow is shown in Table 2 whereas hemodynamic alterations are shown in Figure 1. The data on serum enzymes are given in Figure 2.

Early and late mortality are shown in Table 3. Incidence of perioperative myocardial infarction (PMI) and requirement of Intraaortic Balloon Pumping (IABP) are illustrated in Table 4. Late changes in saphenous

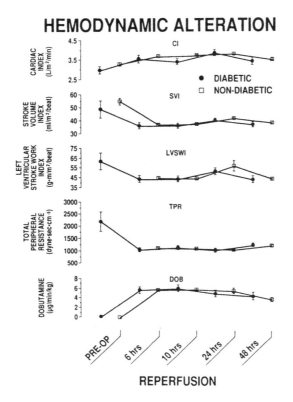

Figure 1. Hemodynamic alteration.
Values are means ± S.E. No significant difference is demonstrated.

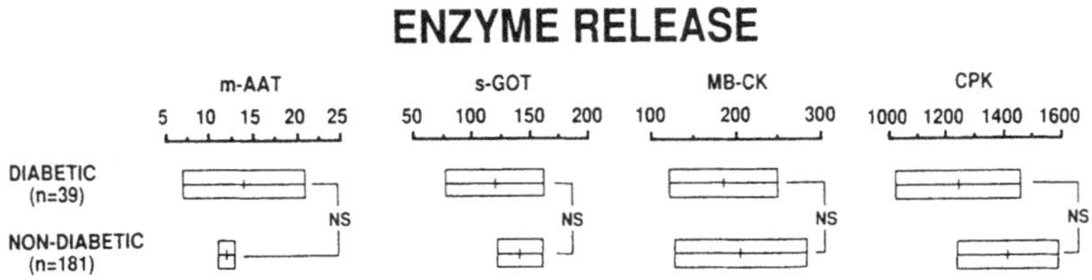

Figure 2. Serum enzymes.
Values are means ± S.E. No significant difference is shown in each parameter.
m-AAT = mitochondrial aspartate amino-transferase.

Table 3. Mortality.

	Diabetic	Non-diabetic	
Early	0/39	0/81	
Late	3/39	6/181	p=0.22

No significant difference in both early and late mortality among two groups.

Table 4. Incident of PMI and requirement of IABP.

	DM	N-D	
PMI (%)	20.5	13.8	p = 0.33
LABP (%)	20.5	12.7	p = 0.24

No significant difference is demonstrated among two groups.

vein graft demonstrated proliferation of smooth muscle cells and infiltration of macrophages in the intimal layers. These findings are qualitatively more remarkable in the diabetic heart. Some of the post-operative complications are given in Table 5.

Discussion

It is known that coronary lesion is observed in diffuse fashion and significantly in the coronary arterioles. Therefore, we anticipated difficulty in achievement of complete revascularization and satisfactory intraoperative myocardial protection. There was no significant difference in pre-operative cardiac function such as left ventricular end-diastolic pressure and ejection fraction between diabetic and non-diabetic heart. And overall hemodynamic alterations did not differ among two groups throughout early reperfusion for 48 hours in this study, however, incidence of cardiac low output was significantly higher in the diabetic heart. Myocardial damage assessed by enzyme release or operative mortality was not different among two groups. These results suggest that the diabetic heart has either the same or

Table 5. Variety and Incidence of Post-op Complication

	Diabetic	Non-Diabetic	x^2
Cardiac			
Arrhythmia	1/39	9/181	p=0.52
Low output	5/39	7/181	p=0.03
Hepatic			
Dysfunction	4/39	21/181	p=0.82
Renal			
Polyuria	1/39	3/181	p=0.70
Infectious			
Wound	2/39	8/181	p=0.85
MOF	2/39	2/181	p=0.09
GI Bleeding	2/39	3/181	p=0.19
Erythroderma	2/39	0/181	p=0.02

Incidence of cardiac low output syndrome and erythroderma is significantly higher in the diabetic groups than that in the non-diabetic heart. Multi-organ failure (MOF) tended to occur in higher incidence in the diabetic heart.

less tolerance to intra-operative ischemic insult as compared to the non-diabetic heart.

Johnson et al. (1) reported that effective relief of angina pectoris following CABG was 62% in DM, 65% in non-DM regarding complete disappearance, while, partial relief was 26% in DM and 25% in non-DM. Furthermore, aggravation of angina was 12.3% in DM and 9.7% in non-DM.

Late result may be involved by diabetes mellitus in survival because DM results in coronary artery stenosis and pathohistological lesion in the myocardial interstitium (2). Five year survival following CABG clearly demonstrated lower rate in DM compared with non-DM with both good and bad left ventricular function (1).

Chychota et al. (3) reported that early patency of graft did not differ between DM heart and non-DM heart, although graft flow was lower in the DM heart, while no difference in graft flow was observed by Verska et al. (4) between DM and non-DM. As we found saphenous vein graft in late stage proliferated with smooth muscle cells and infiltrated with macrophage, which is remarkable in the DM heart. It is in general agreement that bypass graft in the DM heart has a lower patency rate because DM is highly associated with hyperlipidemia and hypertension. Special attention has been paid on the female DM heart in which operative risk and post-operative complication are higher and graft patency rate is lower than male (1, 5-8).

Summary
Our limited clinical experience on CABG for DM heart suggested that myocardial tolerance to intraoperative ischemia and late result were same or less in DM heart as compared to non-DM heart.

References
1. Johnson DW, Pedraza PM, and Kayser KL. Coronary artery surgery in diabetics: 261 consecutive patients followed four to seven years. Am Heart J 1982;104:823-827.
2. Factor SM, Minase T and Sonnenblick EH. Clinical and morphological features of human hypertensive-diabetic cardiomyopathy. Am Heart J 1980;99:446-458.
3. Chychota NC, Gau GT, Pluth JR, Wallace RB, Danielson GK. Myocardial revascularization, comparison of operability and surgical results in diabetic and non-diabetic patients. J Thorac Cardiovasc Surg 1973;65:856-862.
4. Verska JL, and Walker WJ. Aortocoronary bypass in the diabetic patient. Am J Cardiol 1975;35:774-777.
5. Tyras DH, Barner HB, Kaiser GC, Codd JE, Laks H, Willman VL. Myocardial revascularization in woman. Ann Thorac Surg 1978;25:449-453.
6. Douglas JS Jr, King SB, Jones EL, Craver JM, Bradford JM, Hatcher CR. Reduced efficacy of coronary bypass surgery in women. Circ 1981;64 (Suppl 2):11-16.
7. Bolooki H, Vargas A, Green R, Kaiser GA, Ghahramani A. Results of direct coronary artery surgery in women. J Thorac Cardiovasc Surg 1975;69:271-277.
8. Killen DA, Reed WA, Arnold M, McCullister BD, Bell HH. Coronary artery bypass in women: Long-term survival. Ann Thorac Surg 1982;34:559-563.

B. INTERACTIONS OF DIABETES AND HYPERTENSION

The Influence of Diabetes on Myocardial Contractility and Energetics in Spontaneously Hypertensive Rats

N. Takeda, I Nakamura, T. Ohkubo, A. Tanamura, T. Iwai, M. Kato, K. Noma and M. Nagano.

Department of Internal Medicine, Aoto Hospital, Jikei University School of Medicine, Aoto 6-41-2, Katsushika-ku, Tokyo 125, JAPAN.

Introduction

Diabetic patients with hypertension show a high incidence of the development of heart failure. The mechanisms involved in heart failure at the myocardial cellular level remain unclear. To elucidate the myocardial alterations occurring in hypertension associated with diabetes, we examined myocardial contractility and ventricular myosin isoenzymes in diabetic spontaneously hypertensive rats (SHR). Myocardial contractility was assessed by measuring the isometric tension developed in isolated left ventricular papillary muscles, and ventricular myosin isoenzymes were separated by pyrophosphate gel electrophoresis.

Methods

Male SHR were used at the age of 25 to 26 weeks. Age-matched Wistar-Kyoto rats (WKY) were also used. Diabetes was induced in the rats by the intravenous injection of streptozotocin (50 mg/kg), and the hearts were excised 5 to 6 weeks later. Fasting blood glucose levels were measured by the glucose oxidase method a few days before the hearts were excised.

The myocardial contractility study was performed using isolated left ventricular papillary muscles. Muscles were stimulated at a frequency of 0.2 Hz with a voltage 30% above the threshold level, and were perfused with Tyrode solution containing 1.1 mM Ca^{2+} at 32°C. After a steady state was obtained at the muscular length of Lmax, the developed tension and its first derivative curves were recorded. The response to isoproterenol (10^{-7}M) was determined, and then after the interposition of Tyrode solution for 25-30 min,

Nagano, M., Mochizuki, S., Dhalla, N.S. (eds.), CARDIOVASCULAR DISEASE IN DIABETES. Copyright © 1992. Kluwer Academic Publishers, Boston. All rights reserved.

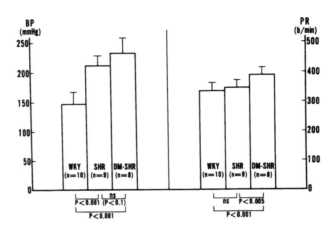

Figure 1. Comparisons of blood pressure and pulse rate.
Vertical lines indicate SD. ns: not significant

the response to dibutyryl cAMP (DBcAMP, 10^{-5} M) was examined. Myocardial contractile responses were obtained by comparing two pairs of values. One was the values measured in the steady state prior to isoproterenol or DBcAMP administration and the other was the maximum values measured after isoproterenol or DBcAMP administration.

Polyacrylamide gel electrophoresis using pyrophosphate was performed according to the method reported elsewhere (1-3). The gel contained 3.8% acrylamide and 0.12% N,N'-methylene-bis-acrylamide. The electrophoresis buffer was 20 mM $Na_4P_2O_7$ (pH 8.8) containing 10% glycerol. Native myosin was extracted from the left ventricle with a solution consisting of 100 mM $Na_4P_2O_7$ (pH 8.8), 5 mM 1,4-dithiothreitol, 5 mM EGTA, and 5 ug/ml leupeptin. Electrophoresis was carried out for 30 h at 2°C and a voltage gradient of 13.3 V/cm.

Student's t-test was used for statistical comparisons.

Results

The blood pressures, pulse rates, and blood glucose levels for the 3 groups are shown in Fig. 1, and 2. Diabetic SHR (DM-SHR) had a significantly higher blood pressure and significantly lower body and ventricular weights. The reduction in body weight was greater than that in ventricular weight (Table 1). There were no significant differences in the developed and resting tensions among the groups, but ± dT/dtmax was significantly decreased in DM-SHR as compared with SHR and WKY (Table 2). Time to peak tension, total contraction time and time to half relaxation were also significantly prolonged in diabetic SHR (Table 3). The myocardial response to isoproterenol was significantly decreased in DM-SHR (Fig.3), as was the response to DBcAMP (Fig. 4). The left ventricular myosin isoenzyme pattern showed a predominance of VM-3 in DM-SHR (Fig.5).

Discussion

When compared with untreated WKY, SHR showed no significant difference in maximum developed tension (T), but ± dT/dtmax decreased in association with the increase of VM-3 in the ventricular myosin isoenzyme pattern. This is similar to the findings in pressure-overload cardiac hypertrophy due to aortic constriction (4), where changes in the ventricular myosin isoenzyme pattern are considered to reflect adaptations made to maintain sufficient force development economically. The extent of the decrease in ± dT/dtmax and the shift of ventricular myosin isoenzyme were both greater in DM-WKY than in untreated SHR. This suggested that diabetes might influence myocardial contractility and energetics more than hypertension in rats. In DM-SHR, T did not differ from that in untreated SHR but ± dT/dtmax was decreased in comparison. T is related to the Ca^{2+} release or uptake by the sarcoplasmic reticulum. There have been reports of depressed function of the sarcoplasmic reticulum in diabetic animals (5-7). The present results are consistent with the speed of contraction being more affected by myocardial transformation than the developed tension and the working capacity (8,9). The myocardial response to isoproterenol and DBcAMP were depressed in DM-SHR in comparison with WKY or SHR. DBcAMP passes through the myocardial cell membrane without stimulating ß-receptors (10), and as we have previously reported with respect to post ß-receptor processes (4,11,12), changes in such processes might also contribute to the depressed myocardial catecholamine responsiveness seen in DM-SHR.

Table 1. Body weight, ventricular weight and papillary muscle size.

mean±SD

	BW (g)	VW (mg)	VW/BV	Papillary muscle size	
				L (mm)	CSA (mm²)
(a) WKY (n=10)	325.0 ±22.9	866.1 ±75.0	2.67 ±0.18	5.4 ±0.5	0.80 ±0.17
(b) SHR (n=9)	356.7 ±14.1**a	1512.3 ±75.7***a	4.24 ±0.10***a	5.6 ±0.5	1.01 ±0.15*a
(c) DM-SHR (n=8)	268.4 ±29.0***a ***b	1056.1 ±82.1***a ***b	3.93 ±0.18***a ***b	5.4 ±0.8	0.76 ±0.22*b

BW : body weight, VW : ventricular weight, L : length, CSA : cross sectional area,
*: $p<0.02$, **: $p<0.005$, ***: $p<0.001$

Table 2. Comparisons of mechanical parameters (I).

means±SD

	AT (g/mm²)	RT (g/mm²)	+dT/dtmax (g/mm²·s)	−dT/dtmax (g/mm²·s)
(a) WKY (n=10)	2.6 ±0.8	0.9 ±0.3	32.3 ±8.4	22.8 ±7.4
(b) SHR (n=9)	2.5 ±0.5	0.9 ±0.2	27.9 ±5.2	20.1 ±4.1
(c) DM-SHR (n=8)	2.5 ±0.7	0.8 ±0.2	23.7 ±4.5**a	15.6 ±3.7*a *b

AT : active tension, RT : resting tension, *: $p<0.05$, **: $p<0.02$

Table 3. Comparisons of mechanical parameters (II)

means±SD

	TPT (msec)	TCT (msec)	T1/2R (msec)
(a) WKY (n=10)	121.5 ±9.4	402.0 ±34.3	84.0 ±9.4
(b) SHR (n=9)	141.1 ±8.6**a	437.0 ±32.3*a	90.6 ±5.8
(c) DM-SHR (n=8)	150.0 ±6.5**a *b	470.0 ±22.9**a *b	102.5 ±2.7**a **b

TPT : time to peak tension, TCT : total contraction time, T1/2R : time to half relaxation. *: $P<0.05$, **: $P<0.001$

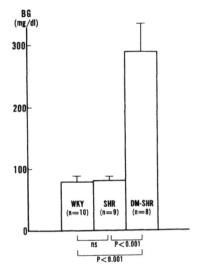

Figure 2. Comparisons of blood glucose.
Vertical lines indicate SD; ns: not significant

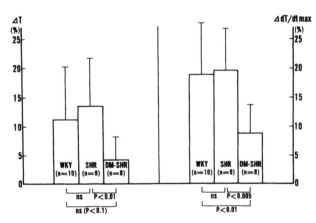

Figure 3. Comparisons of myocardial mechanical responsiveness to isoproterenol.
Vertical lines indicate SD; ns: not significant

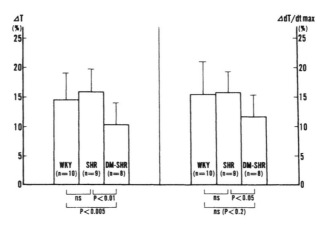

Figure 4. Comparisons of myocardial mechanical responsiveness to DBcAMP. Vertical lines indicate SD; ns: not significant.

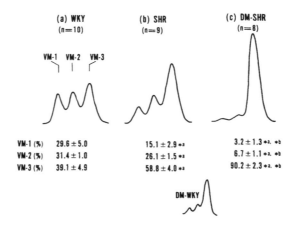

Figure 5. Left ventricular myosin isoenzyme pattern. Values are means ± SD; *:p<0.001

Summary

The influence of diabetes on myocardial contractility and myocardial energetics was investigated in the hypertrophic myocardium of spontaneously hypertensive rats (SHR). Diabetes was induced in 25- to 26- week-old male SHR by intravenous injection of streptozotocin. The body and ventricular weights of diabetic SHR (DM-SHR) were markedly reduced as compared with those of untreated SHR at 5 to 6 weeks after the injection of streptozotocin. There was no significant difference between the two groups with respect to isometric developed tension (T) in isolated left ventricular papillary muscles. However, +dT/dtmax showed a tendency to decrease, -dT/dtmax decreased significantly, and time to half relaxation was significantly prolonged in DM-SHR. Myocardial responses to isoproterenol and dibutyryl cAMP were significantly depressed in DM-SHR. In addition, the left ventricular myosin isoenzyme pattern, which was obtained by pyrophosphate gel electrophoresis, shifted towards VM-3, in DM-SHR. VM-3 has the slowest electrophoretic mobility and the lowest ATPase activity of the isoenzymes. Thus, diabetes compounded myocardial functional alterations in the hypertensive hypertrophic myocardium of SHR in association with changes of energetics.

Acknowledgement

This study was supported in part by the "Chiyoda Mutual Life Foundation".

References

1. Hoh JFY, McGrath PA, Hale PT. Electrophoretic analysis of multiple forms of rat cardiac myosin: Effects of hypophysectomy and thyroxin replacement. J Mol Cell Cardiol 1978;10:1053-1076.
2. d'Albis A, Pantaloni C, Becher JJ. An electrophoretic study of native myosin isoenzymes and of their subunit content. Eur J Biochem 1979;99:261-272.
3. Rupp H, Jacob R. Response of blood pressure and cardiac myosin polymorphism to swimming training in the spontaneously hypertensive rat. Can J Physiol Pharmacol 1982;60:1098-1103.
4. Takeda N, Ohkubo T, Nakamura I, Suzuki H, Nagano M. Mechanical catecholamine responsiveness and myosin isoenzyme pattern of pressure-overloaded rat ventricular myocardium. Basic Res Cardiol 1987;82:370-374.

5. Penpargkul S, Fein F, Sonnenblick EH, Scheuer J. Depressed cardiac sarcoplasmic reticular function from diabetic rats. J Mol Cell Cardiol 1981;13:303-309.
6. Ganguly PK, Pierce GN, Dhalla KS, Dhalla NS. Defective sarcoplasmic reticular calcium transport in diabetic cardiomyopathy. Am J Physiol 1983;244:E528-E535.
7. Lopaschuk GD, Katz S, McNeill JH. The effect of alloxan- and streptozotocin-induced diabetes on calcium transport in rat cardiac sarcoplasmic reticulum. The possible involvement of long chain acylcarnitines. Can J Physiol Pharmacol 1983;61:439-448.
8. Ebrecht G, Rupp H, Jacob R. Alterations of mechanical parameters in chemically skinned preparations of rat myocardium as a function of isoenzyme pattern of myosin. Basic Res Cardiol 1982;77:220-234.
9. Jacob R, Kissling G, Rupp H, Vogt M. Functional significance of contractile proteins in cardiac hypertrophy and failure. J Cardiovasc Pharmacol 1987;10(suppl 6):2-12.
10. Imai S, Otorii T, Takeda K, Katano Y, Horii D. Effects of cyclic AMP and dibutyryl cyclic AMP on the heart and coronary circulation. Jpn J Pharmacol 1974;24:499-510.
11. Takeda N, Dominiak P, Türck D, Rupp H, Jacob R. The influence of endurance training on mechanical catecholamine responsiveness, ß-adrenoceptor density and myosin isoenzyme pattern of rat ventricular myocardium. Basic Res Cardiol 1985;80:88-99.
12. Takeda N, Dominiak P, Türck D, Rupp H, Jacob R. Myocardial catecholamine responsiveness of spontaneously hypertensive rats as influenced by swimming training. Basic Res Cardiol 1985;80:384-391.

Hypertensive- Diabetic Cardiomyopathy in Rats

A. Malhotra

Department of Medicine, Montefiore Medical Center and
Albert Einstein College of Medicine, Bronx, NY, USA

Introduction

Hypertension and diabetes have been demonstrated to increase the risk of developing a cardiomyopathy in man (1,2). Our group previously described contractile, biochemical and ultrastructural properties of myocardium in rats with diabetes or renovascular hypertension (3-6). There were no direct biochemical comparisons made in the hearts of hypertensive, diabetic, hypertensive-diabetic and control rats derived from the same overall group of animals. Histological studies in a rat model with combined renovascular hypertension and diabetes show significant myocardial pathology with evidence of myocyte necrosis, replacement and interstitial fibrosis and possible microvascular spasm (7,8). Recent studies of isolated perfused heart function in spontaneously hypertensive and normotensive rats with and without diabetes strongly suggest that a combination of hypertension and diabetes results in greater cardiac dysfunction than that which occurs with hypertension or diabetes alone (9-11). Contractile protein biochemistry (myosin ATPase from left ventricular samples and myosin isoenzyme distribution from both left and right ventricular samples) was correlated to the papillary muscle function in these animals (12). The relative contribution of hypertension and diabetes to myocardial dysfunction in hypertensive-diabetic rats could be assessed from the present biochemical studies.

Materials and Methods

Animal Models: A single group of female Wistar rats (Charles River), 175 to 200 g in weight, was used to produce hypertensive (H), diabetic (D), hypertensive-diabetic (HD) and control (C) rats. Animals were made hypertensive by placing silver clips (0.24 mm inner diameter) around the left

Nagano, M., Mochizuki, S., Dhalla, N.S. (eds.), CARDIOVASCULAR DISEASE IN DIABETES. Copyright © 1992. Kluwer Academic Publishers, Boston. All rights reserved.

renal artery as described previously (3). Rats were considered hypertensive when systolic blood pressure was 150 mmHg or greater by 4 weeks after surgery. For diabetic animals, a single injection of 60 mg/kg streptozotocin (UpJohn Company) was administered intravenously by tail vein. Rats were considered diabetic when serum glucose concentration was 300 mg/100 ml or greater. To obtain combined hypertensive and diabetics, left renal artery clipping was performed 1 to 2 weeks before the streptozotocin injection (12). The criteria for development of hypertension and diabetics were the same as described above for hypertensives and diabetes individually. After initial determinations, blood pressure and heart rate were monitored (using ether anesthesia) every 2 to 4 weeks in H and HD rats and every 1 to 2 months in D and C rats. Two to 4 months after the renal artery clipping or streptozotocin injection, animals were sacrificed under ether anesthesia, at which time animals were weighed and blood for serum glucose was obtained (12).

Biochemical Measurements: The left and right ventricles were separately weighed and frozen in 50% glycerol (containing 50mM KCl and 10mM K_3PO_4, pH 7.0) at -80°C for contractile protein studies. Myosin from individual hearts was purified as described previously (5). Actin was extracted from rabbit skeletal muscle powder and purified as described by Spudich and Watt (13). Myosin preparations were checked for purity on polyacrylamide SDS slab gel gradients (5-16.5%) containinig 0.1% SDS according to the method of Laemmli (14). Myosin obtained in this manner was shown by SDS gel electrophoresis to be free of actin, troponin and tropomyosin and to be without evidence of proteolytic degradation. Protein concentrations were measured by the Biuret technique, using bovine serum albumin as a standard. Myosin ATPase activity measurements were performed in a final volume of 1.0ml at pH 7.6 and 30°C (5). All ATPase activity measurements were initiated by the addition of Na_2-ATP and terminated after 10 min by the addition of 0.5 ml or 1 ml of 10% tricholoroacetic acid. Inorganic phosphate (Pi) for Ca^{2+} - myosin ATPase was determined by the method of Fiske and Subbarow (15). Actin activated Mg^{2+}-ATPase activity of myosin was measured in a final volume of 1 ml containing 50 mM KCl, 20 mM Imadazole (pH 7.0), 3 mM $MgCl_2$, 2mM Na_2-ATP, 0.1 mg/ml of myosin, and 0.46 mg/ml of actin at 25°C. Microphosphate estimation of Pi for actin-activated Mg^{2+}-ATPase of myosin was determined by the method of Zak and co-workers (16). Results are expressed as micromoles of phosphate liberated per milligram of protein per minute.

For isoenzyme distribution, pyrophosphate gels of different myosin preparations under non-disassociating conditions were analyzed as described previously (17,18). Densitometric scans were recorded at 595 nm on a Beckman Acta MVI spectrophotometer, and the content of each isoenzyme was calculated from area under each peak by planimetry or by a Hewlett Packard integrator (3390 A) attached to an E-C apparatus densitometer.

Statistical Analysis: Statistical comparisons between two groups were performed using the unpaired Student's T-test. When three or more groups were compared, multiple analysis of variance by Newman Keul's test (19) was used. For correlation of mechanical and contractile protein data linear regression was performed using the method of least squares. Statistical significance was defined at P<0.05.

Results

Systolic blood pressure (BP; in mmHg) was increased in both hypertensives (187±4) and hypertensive-diabetics (171±3) when compared to controls (126±3) and diabetics (125±4). Serum glucose concentration was elevated significantly in D and HD rats (590-620 mg/100 ml vs 200-210 mg/100 ml in C and H groups). Body weight was significantly decreased in HD rats as compared to the controls (C = 297±7 g and HD = 227±15 g, N = 10 animals). Left ventricular (LV) weight increased significantly in hypertensives as compared to the controls (C = 0.61±0.02 g and H = 0.81±0.05 g; N = 10). There was a minimal increase of LV mass in HD's (0.68±0.05 g) but a small decrease of LV mass was observed in D's (0.55±0.01 g). Right ventricular (RV) weight was increased in HD rats (0.15±0.01 g) when compared to controls (0.12±0.01 g). Both hypertensives (0.15±0.02 g) and diabetics (0.14±0.01 g) were associated with an increase in relative RV mass.

Figure 1 shows that cardiac Ca^{2+} myosin ATPase in LV decreased progressively in preparations from hypertensives (H), diabetics (D) and hypertensive-diabetic (HD) rats as compared to the controls (C). The decline in myosin ATPase reflected the additive effects of hypertension and diabetes.

In Figure 2, the actin activated Mg^{2+}-myosin ATPase demonstrates similar trends as seen with Ca^{2+} myosin ATPase data although only the differences between C and either H, D or HD groups were statistically different using a one way analysis of variance. Both hypertension and diabetes were associated with a decrease in actin activated Mg^{2+}-myosin

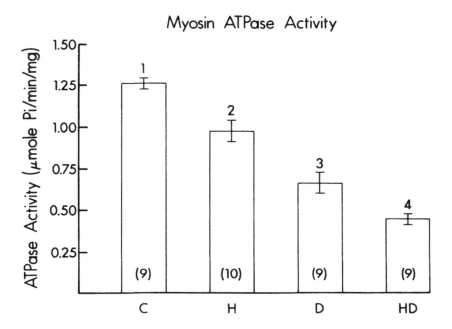

Figure 1. Ca^{2+}- myosin ATPase is shown as u mole of inorganic phosphate per mg per min at 30°C. C, controls; H, hypertensives; D, diabetics and HD, hypertensive-diabetics. No. of preparations are shown in parenthesis in the bar graph. Statistics 1-2, 1-3, 1-4, 2-3, 2-4. Pairs of numbers given in statistics signify group differences for which $P \leq 0.05$.

ATPase. Figure 3 shows the relative percentage of V_1 isoenzyme distribution in the LV's and RV's of C, H,D and HD groups. The decline in percent of V_1 isomyosin was progressive in parallel with the myosin ATPase data in Figure 1. There was a complete shift in V_1 to V_3 in HD's except in the heart of 1 animal (HD). The decline in percent V_1 isomyosin in HD's was reflected by the additive effects of hypertension and diabetes. Distribution of V_1 isomyosin in the RV's is shown on the right panel of Figure 3. Only myosin isoenzyme studies were performed on RV samples because of the lack of availability of larger muscle tissue. There was no significant decrease in percentage of V_1 isoenzyme in hypertensives when compared to controls, but D's and HD's exhibited a similar profound decrease in V_1 isoenzyme percent as observed in the LV of these animals.

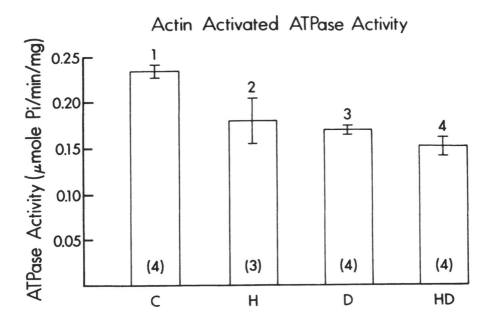

Figure 2. Actin activated Mg^{2+} - myosin ATPase activity shown is expressed as u mole Pi per min per mg at 25°C. C, controls; H, hypertensives; D, diabetics and HD, hypertensive-diabetics. No. of preparations are shown in parenthesis in the bar graph. Statistics 1-3, 1-4. Pairs of number in statistics signify group differences for which $P \leq 0.05$.

Discussion

The present study was focussed on the individual and combined effects of hypertension and diabetes on myocardial contractile proteins. While the severity of diabetes was comparable in diabetic and hypertensive-diabetic rats, the magnitude of hypertension was somewhat greater in hypertensives than HD rats. A hypotensive effect of diabetes has been previously shown in spontaneously hypertensive rats (9,10). The marked decline in body weight in HD rats might reflect additive effects of both hypertension and diabetes and may be a manifestation of congestive heart failure. This is suggested by the higher relative lung and liver weights observed in this group (12). The increase in relative right ventricular weight in HD rats raises the possibility of pulmonary hypertension and/or right ventricular failure in these animals.

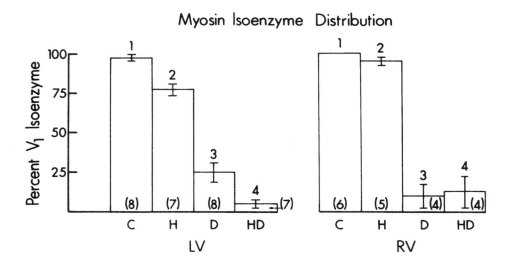

Figure 3. Myosin isoenzyme distribution is shown as percent V_1 isomyosin in LV (left panel) and RV (right panel) in the hearts of C, controls; H, hypertensives; D, diabetics and HD, hypertensive-diabetics. No. of preparations are shown in parenthesis in the bar graphs. Statistics for LV (%V_1) 1-2, 1-3, 1-4, 2-3, 2-4, 3-4; statistics for RV (%V_1) 1-3, 1-4, 2-3, 2-4. Pairs of numbers in statistics signify group differences for which $P \leq 0.05$.

Earlier studies from our group (4,5,20,21) and others (22,23) have shown alterations in contractile proteins, depressed cardiac SR function, alteration in sarcolemmal Na^+-K^+ ATPase and changes in mechanical function only in diabetics or in renal hypertensive animals. Contractile protein biochemistry has not been previously reported in this model of hypertensive-diabetic rat. In the present study, we analyzed left ventricular myosin ATPase activity and isoenzyume distribution in the LV's and RV's of C, H, D and HD rats. With respect to the left ventricle, there was a progressive decline in the myosin ATPase and in the percent content of V_1 myosin isozyme while comparing C to H, D and HD rats. The contractile protein changes in left ventricular preparations from H and D rats were similar to those previously described

(5,6). The effects of hypertension and diabetes were nearly additive in HD's. There was a complete transformation to V_3 in all but one HD rat. The decrease in myosin ATPase activity was approximately proportional to the shift from V_1 with higher specific activity to V_3 with slower ATPase activity. The decrease in peak velocity of shortening correlated very well with the changes in contractile protein ATPase activity (R =0.77) and isoenzyme shift (R = 0.82) in this model as reported by Fein et al. (12). This relationship has been well-documented earlier in skeletal muscle and in cardiac muscle. With respect to the right ventricle, the absence of any significant effect of systematic hypertension does not seem surprising and suggest that there is no substantial right ventricular pressure overload in H's. Conversely, the profound effect of diabetes is also expected since the metabolic disorder should influence both ventricles.

Summary

The combination of hypertension and diabetes has been shown to increase the risk of developing cardiomyopathy in man. Ventricular myosin ATPase and isoenzyme distribution were studied in hypertensive (H), diabetic (D), hypertensive - diabetic (HD) and control (C) rats. Left ventricular myosin ATPase activity showed an evidence for a progressive decline when comparing C with H, D and HD rats. The effects of hypertension and diabetes were nearly additive in HD's. Analysis of myosin isoenzyme distribution demonstrated a complete transformation to V_3 isomyosin in all but 1 HD rat. The decrease in myosin ATPase activity was roughly proportional to the shift from V_1 to V_3 isoenzyme. The absence of any significant change in V_1 isomyosin in the right ventricle (RV) suggests that there was no substantial RV pressure overload in H's. The decrease in peak velocity of shortening correlated with the changes in contractile protein ATPase activity and the myosin isoenzyme distribution (Data not shown; see ref. 12). These data suggest that the combination of myocardial pathology (due mainly to hypertension and diabetes) results in a further decline in cardiac contractile protein activity in HD rats when compared to H or D alone.

Acknowledgements

The author wishes to thank Dr. James Scheuer, Chairman, Department of Medicine, Montefiore Medical Center and Albert Einstein College of Medicine,

Bronx, NY for the encouragement and advice during the preparation of this manuscript. I would like to express my sincere thanks and profound gratitude to my collaborators - Drs. Frederick S. Fein, Edmund H. Sonnenblick and Stephen Factor. Expert secretarial assistance by Ms. Janice Brewton is deeply appreciated. This work was supported by the National Heart, Lung and Blood Institute Grants HL33240 and HL37412.

References

1. Factor SM, Minase T, Cho S, Fein F, Capasso JM and Sonnenblick EH. Coronary microvascular abnormalities in the hypertensive-diabetic rat. A primary cause of cardiomyopathy? Amer J Pathol 1984;116:9-20.
2. Shapiro LM, Howat AP, Calter MM. Left ventricular function in diabetes mellitus: I. Methodology and prevalence and spectrum of abnormalities. Br Heart J 1981;45:122-128.
3. Capasso JM, Strobeck JE, Malhotra A, Scheuer J and Sonnenblick EH. Contractile behaviour of rat myocardium after reversal of hypertensive hypertrophy. Amer J Physiol 1982;242:H882-H889.
4. Capasso JM, Strobeck JE and Sonnenblick EH. Myocardial mechanical alterations during gradual onset long-term hypertension in rats. Amer J Physiol 1981;241:H435-H441.
5. Malhotra A, Penpargkul S, Fein FS, Sonnenblick EH and Scheuer J. The effect of streptozotocin-induced diabetes in rats on cardiac contractile proteins. Circ Res 1981;49:1243-1250.
6. Capasso JM, Malhotra A, Scheuer J and Sonnenblick EH. Myocardial biochemical, contractile and electrical performance after imposition of hypertension in young and old rats. Circ Res 1980;58:445-460.
7. Factor SM, Minase T and Sonnenblick EH. Clinical and morphological features of human hypertensive-diabetic cardiomyopathy. Amer Heart J 1980;99:446-458.
8. Factor SM, Bhan R, Minase T, Wolinsky H and Sonnenblick EH. Hypertensive-diabetic cardiomyopathy in the rat: An experimental model of human disease. Amer J Pathol 1981;102:219-228.
9. Rodgers RL. Depressor effect of diabetes in the spontaneously diabetic rat: Associated changes in heart performance. Can J Physiol Pharmacol 1985;64:1177-1184.

10. Rodrigues B and McNeill JH. Cardiac function in spontaneously hypertensive-diabetic rats. Amer J Physiol 1986;251:H571-H580.
11. Fein FS, Capasso JM, Aronson RS, Cho S, Nordin C, Miller-Green B and Sonnenblick EH. Combined renovascular hypertension and diabetes in rats: A new preparation of congestive cardiomyopathy. Circ 1984;70:318-330.
12. Fein FS, Zola BE, Malhotra A, Cho S, Factor SM, Scheuer J and Sonnenblick EH. Hypertensive-diabetic cardiomyopathy in rats. Amer J Physiol 1991 (In Press).
13. Spudich JA and Watt S. The regulation of rabbit skeletal muscle contraction. J. Biol. Chem. 1971;246:4866-4871.
14. Laemmli UK. Cleavage of structural proteins during the assembly of the head of bacteriophage T_4. Nature (London), 1970;227:680-685.
15. Fiske CH, Subbarow Y. The colorimetric determination of phosphorous. J Bio Chem 1925;66:375-400.
16. Zak BE, Epstein E and Baginski ES. Determination of liver microsomal glucose-6-phosphatase. Ann Clin Lab Sci 1977;7:169-177.
17. Hoh JFY, McGrath PA, Hale PT. Electrophoretic analysis of multiple forms of rat cardiac myosin: Effects of hypophysectomy and thyroxine replacement. J Mol Cell Cardiol 1977;10:1053-1076.
18. Malhotra A, Karell M, Scheuer J. Multiple cardiac contractile protein abnormalities in myopathic Syrian hamsters (Bio 53:58) J Mol Cell Cardiol 1985;17:95-107.
19. Zar JH. Biostatistical Analysis. Prentice Hall, Englewood Cliffs, New Jersey, USA, 1974;151-155.
20. Penpargkul S, Fein FS, Sonnenblick EH and Scheuer J. Depressed cardiac sarcoplasmic reticular function from diabetic rats. J Mol Cell Cardiol 1981;13:303-309.
21. Fein FS, Kornstein LB, Strobeck JE, Capasso JM and Sonnenblick EH. Altered myocardial mechanics in diabetic rats. Circ Res 1980;47:922-933.
22. Dillman WH. Diabetes mellitus induced changes in cardiac myosin in the rat. Diabetes 1980;29:579-582.
23. Pierce GN, Dhalla NS. Sarcolemmal Na^+-K^+-ATPase activity in diabetic rat heart. Amer J Physiol 1983;245:C241-C247.

Combined Effects of Hypertension and Diabetes on Myocardial Contractile Proteins and Cardiac Function in Rats

M. Kato, N. Takeda, E. Kazama, J. Yang, T. Asano, H.Q. Yin and M. Nagano

Department of Internal Medicine, Aoto Hospital, Jikei University School of Medicine, Aoto 6-41-2, Katsushika-ku, Tokyo 125, JAPAN.

Introduction

Hypertension occurs with greater frequency in diabetic than in non-diabetic patients, and when heart failure develops in these patients it is occasionally resistant to therapy. Clinically, numerous reports have indicated a close relationship between diabetes and hypertension. Hypertension and diabetes mellitus (DM) both show a wide prevalence in humans; they can cause a number of myocardial deficiencies, resulting in a strikingly increased incidence of heart failure. The present study investigated the influence of hypertension, diabetes, and their combination on cardiac function and cardiac contractile proteins in Wistar rats.

Materials and Methods

Animals; Hypertension was induced by the Type II Goldblatt method in normotensive male Wistar rats (1) weighing 150-160 g, using silver clips placed on the left renal artery. Blood pressure was determined by tail plethysmography (Natsume KN-210-1) every week for 12 weeks post-operatively. Rats which showed a systolic blood pressure greater than 180 mmHg were defined as hypertensive. Hearts were removed for the isolation of actomyosin, and hearts of normal male Wistar rats of the same age were used as the control (C rats).

Diabetic rats (DM rats) were produced by the intravenously injecting C rats with alloxan at a dose of 45 mg/kg of body weight. Rats which had a fasting blood glucose over 250 mg/100 ml were defined as hyperglycemic, and their hearts were removed for isolation of actomyosin 4 weeks after the injection of alloxan. H+DM rats were produced by the intravenous injection of alloxan (45 mg/kg) into Goldblatt rats at 6 weeks after the operation to induce hypertension, and the hearts were removed for experimentation 4 weeks after the injection of alloxan. At the end of the experimental period, each animal of the four groups was weighed and anesthetized with sodium pentobarbital, and the the hearts were removed rapidly for experimentation.

Actomyosin extraction; Ventricles were minced and homogenized in Weber's solution (0.6 M KCl, 0.04 M $NaHCO_3$, and 0.01 M Na_2CO_3) and incubated for 20 hours at 4°C. The homogenate was centrifuged at 20,000 g for 60 minutes, distilled water was added to the supernatant and then this was centrifuged at 8,000 g for 15 minutes. The supernatant was discarded and the infranatant was added 1.2 M KCl to a final concentration of 0.6 M, followed by centrifugation at 20,000 g for 60 minutes. The supernatant was then recentrifuged at 8,000 g for 15 minutes, and the pellet was dissolved in 0.6 M KCl to obtain natural actomyosin (2).

Measurement of Ca^{2+}ATPase activity; Ca^{2+} ATPase activity was measured at pH 7.4 and pH 6.8 at 25°C (3). For the measurement of myosin Ca^{2+} ATPase activity, the actomyosin solution mixture was preincubated at 25°C, and reaction was initiated by the addition of the substrate. Aliquots of solution were incubated at 25°C for 5 minutes, then the reaction was stopped by the addition of trichloracetic acid. After centrifugation, the inorganic phosphate content of the supernatant was measured by the method of Fiske and Subbarow.

Other Methods

Left ventricular myosin isoenzymes were separated by the method of Hoh et al. (4), and left ventricular function was measured by Dowell's method (5). Rats were anesthetized and the right carotid artery was exposed via an incision in the neck. A Millar micro-tip catheter pressure transducer was advanced into the left ventricle, and the systolic and end-diastolic ventricular pressures were measured. Simultaneously, an electrocardiogram was recorded and the maximum rate of left ventricular (LV) pressure development was determined, and the the LV dP/dt max was derived using an analog differentiator.

Results

Figure 1 shows blood pressure curves for the four groups of rats. The blood pressure was constant throughout the experimental period in C rats. DM rats exhibited a slight but not significant elevation of blood pressure after the alloxan injection. H rats showed a significant increase of blood pressure at 10 days after the operation, and the blood pressure in H + DM rats was almost the same as in H rats. H and H+DM rats had a 10-week history of hypertension with or without a 4-week history of diabetes. Blood glucose levels in the four groups are shown in Fig. 2. The mean ± S.D. of the blood glucose values was comparable in the DM and H+DM rats.

Fig. 3 shows the relationship between heart weight and body weight in the rats. For DM rats, both the body weight and the heart weight was lower than in C rats. The heart weight of H rats was markedly increased and the body weight was moderatley reduced compared with C rats. Fig. 4 shows the heart/body weight ratios for the four groups. H rats and H+DM rats revealed a marked increase in heart/body weight ratio compared with C rats and DM rats.

Figs. 5 and 6 show myosin Ca^{2+} ATPase activity at pH 7.4 and pH 6.8, respectively. The ventricular myosin Ca^{2+} ATPase activity level at pH 7.4 was significantly lower in H rats (0.27 ± 0.03 Pi umol/mg/min) than in C rats (0.42 ± 0 .03 Pi umol/mg/min). DM rats exhibited an even lower value of 0.13 ± 0.02 Pi umol/mg/min, and H+DM rats had the lowest value at 0.06 ± 0.03 Pi umol/mg/min).

The myosin Ca^{2+} ATPase activity at pH 6.8 was also significantly lower in H rats (0.55 ± 0.08 Pi umol/mg/min) than in C rats (0.82 ± 0.08 Pi umon/mg/min). DM rats exhibited a value of 0.30 ± 0.09 Pi umol/mg/min, and H+DM rats again showed the lowest value at 0.17 ± 0.06 Pi umol/mg/min.

Figs. 7 and 8 depict actomyosin Ca^{2+} ATPase activity levels at pH 7.4 and pH 6.8 in the four groups of rats. These data showed essentially the same trend as seen for myosin Ca^{2+} ATPase activity, but there was a disparity between the level of myosin and actomyosin activity at the same pH.

Table 1 shows LV dP/dt max in the four rat groups. LV dP/dt max was increased to 14,130 ± 3,046 mmHg in H rats, against 8,901 ± 1,436 mmHg in C rats. DM rats showed a significantly lower value of 6, 254 ± 2,292 mmHg in comparison with C rats, while H+DM rats showed a value of 8,115 ± 2,158 mmHg, which was intermediate between the DM and H groups and differed little from the control level.

Fig. 9 shows the electrophoretic profiles of left ventricular myosin isoenzymes from rats of the four groups. Myosin isoenzymes were prepared as described in Methods.

Fig. 10 shows polyacrylamide SDS gel patterns for myosin isoenzymes in the four groups, and Table 2 shows the relative percentages of myosin isoenzymes determined in several rats from each group by electrophoretic analysis. As can be seen, fraction V_1 contained 72.9%, fraction V_2 contained 13.5%, and fraction V_3 contained 13.6% in the analysis of the left ventricular myocardium of C rats. In contrast, marked changes in the myosin isoenzyme pattern were noted in H rats (V_1, 40.4%; V_2, 27.8% and V_3, 31.7%). DM rats (V_1, 13.5%; V_2, 22.8%, and V_3, 63.4%) and H+DM rats (V_1, 9.9%; V_2, 18.9%, and V_3, 70.9%). A shift towards the situation $V_1<V_2<V_3$ was observed to a varying extent in the different groups.

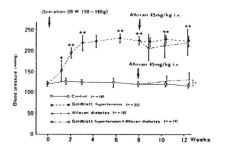

Figure 1. Blood pressure curves for the four groups of rats. Rats which showed a systolic blood pressure greater than 180 mmHg were defined as hypertensive. The blood pressure was constant throughout the experimental period in C rats. H rats showed a significant increase of blood pressure at 10 days after the operation, and the blood pressure in H+DM rats was almost the same as in H rats. P values denoted by asterisks indicate a comparison between C rats and H or H + DM rats. *P<0.05 **P<0.01 mean ± S.D.

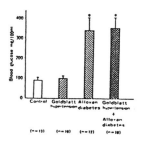

Figure 2. Blood glucose levels in the four rat groups. The mean ± S.D. of the blood glucose values was comparable in the DM and H+DM rats. *P<0.001.

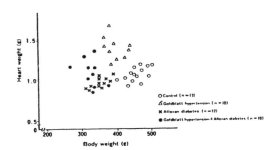

Figure 3. The relationship between heart weight and body weight in the rats. In DM rats, both the body weight and the heart weight was lower than in C rats. The heart weight of H rats was markedly increased and the body weight was moderatley reduced compared with C rats.

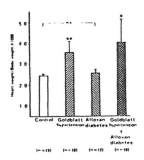

Figure 4. Heart/body weight ratios for the four groups. H rats and H+DM rats revealed a marked increase in heart/body weight ratio compared with C rats and DM rats. *$P<0.05$ **$P<0.01$ mean ± S.D.

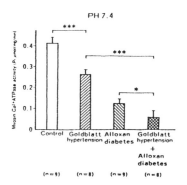

Figure 5. Myosin Ca^{2+} ATPase activity at pH 7.4. The ventricular myosin Ca^{2+} ATPase activity level at pH 7.4 was significantly lower in H rats than in C rats. DM rats exhibited an even lower value, and H+DM rats had the lowest value. *P<0.05, ***P< 0.001 mean ± S.D.

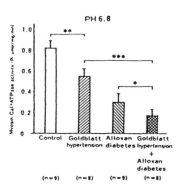

Figure 6. Myosin Ca^{2+} ATPase activity at pH 6.8. *P<0.05, **P<0.01, ***P<0.001 mean ± S.D.

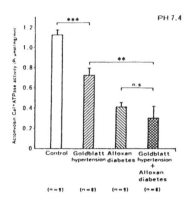

Figure 7. Actomyosin Ca^{2+} ATPase activity levels at pH 7.4. Ca^{2+} ATPase activity levels at pH 7.4 showed essentially the same trends as seen for myosin Ca^{2+} ATPase activity, but there was a disparity between the level of myosin and actomyosin activity. **$P<0.01$, ***$P<0.001$ mean ± S.D.

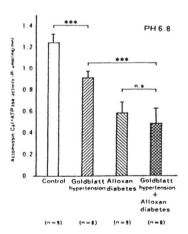

Figure 8. Actomyosin Ca^{2+} ATPase activity levels at pH 6.8. ***$P<0.001$ mean ± S.D.

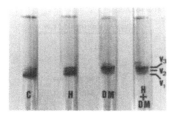

Figure 9. Electrophoretic profiles of left ventricular myosin isoenzymes. Comparison of left ventricular cardiac myosin from control rats (C), Goldblatt hypertensive rats (H), diabetic rats (DM), hypertensive-diabetic rats (H + DM).

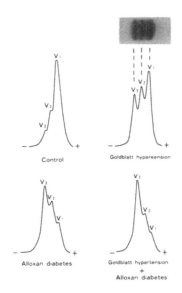

Figure 10. Myosin isoenzyme patterns of four rat groups. Densitometric patterns of PAG disc electrophoresis of rat myosin isoenzyme.

Table 1. LV dP/dt max in the four rat groups.

Rats		LV dP/dt max (mmHg/sec)
Control	n=8	8,901 ± 1,436
Goldblatt hypertension	n=4	14,130 ± 3,046*
Alloxan diabetes	n=5	6,254 ± 2,292**
Goldblatt hypertension + Alloxan diabetes	n=9	8,115 ± 2,158

LV dP/dt max was increased in H rats. DM rats showed a significantly lower value in comparison with C rats, while H+DM rats showed intermediate between the DM and H groups and differed little from the control level. Mean ± S.D.

Table 2. The relative percentages of myosin isoenzymes in the four groups.

Rats		V_1	V_2	V_3
Control	n=5	72.9 ± 3.1	13.5 ± 1.5	13.6 ± 3.4
Goldblatt hypertension	n=9	40.4 ± 9.0*a	27.6 ± 4.3	31.7 ± 7.5*a
Alloxan diabetes	n=5	13.5 ± 6.2*b,c	22.8 ± 3.6	63.4 ± 8.4*b,c
Goldblatt hypertension + Alloxan diabetes	n=6	9.9 ± 2.4*b,d	18.9 ± 4.3	70.9 ± 4.9*b,d

*Significant difference from control, P<0.001. a and b denotes significant difference from each other by a vertical line, P<0.001. c and d denotes no difference from each other. Mean ± S.D.

Discussion

Heart disease accompanying diabetes mellitus is a very important prognostic factor, due to its high incidence and the high percentage of cardiac deaths in diabetes patients. Furthermore, if hypertension is present in a diabetic patient, the risk of heart failure is high, and such heart failure is often resistant to therapy. Thus, the combination of diabetes mellitus and hypertension requires special care in its treatment.

It was shown that the combination of diabetes and hypertension could enhance myocardial damage by Sonnenblick et al. (6,7,8,9), Mall (10), and Rodgers (11) among others. The effects of diabetes and hypertension on the myocardium may be divided into those due to ischemic and those due to metabolic abnormalities. Concerning the metabolic abnormalities, many studies have been performed in laboratory animals from a biochemical perspective.

In our experimental animal models of diabetes mellitus, alloxan or STZ have been administered to rats to produce diabetes, and investigations have been conducted into the causes of impaired myocardial function. Takeda et al. (12) working at our laboratories, found that the maximum rate of tension increase (+dT/dt max) and maximum rate of tension decrease (-dT/dt max) were reduced and the time to peak tension was prolonged in the isometric contraction of isolated left ventricular papillary muscles obtained from diabetic rats. In the case of pressure overload myocardial hypertrophy, for both Goldblatt hypertensive rats and SHR, the maximum rates of tension increase and decrease have been shown to be reduced and the time to peak tension to be prolonged, as was the case with diabetes mellitus. However, in both diabetic rats and Goldblatt hypertensive rats, the maximum tension developed was not always decreased.

It has been shown that the myosin isoenzyme distribution varies with species (13), age (14), hormonal abnormalities (4,10), and stress (15). Isoenzymic changes of myosin, which could account for the enzymatic alterations, have been described in hypophysectomised rats (4). Hoh et al. have identified three isoenzymes of rat ventricular myocardial myosin on the basis of their mobility in non-dissociating gel electrophoresis. We assumed that in normal rats the isoenzyme from fraction V_1 predominated and myosin Ca^{2+} ATPase activity was relatively high. Under chronic pressure overload or in a hyperglycemic state, type V_1 myosin changes to type V_3 myosin, resulting in reduced shortening velocity. This evidence has been obtained from rats with myocardial alterations associated with long-term renal hypertension and diabetes.

In this study, as shown in Table 2, myosin isoenzyme analysis revealed a predominance of type V_1 in C rats, wyhile the isoenzyme pattern in H rats showed a shift to a predominance of type V_3. A more pronounced shift (with the pattern of $V_1<V_2<V_3$) was observed in DM rats, and H+DM rats

displayed the most conspicuous charge to the predominance of V_3. It is well known that decreased myocardial contractility in hypertensive or diabetic rats is associated with reduced myofibrillar ATPase activity (3,16). In DM rats, a decrease occurs in the maximum velocity of ventricular contraction, accompanied by a decrease in myosin Ca^{2+} ATPase activity (17,18).

There is evidence that various forms of hemodynamic stress are associated with changes in the ATPase activity of myocardial myosin and actomyosin (16). Cardiac hypertrophy induced by pressure overload is associated with a decrease in the myofibrillar ATPase activity and the maximum unloaded shortening velocity, while the hypertrophy induced by several weeks of swimming training (19) or experimental thyrotoxicosis increase both the ATPase activity and unloaded shortening velocity (20). Comparative assessments have been made concerning cardiac performance by taking LV dP/dt max as a parameter of left ventricular function in rats with various alterations in myosin isoenzyme patterns and enzymatic activity.

It is empirically known that the use of a cardiotonic which augments cardiac contractility is associated with a steepening of the gradient of the rise in left ventricular pressure during the isovolumic contraction phase, whereas administration of drugs that diminsh cardiac contractility results in a gentle slope of the left ventricular pressure curve during the same phase of the cardiac cycle. Reports on LV dP/dt max changes in spontaneously hypertensive rats (SHR), have revealed that the mechanical performance of the left ventricle is depressed even in the early stages of hypertension in SHR (21). In contrast, Pfeffer et al. have reported that the compensation phase in moderate ventricular hypertrophy was associated with a normal cardiac pumping ability (22), although older male SHR did not sustain this pumping ability and demonstrated a depressed cardiac performance which was not evident in age-matched 18-month-old female SHR (22). We found that H rats exhibited a moderate elevation of LV dP/dt max, while DM rats showed a slight fall compared with C rats, and there was no significant difference between H+DM rats and C rats. Thus, there was no substantial fall below the control LV dP/dt mkax in any of the experimental groups, except in some H+DM rats that developed heart failure.

Under hypertensive cardiac overload or in the diabetic state, the heart is placed in a noticeably unfavorable situation with respect to energy utilization. The myosin isoenzyme shift from V_1 to V_3, i.e., the change to ATPase with a lower activity, has advantages for the myocardium under such circumstances from the aspect of energy utilization efficiency. Thus, this isoenzyme shift can be seen as representing myocardial adaptation.

In conclusion, we found that hypertension and diabetes induced alterations in myocardial myosin isoenzyme patterns and Ca^{2+} ATPase activity. In hypertensive-diabetic rats, the changes of myocardial contractile proteins were more marked than with either hypertension or diabetes alone. Finally, other hypertension and diabetes exerted adverse effect upon myocardial function by inducing structural changes of the contractile proteins.

Summary

The effects of hypertension and diabetes on myocardial contractile proteins and cardiac functions were investigated in Wistar rats. Hypertension was induced by left renal artery banding (H rats), and diabetes by the injection of 45 mg/kg of alloxan (DM rats). The combination of hypertension and diabetes (H+DM rats) was produced by injecting alloxan into H rats. Myosin and actomyosin Ca^{2+} ATPase activities were measured and the myocardial myosin isoenzymes were compared in 4 groups of rats. The LV dP/dt max was also measured using a compared Millar micro-tip transducer inserted via the right carotid artery. The V_3 isoenzyme fraction increased from 13.6% in C rats to 31.7% in H rats, and then to 63.4% in DM rats. H+DM rats had the highest V_3 fraction at 70.9%. Myosin and actomyosin Ca^{2+} ATPase activities were decreased significantly in H and DM rats compared with C rats, and also in H+DM rats compared with H or DM rats. LV dP/dt max increased by 59% in H rats compared with C rats. DM rats displayed a significant decrease of 30% compared with C rats, and H + DM rats showed a 9% decline.

Contractile proteins from hypertensive-diabetic rat myocardium were markedly affected when compared with proteins from rats with either hypertension or diabetes alone. The decrease in myosin or actomyosin Ca^{2+} ATPase activity was accompanied by a progressive change of the predominant myosin isoenzyme from V_1 to V_3. Thus, combination of hypertension and diabetes exerted adverse effects upon myocardial function by producing structural changes of the contractile proteins.

Acknowledgements

This study was partly supported by a Grant-in-Aid for Scientific

Research (No. 01770872) from the Ministry of Education, Culture and Science, Japan, 1989.

References

1. Kaplan NM. The Goldblatt Memorial Lecture, Part II. The role of the kidney in hypertension. Hypertension 1979;1:456-461.
2. Stracher A. Evidence for the involvement of light chains in the biological functioning of myosin. Biochem Biophys Res Commun 1969;35:519-525.
3. Medugorac I. Characteristics of the hypertrophied left ventricular myocardium in Goldblatt rats. Basic Res Cardiol 1977;72:261-267.
4. Hoh JFY, McGrath PA and Hale PT. Electrophoretic analysis of multiple forms of rat cardiac myosin: Effects of hypophysectomy and thyroxine replacement. J Mol Cell Cardiol 1977;10:1053-1076.
5. Dowell RT, Cutilletta AF and Sodt PC. Functional evaluation of the rat heart in situ. J Appl Physiol 1975;39:1043-1047,
6. Fein FS, Cho S, Zola BE, Miller B and Factor SM. Cardiac pathology in the hypertensive diabetic rat. Biventricular damage with right ventricular predominance. Am J Pathol 1989;134:1159-1166.
7. Factor SM, Minase T, Cho S, Fein F, Capasso JM and Sonnenblick EH. Coronary microvascular abnormalities in the hypertensive-diabetic rat. A primary case of cardiomyopathy? Am J Pathol 1984;116:9-20.
8. Fein FS, Capasso JM, Aronson RS, Cho S, Nordin C, Miller-Green B, Sonnenblick EH and Factor SM. Combined renovascular hypertension and diabetes in rats: A new preparation of congestive cardiomyopathy. Circulation 1984;70:318-330.
9. Factor SM, Bhan R, Minase T, Wolinsky H and Sonnenblick EH. Hypertensive-diabetic cardiomyopathy in the rat. An experimental model of human disease. Am J Pathol 1981;102:218-228.
10. Mall G, Klingel K, Baust H, Hasslacher Ch, Mann J, Mattfeldt T and Waldherr R. Synergistic effects of diabetes mellitus and renovascular hypertension on the rat heart-stereological investigations on papillary muscles. Virchows Arch A 1987;411:531-542.
11. Rodgers RL. Depressor effect of diabetes in the spontaneously hypertensive rat: Associated changes in heart performance. Can J Physiol Pharmacol 1985;64:1177-1184.

12. Takeda N, Nakamura I, Hatanaka T, Ohkubo T. and Nagano M. Myocardial mechanical and myosin isoenzyme alterations in streptozotocin-diabetic rats. Jap Heart J 1988;29:455-463.
13. Rupp H, Kissling G and Jocob R. Hormonal and hemodynamic determinants of polymorphic myosin. In: Perspectives in Cardiovascular Research, Vol. 7. Katz, AM (ed). Raven Press, New York, 1983, pp.373-383.
14. Schwartz K, Lompre AM, Lacombe G, Bouveret P, Wisnewsky C, Whalen RG, D'Albis A and Swynghedauw B. Cardiac myosin isoenzymic transitions in mammals. In: Perspectives in Cardiovascular Research, Vol 7. Katz, AM (ed). Raven Press, New York, 1983, pp.345-358.
15. Carey RA, Natarajan G, Bove AA, Coulson RL and Spann JF. Myosin adenosine triphosphatase activity in the volume-overloaded hypertrophied feline right ventricle. Circ Res 1979;45:81-87.
16. Scheuer J and Bahn AK. Cardiac contractile proteins. Adenosine triphosphatase activity and physiological function. Circ Res 1978;45:1-12.
17. Fein FS, Kornstein LB, Strobeck JE, Capasso JM and Sonnenblick EH. Altered myocardial mechanics in diabetic rats. Circ Res 1980;47:922-933.
18. Pierce GN and Dhalla NS. Cardiac myofibrillar ATPase activity in diabetic rats. J Mol Cell Cardiol 1981;13:1063-1069.
19. Takeda N, Nakamura I, Ohkubo T, Hatanaka T and Nagano M. Effects of physical training on the myocardium of streptozotocin-induced diabetic rats. Basic Res Cardiol 1988;83:525-530.
20. Jacob R, Ebrecht G, Holubarsch CH, Rupp H and Kissling G. Mechanics and energetics in cardiac hypertrophy as related to the isoenzyme pattern of myosin. Perspectives in Cardiovascular Research, Vol. 7. Katz, AM. (ed.) Raven Press, New York, 1983, pp. 553-569.
21. Spech MM, Ferrario CM and Tarazi RC. Cardiac pumping ability following reversal of hypertrophy and hypertension in spontaneously hypertensive rats. Hypertension 1980;2:75-82.
22. Pfeffer JM, Pfeffer MA and Braunwald E. Development of left ventricular dysfunction in the female spontaneously hypertensive rats. In: Perspectives in Cardiovascular Research, Vol. 7. Katz, AM. (ed.) Raven Press, New York, 1983, pp.73-84.

Diabetes Does Not Accelerate Cardiac Hypertrophy In Spontaneously Hypertensive Rats (SHR)

T. Sato, Y. Nara, Y. Kato, Y. Yamori

Departments of Internal Medicine & Pathology, Shimane Medical University
Izumo, JAPAN.

Introduction

Spontaneously hypertensive rats (SHR) develop various cardiovascular changes including cerebral hemorrage and/or infarction, nephrosclerosis and cardiac hypertrophy. Hypertension, which is present in 40-80% of patients with long standing diabetes mellitus (1) has been implicated in the development of diabetic cardiac complications. The aim of this study is to investigate the effect of diabetes on cardiac hypertrophy in SHR.

Methods

Diabetes was developed in SHR by neonatal injection of streptozotocin as previously described (2). Five female hypertensive diabetic rats (SHR-D) and hypertensive non-diabetic rats (SHR-C) were sacrificed at the age of 8 months, and the heart was removed and weighed. The left ventricle and coronary vessels were examined histologically. Cardiac hypertrophy was estimated by the size of myocardial cell nuclei (MCN) and the number of MCN per test area with an automatic image analyzer. Narrowing rate of each coronary artery whose diameter was 50-200 um was calculated by the formula of 1-luminal area/total cross section area.

Results

General characteristics of each group are summarized in Table 1. Body weight of SHR-D increased less than that of SHR-C. Blood pressure of SHR-D was significantly higher than that of controls. FBS was significantly higher and F-IRI was significantly lower in SHR-D than in SHR-C. There was no significant difference in plasma lipids level between in SHR-C and SHR-D.

Nagano, M., Mochizuki, S., Dhalla, N.S. (eds.), CARDIOVASCULAR
DISEASE IN DIABETES. Copyright © 1992. Kluwer Academic Publishers,
Boston. All rights reserved.

Table 1. General Characteristics of Groups

Group (number)	Body Weight (g)	Blood Pressure (mmHg)	FPG (mg/dl)	F-IRI (uU/ml)	Trigly-ceride (mg/dl)	Total chol. (mg/dl)	HDL chol. (mg/dl)
SHR-C (5)	225 ± 6	198 ± 4	110 ± 10	33 ± 4	41 ± 3	52 ± 4	36 ± 4
	$p<0.01$	$p<0.01$	$p<0.01$	$p<0.01$	NS	NS	NS
SHR-D (5)	192 ± 6	213 ± 3	201 ± 29	21 ± 2	45 ± 16	47 ± 6	34 ± 6

Results are expressed as mean ± SD

Table 2. Quantification of Myocardial Hypertrophy

Group (number)	Heart Weight (g)	Relative Heart Weight (/100g Body Weight)	Myocardial cell nucleus	
			Number (/$10^3 um^2$)	Size (um^2)
SHR-C (5)	1.02 ± 0.08	4.52 ± 0.33	1.06 ± 0.09	18.9 ± 7.3
	$p<0.01$	NS	$p<0.01$	$p<0.01$
SHR-D (5)	0.87 ± 0.03	4.52 ± 0.05	1.26 ± 0.07	16.0 ± 5.4

Table 2 shows absolute and relative heart weight, and also shows the number of myocardial cell nuclei (MCN) and the size of MCN per test area in both groups. Absolute heart weight of SHR-D was significantly lower than that of SHR-C, however there was no significance in relative heart weight between SHR-C and SHR-D. The number of MCN was significantly increased and the size of MCN was significantly smaller in SHR-D than SHR-C, indicating a reduced myocardial cell size.

Histologically, the myocardial fibers of SHR-D appeared constantly reduced in size when compared with those of SHR-C. Differences in interstitial fibrosis between SHR-C and SHR-D were not significant. The results of quantification of intramyocardial vascular alterations are shown in Table 3.

Table 3. Quantification of Intramyocardial Vascular Alterations

Group (number)	Observed Vessel Number	Total Cross Section Area (T) um^2	Luminal Area (L) um^2	Narrowing Rate (1-L/T) %
SHR-C (5)	85	2746 ± 2135	1136 ± 1047	59.9 ± 14.4
		NS	p<0.01	p<0.01
SHR-D (5)	92	2936 ± 2088	760 ± 669	75.5 ± 9.7

Results are expressed as mean ± SD

The luminal area was significantly smaller and the narrowing rate was significantly higher in SHR-D than in SHR-C, indicating a thickening of the media.

By comparing the histograms compiled from narrowing rate of SHR-C and SHR-D (Fig. 1), we observed for the latter, a clear shift to the right. The media and adventitia and/or perivascular fibrosis of SHR-D were generally thicker than those of SHR-C. Amount of PAS-positive material in vascular walls was greater in SHR-D than SHR-C. Intimal thickening or duplication of lamina elastica was not clear in both groups.

Discussion

By investigating the relative number and size of cell nuclei, it was found that myocardial fibers were hypotrophic in SHR-D. The hypertrophy in SHR is most likely dependent on a higher dynamic load whereas hypotrophy in diabetics is probably related to a more generalized negative effect of diabetes on striated muscle, as found in the diaphragm of Wistar rats (3).

Diabetic cardiomyopathy manifested by myocardial cell degeneration and fibrosis has been described in normotensive (4) and Goldblatt-hypertensive (5) rats. Fibrosis was greater in hypertensive diabetic than in hypertensive non-diabetic rats but absent in normotensive diabetic rats (5). Only a slight diffuse and/or localized fibrosis and perivascular fibrosis were present in our animals, particularly in SHR-D. The media and adventitia of SHR-D were thicker than those of control. Diabetes and hypertension are considered to predisposing factors in arteriosclerosis. Progressive medial thickening and

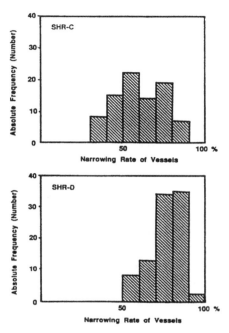

Figure 1. Distribution of Narrowing Rate of SHR-C (top) and SHR-D (bottom).

re-orientation of smooth muscle cells in the absence of intimal lesions have been described in the intrarenal arteries of SHR from 10 weeks on (6). Medial thickening was found in coronary vessels of stroke-prone SHR (7) and the epicardial vessels of SHR were affected by medial degeneration (8). Diabetes accelerates these medial thickenings in SHR.

Summary

Diabetes mellitus was induced in spontaneously hypertensive rats (SHR) by neonatal injection of streptozotocin. At the age of 8 months, the left ventricle and coronary vessels were examined histologically. Body weight of hypertensive diabetic rats (SHR-D) increased less than that of hypertensive non-diabetic rats (SHR-C). Blood pressure of SHR-D was significantly higher than that of controls. FBS was significantly higher and F-IRI was significantly lower in SHR-D than in SHR-C. There was no significant difference in plasma lipids level between SHR-C and SHR-D. Absolute heart weight of SHR-D was significantly lower than that of SHR-C, however, there was no significance in relative heart weight between SHR-C and SHR-D. The number of myocardial cell nuclei (MCN) was significantly increased and the size of MCN was significantly smaller in SHR-D than SHR-C, indicating a reduced myocardial cell size. The luminal area was significantly smaller and the narrowing rate was significantly smaller and the narrowing rate was significantly higher in SHR-D than in SHR-C, indicating a thickening of the media.

References

1. Christlieb AR. Diabetes and hypertensive vascular disease. Mechanisms and treatment. Am J Cardiol 1973;32:592-606.
2. Sato T, Nara Y, Note S, and Yamori Y. New establishment of hypertensive diabetic animal models: Neonatally streptozotocin-treated spontaneously hypertensive rats. Metabolism 1987;36:731-737.
3. Bestetti G, Zemp C, Probst D, and Rossi GL. Neuropathy and myopathy in the diaphragm of rats after 12 months of streptozotocin-induced diabetes mellitus. A light-, electron-microscopic and morphometric study. Acta Neuropathol 1981;55:11-20.
4. Baandrup U, Ledet T, and Rasch R. Experimental diabetic cardiopathy preventable by insulin treatment. Lab Invest 1981;45:169-172.
5. Factor SM, Bhan R, Minase T, Wolinsky H and Sonnenblick EH. Hypertensive-diabetic cardiomyopathy in the rat. An experimental model of human disease. Am J Pathol 1981;102:219-228.
6. Limas C, Westrum B and Limas CJ. The evolution of vascular changes in the spontaneously hypertensive rat. Am J Pathol 1980;98:357-384.
7. Yamori Y, Kihara M, Fujishin S, Nara Y and Ooshima A. Structural alteration in relation to cardiac hypertrophy in SHR. Jpn Heart J 1980;21:568.
8. Saer JB, Chen I, Yates RD and Ichinose H. Age-related alterations in epicardial arteries of spontaneously hypertensive rats. Virch Arch [Cell Pathol] 1981;36:77-86.

A Close Correlation of Fasting Insulin Levels to Blood Pressure in Obese Children

H. Kanai, Y. Matsuzawa, S. Fujioka, K. Tokunaga and S. Tarui

The Second Department of Internal Medicine, Osaka University Medical School, Osaka, JAPAN

Introduction

Many epidemiologic studies suggest that obesity is an important factor in the development of hypertension (1,2). However, the mechanism linkage of obesity to hypertension has not been fully elucidated (3,4). Especially in adult obese subjects, they have various degrees of arteriosclerosis in each case because the severity of metabolic disorders and the duration of obesity were different in each case, and it may be related with hypertension or cardiac function in obesity (5). However, it is difficult to estimate the effect of arteriosclerosis on blood pressure quantitatively. Therefore, we studied the relationship between blood pressure and obesity in school children in order to exclude the effects of aging and arteriosclerotic factors and clarify the direct effect of obesity on blood pressure in this population.

Methods

Our study comprised 324 (216 males and 108 females) obese school children living in Osaka, aged 11.2 ± 2.1 years (mean ± standard deviation). Children with a body weight more than 40% above the standard body weight (SBW) were classified as obese. The SBW was estimated by Hibi's nomogram (6), which was a weight-for-height chart for children, decided by the statistical data on national wide scales. Systolic and diastolic blood pressure (mmHg), defined by the first and the fifth phase of Korotkoff's sound, were measured using a sphygmomanometer with a 12 cm cuff after a 10 minute rest in supine position. The mean of two measurements was used in analysis. This cuff, which is ordinarily used for non-obese adults, is adequate for blood pressure measurement in obese children, because overestimation of blood pressure due

Nagano, M., Mochizuki, S., Dhalla, N.S. (eds.), CARDIOVASCULAR DISEASE IN DIABETES. Copyright © 1992. Kluwer Academic Publishers, Boston. All rights reserved.

to short cuff width is excluded by this method (7). Blood pressure was also measured in 2629 non-obese school children in the same generation using a 9 cm cuff in the same way. The criteria of hypertension in children were decided by the data of blood pressure in these control children as follows. Namely, the subjects with a systolic blood pressure level more than the mean value plus twice the standard deviation and/or with a diastolic blood pressure level more than the mean value plus twice the standard deviation were classified as hypertensive.

Height, weight, waist circumference (umbilical portion) and hip circumference (over greater trochanters) were measured in all obese children and 97 control children. Skinfold thickness of the triceps (the middle of upper arm), subscapular and periumbilical area was also estimated using calipers. We used triceps skinfold thickness as a measure of peripheral body fat and subscapular and periumbilical skinfold thickness as a measure of central body fat. Waist to hip circumference ratio (WHR), which is commonly used to differentiate lower body obesity and upper body obesity, was also calculated.

Blood samples were collected after an overnight fast from 50 obese children and 97 control children. Serum levels of total cholesterol, triglyceride and uric acid were measured by enzymatic methods. Plasma glucose levels were measured by a glucose oxidase method and serum immunoreactive insulin (IRI) levels were measured by a double antibody radioimmunoassay. Blood samples for the assay of plasma adrenaline and noradrenaline were collected in cold tubes containing EDTA2Na (1.5 mg/ml). Plasma levels of adrenaline and noradrenaline were measured using a high performance liquid chromatography.

Statistics. Results were expressed as mean ± standard deviation. The significance of differences between means of measurement for two groups was determined by Student's t-test for unpaired data. Linear regression analysis was used to study the relationship between the variables.

Results

The obese children had significantly high blood pressure levels compared with the non-obese children (systolic blood pressure: 121 ± 14 mmHg vs. 112 ± 11 mmHg, $p < 0.001$; diastolic blood pressure: 72 ± 9 mmHg vs. 66 ± 7 mmHg, $p < 0.001$).

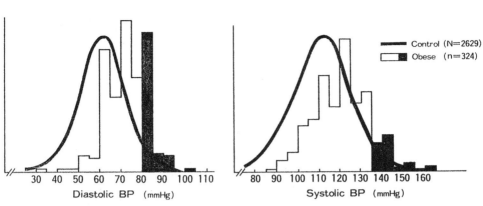

Figure 1. Distribution pattern of blood pressure (BP) in obese and non-obese control children.

Figure 1 shows the distribution pattern of blood pressure in the obese and the non-obese controlled children. The systolic or diastolic blood pressure in 2629 control children followed a normal distribution very closely. In this figure, the distribution pattern of blood pressure in the control children was indicated schematically as a normal probability curve determined by the mean and standard deviation. The distribution pattern of systolic or diastolic blood pressure in the obese children shifted to a right zone (higher blood pressure zone) compared with that in controlled children. The criteria of hypertension in children were defined to be more than 135 mmHg of systolic blood pressure and/or 80 mmHg of diastolic blood pressure, because the mean of systolic or diastolic blood pressure plus twice the standard deviation in the non-obese children was 135 mmHg or 80 mmHg, respectively. Consequently, 34% of the obese children were classified as hypertensive.

Anthropometric and metabolic features of the obese children and the non-obese children are shown in Table 1. They had different topography (high WHR and thick skinfolds) and metabolic disorders compared with the non-obese children, although the mean WHR in the obese children was considerably low in contrast with the WHR reported in adult subjects with the same degree of obesity. The levels of fasting serum IRI, triglyceride and uric acid in the obese children were also significantly higher than those in the non-obese children. Moreover, we compared the anthropometric and metabolic features between the hypertensive and the normotensive obese groups by our criteria, as was shown in Table 2.

Table 1. Clinical features of obese and non-obese children.

	Obese (n=324)	Non-obese (n=97)
Age (years)	11.2 ± 2.1	11.1 ± 2.2
Skinfold thickness		
Triceps (mm)	27 ± 12=	14 ± 4
Subscapular (mm)	35 ± 13=	8 ± 3
Periumbilical (mm)	37 ± 13=	10 ± 5
Waist / Hip ratio	0.92 ± 0.12=	0.81 ± 0.09
Metabolic factors[a]		
Fasting plasma glucose (mg/dl)	90 ± 7	94 ± 8
Fasting serum IRI (uU/ml)	15.2 ± 7.5†	4.8 ± 1.6
Total cholesterol (mg/dl)	184 ± 32	177 ± 29
Triglyceride (mg/dl)	130 ± 46†	110 ± 44
Uric acid (mg/dl)	4.4 ± 0.6*	4.0 ± 1.1

[a] in obese subjects were measured in 50 subjects.
The values are mean ± standard deviation.
*$p < 0.02$; †$p < 0.01$; =$p < 0.001$.
IRI = immunoreactive insulin.

The distribution patterns of blood pressure and % of SBW and anthropometric factors in 50 obese subjects who had blood drawn were almost similar to those in 324 obese subjects (data not shown). There were no differences in the degree of obesity (% of SBW), WHR and each subcutaneous fat thickness between the hypertensive and normotensive groups. There were also no significant differences in the levels of fasting plasma glucose, serum total cholesterol, triglyceride, uric acid, plasma adrenaline and noradrenaline between the two groups. On the other hand, there was a significant difference in the levels of fasting serum IRI between the two groups. The relationship between systolic or diastolic blood pressure and fasting serum IRI in these obese children was shown in Figure 2. The systolic blood pressure was closely correlated to the fasting serum IRI levels ($r=0.63$, $p < 0.001$). The diastolic blood pressure was also correlated to the fasting serum IRI levels, but the correlation coefficient was lower ($r=0.44$, $p < 0.01$).

Discussion

The blood pressure in the obese children was significantly higher than that in the non-obese children. In topography, the obese children had

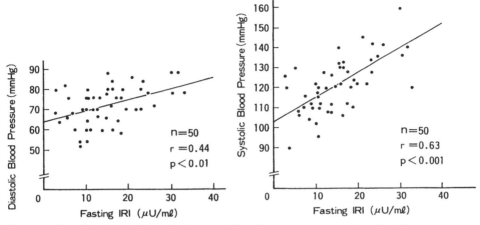

Figure 2. Relationship between blood pressure and fasting serum immunoreactive insulin (IRI) in obese children.

significantly high WHR, thick skinfolds compared with the non-obese children. In metabolic factors, they also had high serum insulin, triglyceride and uric acid levels compared with the non-obese children. These results are in agreement with our previous paper (8). Dividing the obese children into a hypertensive group and a normotensive group, we compared these anthropometric and metabolic factors between the two groups in order to clarify the effects of these factors on blood pressure. We found that the fasting serum insulin levels in the hypertensive group were significantly higher than those in the normotensive group. On the other hand, there were no significant differences in the degree of obesity, WHR, each skinfold thickness (regional fat accumulation) and any other metabolic factors measured here between the two groups. Moreover, we also found that both of the systolic and diastolic blood pressure in the obese children were closely correlated with their fasting serum insulin levels. The results suggested that hyperinsulinemia played an important role in the pathogenesis of hypertension in obese children independent of degree of obesity. Some studies on serum insulin levels in obese adults have been reported (9-13), but they did not present a close or independent correlation between insulin and blood pressure. Adult obese subjects have various degree of arteriosclerosis accelerated by hyperlipidemia, hyperuricemia and diabetic complications such as macro-and microangiopathy and their blood pressure levels may be affected by the arteriosclerosis. As a result, a strong correlation between insulin and blood

Table 2. Clinical features of hypertensive and normotensive obese children.

	Hypertensive (n=110)	Normotensive (n=214)
Systolic blood pressure (mmHg)	135 ± 10†	114 ± 10
Diastolic blood pressure (mmHg)	82 ± 4†	67 ± 7
Heart rate (beats/min)	82 ± 10	81 ± 11
% of standard body weight	149 ± 17	148 ± 10
Skinfold thickness		
Triceps (mm)	28 ± 7	27 ± 12
Subscapular (mm)	36 ± 10	35 ± 14
Periumbilical (mm)	37 ± 11	36 ± 12
Waist / Hip ratio	0.93 ± 0.08	0.92 ± 0.12
Metabolic factors[a]		
Fasting plasma glucose (mg/dl)	90 ± 6	90 ± 7
Fasting serum IRI (uu/ml)	19.3 ± 8.3*	13.0 ± 6.1
Total cholesterol (mg/dl)	186 ± 30	182 ± 33
Triglyceride (mg/dl)	143 ± 53	123 ± 42
Uric acid (mg/dl)	4.6 ± 0.8	4.3 ± 0.5
Adrenaline (pg/ml)	68 ± 33	58 ± 25
Noradrenaline (pg/ml)	271 ± 92	258 ± 75

[a] were measured in 50 (17 hypertensive and 33 normotensive) obese children. Hypertension of children was defined to be more than 135 mmHg of systolic and/or 80 mmHg diastolic blood pressure. The values are mean ± standard deviation. *$p < 0.01$; †$p < 0.001$. IRI = immunoreactive insulin.

pressure would not be indicated in those adult subjects.

On the other hand, we and other investigators (14-16) reported that central deposition of body fat in adults including intra-abdominal fat accumulation might be an important predictive factor for development of hypertension or cardiac dysfunction as originally proposed by Vague (16). However, in the present study for obese children, we did not observe a relationship between blood pressure and body features determined by WHR or subcutaneous skinfold thickness. In addition, there was no significant correlation between WHR and insulin levels in these obese children (r=0.07, not significant). From this data, central fat deposition in obese children would not have a necessarily important role in the pathogenesis of hypertension. Central obesity in adults has been shown to be accompanied more frequently with metabolic disorders including hyperinsulinemia and arteriosclerotic vascular changes (17-20). They may be related to the pathogenesis of hypertension to a high degree (21). However, in our subjects, it may be too early for central fat deposition to produce severe metabolic disorders, arteriosclerotic vascular changes and hypertension.

The mechanism of elevation of blood pressure due to hyperinsulinemia in obesity may be speculated as follows: Hyperinsulinemia is known to stimulate sodium reabsorption by the kidneys and expand extracellular fluid volume (22), and this may lead to an increase in cardiac output and elevation of blood pressure. Insulin may also affect peripheral vascular resistance by influencing sodium and/or calcium uptake by arterial smooth muscle (23). The increased metabolic rate in the central nervous system, which may be associated with insulin, could also raise blood pressure by strengthening the contraction of cardiac muscle or increasing vascular resistance (24), although we could not observe a significant difference in the peripheral levels of plasma adrenaline and noradrenaline.

Another notion is that hyperinsulinemia in obese subjects is known to be related to insulin resistance (25). Hyperinsulinemia may be related to hypertension through insulin resistance (9,11,26). Further investigation would be required concerning the mechanism for linkage of hyperinsulinemia to hypertension.

Summary

The relationship between blood pressure and anthropometric or metabolic factors was studied in 324 obese children aged 11.2 ± 2.1 years. The blood pressure in the obese children was significantly higher than that in the non-obese children (systolic blood pressure: 121 ± 14 mmHg in obese children vs. 112 ± 11 mmHg in non-obese children, $p < 0.001$; diastolic blood pressure: 72 ± 9 mmHg in obese children vs. 66 ± 7 mmHg in non-obese children, $p < 0.001$). When the obese children were divided into hypertensive and normotensive groups, there was a significant difference in fasting serum insulin levels between the two groups (19.3 ± 83 uU/ml in the hypertensive group vs. 13.0 ± 6.1 uU/ml in the normotensive group. A close correlation between fasting serum insulin levels and systolic blood pressure was demonstrated in the obese children ($r=0.63$, $p < 0.0001$).

However, there was no significant correlation between blood pressure and degree of obesity or waist to hip ratio in the obese children. There was also no significant correlation between blood pressure and fasting plasma glucose, serum total cholesterol or triglyceride in the obese children. These results suggested that hyperinsulinemia itself played an important role in the pathogenesis of hypertension in early stages of obesity.

Acknowledgements

We are indebted to Dr. Kazuyuki Hirayama, the Izumiohtsu Medical Association, Izumiohtsu City, Osaka, Japan, for his help to make a plan of this examination in obese children.

References
1. Whyte HM. Blood pressure and obesity. Circulation 1956;19:511-516.
2. Kannel WB, Brand N, Skinner JJ, Jr, Dawber TR, MacNamara PM. Weight and blood pressure. Findings in hypertension screening of 1 million Americans. JAMA 1978;240:1607-1610.
3. Frohlich ED, Messerli FH, Reisin E, Dunn FG. The problem of obesity and hypertension. Hypertension 1983;5 (Suppl. III):III-71-III-78.
4. Dornfeld LP, Maxwell MH, Waks A, Tuck M. Mechanism of hypertension in obesity. Kidney Int 1987;32 (Suppl. 22):S254-S258.
5. Nakajima T, Fujioka S, Tokunaga K, Hirobe K, Matsuzawa Y, Tarui S. Non-invasive study of left ventricular performance in obese patients. Influence of duration of obesity. Circulation 1985;71:481-486.
6. Hibi I. Obesity In: Textbook of Pediatrics, Vol. 4 (in Japanese). Nakayashoten Press, Tokyo, 1968;330-343.
7. Karvonen MJ, Telivuo LJ, Järvinen EJK. Sphygmomanometer cuff size and the accuracy of indirect measurement of blood pressure. Am J Cardiol 1964;13:688-693.
8. Tokunaga K, Ishikawa K, Sudo H, Matsuzawa Y, Yamamoto A, Tarui S. Serum lipoprotein profile in Japanese obese children. Int J Obesity 1981;6:399-404.
9. Manicardi V, Camellini L, Bellodi G, Coscelli C, Ferrannini E. Evidence for an Association of High Blood Pressure and Hyperinsulinemia in Obese Man. J Clin Endocrinol Metab 1986;62:1302-1304.
10. Christlieb AR, Krolewski AS, Warram JH, Soeldner JS. Is insulin the link between hypertension and obesity? Hypertension 1985; 7 (Suppl. II): II-54-II-57.

11. Modan M, Halkin H, Almog S, Lusky A, Eshkol A, Shefi M, Shitrit A, Fuchs Z. Hyperinsulinemia: A link between hypertension obesity and glucose intolerance. J Clin Invest 1985;75:809-815.
12. Lucas CP, Estigarribia JA, Darga LL, Reaven GM. Insulin and blood pressure in obesity. Hypertension 1985;7:702-706.
13. Weinsier RL, Norris DJ, Birch R, Bernstein RS, Pi-Sunyer FX, Yang M, Wang J, Pierson RN, Jr., Van Itallie TB. Serum insulin and blood pressure in an obese population. Int J Obesity 1986;10:11-17.
14. Nakajima T, Fujioka S, Tokunaga K, Matsuzawa Y, Tarui S. Correlation of intra-abdominal fat accumulation and left ventricular performance in obesity. Am J Cardiol 1989;64:369-373.
15. Kanai H, Matsuzawa Y, Kotani K, Nagai Y, Fujioka S, Nakajima T, Tokunaga K, Tarui S. Hypertension and fat distribution in Japanese obese women. Close correlation of visceral fat accumulation to high blood pressure (abstr.). Circulation 1989;80 (Suppl. II):II-284.
16. Vague J. The degree of masculine differentiation of obesities. A factor determining predisposition to diabetes, atherosclerosis, gout and uric calculous disease. AM J Clin Nutr 1956;4:20-34.
17. Kissebah AH, Vydelingum N, Murray R, Evans DJ, Hartz AJ, Kalkhoff RK, Adams PW. Relation of body fat distribution to metabolic complications of obesity. J Clin Endocrinol Metab 1982;54:254-260.
18. Fujioka S, Matsuzawa Y, Tokunaga K, Tarui S. Contribution of intra-abdominal fat accumulation to impairment of glucose and lipid metabolism in human obesity. Metabolism 1987;36:54-59.
19. Matsuzawa Y, Fujioka S, Tokunaga K, Tarui S. Classification of obesity with respect to morbidity. Asian Med J 1989;32:435-441.
20. Tarui S, Fujioka S, Tokunaga K, Matsuzawa Y. Pathophysiology between subcutaneous-type and visceral-type obesity. In: Diet and Obesity. Bray, GA, LeBlanc J, Inoue S, Suzuki M (Eds.). Japan Sci Soc Press, Tokyo, 1988;143-152.
21. Björntorp P. Hypertension and other complications in human obesity. J Clin Hypertens 1986;2:163-165.
22. DeFronzo RA, Cooke CR, Andres R, Faloona GR, Davis PJ. The effect of insulin on renal handling of sodium, potassium, calcium and phosphate in man. J Clin Invest 1975;55:845-855.
23. Birkenhäger WH, De Leeuw PW. Pathophysiological mechanisms in essential hypertension. Pharmac Ther 1979;8:297-319.

24. Young JB, Landsberg L. Diet-induced changes in sympathetic nervous system activity. Possible implications for obesity and hypertension. J Chron Dis 1982;35:879-886.
25. Bonora E, Coscelli C, Butturini U. Relationship between insulin resistance, insulin secretion and insulin metabolism in simple obesity. Int J Obesity 1985;9:307-312.
26. Ferrannini E, Buzzigoli G, Bonadonna R, Giorico MA, Oleggini M, Graziadei L, Pedrinelli R, Brandi L, Bevilacqua S. insulin resistance in essential hypertension. N Engl J Med 1987; 317:350-357.

C. PATHOPHYSIOLOGICAL ASPECTS OF CARDIOVASCULAR DYSFUNCTION IN DIABETES

Cardiovascular Involvements in a New Spontaneously Diabetic (WBN/Kob) Rat

Y. Sakaguchi, S. Kato, A. Fujimoto, S. Tsuruta, M. Tsuchihashi, A. Kawamoto,
S. Uemura, Y. Nishida, S. Fujimoto, T. Hashimoto, T. Kagoshima,
H. Ishikawa and R. Okada*

First Department of Internal Medicine, Nara Medical University, Nara, JAPAN.
*Labo. for Cardiovasc. Research of Internal Medicine, Juntendo University,
Tokyo, JAPAN.

Introduction

Diabetes mellitus is associated with an increased prevalence of congestive heart failure, independent of atherosclerotic coronary artery disease. Recent studies suggest that hypertension increases the incidence of congestive heart failure due to diabetes (1-3). Many experimental studies on chronically diabetic rats, induced by streptozotocin, have been performed regarding the involvement of cardiovascular system (4-7), but diabetic (WBN/Kob) rats have not yet been used for this purpose. We have observed morphological changes indicating the cardiac involvements in WBN/Kob rats at 18 months of age. We obtained the result that the heart weight and percent fibrosis in the myocardium were 25% and 75% greater than those in Wistar control rats, respectively. In addition, hypertrophy and dilatation of the left ventricle and massive fibrosis in ventricles were recognized in WBN/Kob rats at 18 months of age.

In this study we wish to elucidate the progressive process of cardiovascular abnormalities in WBN/Kob rats. The hearts of WBN/Kob rats and controls were examined morphologically, and catecholamine concentrations in the cardiac tissue and serum were determined at intervals from 3 to 18 months of age.

Materials and Methods

Thirty-eight male WBN/Kob rats obtained from Shizuoka Laboratory Animal

Nagano, M., Mochizuki, S., Dhalla, N.S. (eds.), CARDIOVASCULAR DISEASE IN DIABETES. Copyright © 1992. Kluwer Academic Publishers, Boston. All rights reserved.

Center were used as experimental subjects and 25 age-matched male Wistar rats as control. WBN/Kob and Wistar rats were weighed, and systolic blood pressures were measured by the tail cuff method, and glucose tolerance test was performed at 3, 7, 12 and 18 months of age. For the glucose tolerance test, a 10% glucose solution, 2 mg per 100g of weight was injected into the intraperitoneum. After injection, the blood glucose concentration was determined at 30, 60 and 120 minutes by the glucose oxidase method. WBN/Kob and age-matched control rats were killed under mild ether anesthesia at 2, 7, 12 and 18 months of age.

For catecholamine concentrations in serum, rats were slightly anesthetized with pentobarbital and blood was collected from the abdominal aorta by a small catheter. For catecholamine concentrations in the myocardium after thoracotomy, the heart was excised and quick-frozen, and the apex area (about 0.4g) was homogenized for 3 minutes and then centrifuged at 3000xg for 3 minutes. An aliquot of the supernatant was neutralized with 5 M K_2CO_3 and aliquots were taken for determination of epinephrine, norepinephrine and dopamine by high performance liquid chromatography. For histological study, two mid-ventricular rings including both transverse sections of ventricles were embedded in paraffin and stained with hematoxylin-eosin, azan-mallory and PAS stain. To examine quantitative morphology, a color image processor (SPICCA-II) was employed for measuring the cardiac myocytes. The involvements of the cardiac tissue and vascular system were observed by light and electron microscopy.

All values are expressed as the mean ± standard error. Test of significance was performed by the Student's t-test.

Results

Animal profile

The body weight of WBN/Kob rats was more than that of control rats from 3 months of age, and a decrease of body weight was noted at 18 months of age in WBN/Kob rats (Fig. 1). Abnormalities in the glucose tolerance test were observed slightly from 7 months of age in WBN/Kob rats and a definite increase in blood sugar was recognized from 12 months of age in this rat; the degree of abnormalities in blood sugar gradually became severe (Fig.2).

The heart weight in WBN/Kob rats was greater than that of the control rats from 3 months of age and it increased with the age of the animal (Fig. 3). The ratio of heart weight versus body weight was significantly greater in

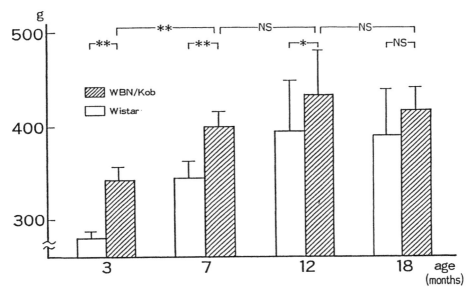

Figure 1. Body weights in WBN/Kob and control rats.

WBN/Kob rats, and this ratio increased with the age (Fig. 4). These rats showed mild hypertension since 3 months of age and the blood pressure value in these rats did not change between 3 and 18 months of age. The systolic blood pressure was about 140 mmHg which was about 20 mmHg higher than the control rats (Fig. 5).

Morphological findings

Diameters of the myocytes increased gradually with the advance of age, and there were significant differences between WBN/kob and control rats in myocytic diameter (Fig. 6). Histologically, in the perivascular area, focal necrosis of the cardiac myocytes was seen at 3 months of age and slight cell infiltration was recognized in the necrotic area in WBN/Kob rats. The infiltrated cells were mostly histiocytes or lymphocytic cells. The replacement fibrosis for focal necrosis appeared from 7 months of age. Since about 12 months of age the diabetes mellitus became apparent, the replacement fibrosis spread into all layers of both ventricles, and hypertrophy and

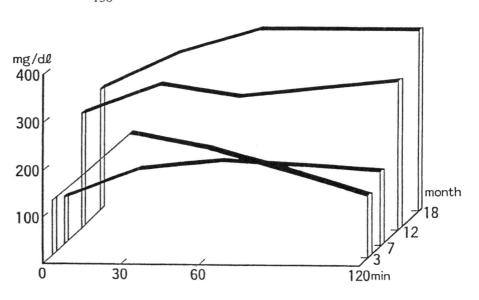

Figure 2. Glucose tolerance test in WBN/Kob and control rats.

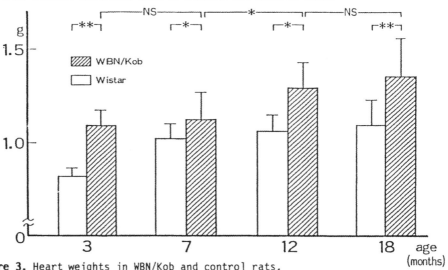

Figure 3. Heart weights in WBN/Kob and control rats.

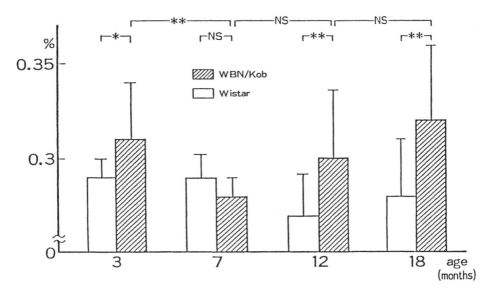

Figure 4. Ratio of heart weight versus body weight in WBN/Kob and control rats.

dilatation of the left ventricle became severe with the advance of age (Fig. 7a-d). The aortic, arterial and arteriolar lesions were not recognized clearly in WBN/Kob rats.

Electron microscopically, swelling and the rough cristae of the mitochondria in the cardiac myocytes of those rats were noted from 3 months of age. These findings revealed by light microscopy corresponded to small vascular degeneration. Although the electron microscopical findings were recognized at the age of 18 months, the degree of these lesions was not significantly different from that at the age of 3 months (Fig. 8).

Catecholamine concentration

In WBN/Kob rats, the catecholamine concentration in the cardiac tissue was lower at the age of 3 months than that in control rats. And this tendency continued from 3 to 18 months of age. Although this tendency was noted in concentrations of epinephrine and norepinephrine, there were no differences in the dopamine concentration in cardiac tissue between WBN/Kob and control rats

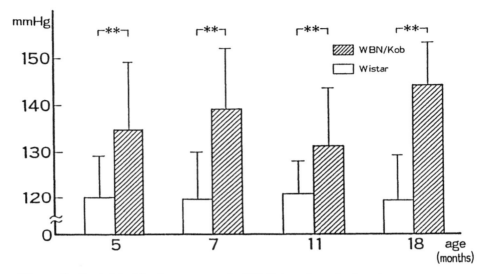

Figure 5. Systolic blood pressures in WBN/Kob and control rats.

(Fig. 9). On the other hand, the catecholamine concentration in serum of WBN/Kob rats was lower at the age of 18 months than in control rats. We were unable to determine the catecholamine concentration in sera at 3, 7 and 12 months of age because not enough sera at these ages were available to determine catecholamine concentrations.

Discussion

WBN/Kob rat is a new spontaneously diabetic animal. We have reported cardiac involvements in this rat at 18 months of age, and we mentioned that focal cardiac myocytic necrosis and replacement fibrosis were noted in the myocardium and the concentration of catecholamine in cardiac tissue of WBN/Kob rats was lower than in control rats.

Capillary and arteriolar lesions in diabetes

The concept of a small vessel disorder involving diffuse organ systems in diabetes is not new (8-10). In WBN/Kob rat, we did not recognize involvements in small vessels. Previous investigators have mentioned the presence of pathologic findings in the vasculature of the myocardium. In this study we demonstrated that there were diffuse lesions throughout the

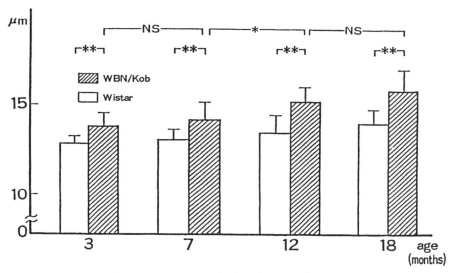

Figure 6. Diameter of myocytes in WBN/Kob and control rats.

myocardium and myocardial hypertrophy from 3 months of age in WBN/Kob rats. But there were no pathologic findings in arterioles and small vessels in the myocardium of WBN/Kob rats. In other organs, for example the kidney, lungs and liver, vascular lesions were not recognized in WBN/Kob rats. From these findings it appears that the myocardial lesion might not be produced by the small vessel disease but the possibility of metabolic derangement associated with diabetes or hypertension cannot be ruled out.

Morphological findings

In this report, we revealed histologically that focal necrosis of the myocytes in WBN/Kob rats was seen from 3 months of age, and the replacement fibrosis for the necrotic area increased in both ventricles since 7 months of age. Since 12 months of age when diabetes mellitus became meanifested, hypertrophy and dilatation in the left ventricle were more severe than those in the period of non-diabetic state. On the basis of these facts, we thought that the myocyte necrosis might have been associated with hypertension and that the progress of the involvement of the myocardium in WBN/Kob rats might depend heavily on the diabetic state without involvement of vessels.

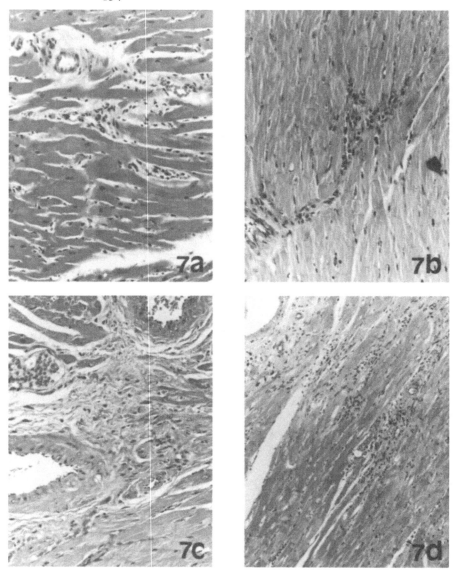

Figure 7. Histological findings in hearts of WBN/Kob rats. (a) Necrosis of the cardiac myocytes in the perivascular area of 3 month-old WBN/Kob rat. HE, x100, (b) Cell infiltration and necrosis in the middle layer of the heart of 7 month-old WBN/Kob rat. HE, x100, (c) Necrosis of the cardiac myocytes and replacement fibrosis in the heart of 12 month-old WBN/Kob rat. HE, x100, (d) Massive fibrosis in the middle and internal layers, and hypertrophy and dilatation in the left ventricle of 18 month-old WBN/Kob rat. HE, x100.

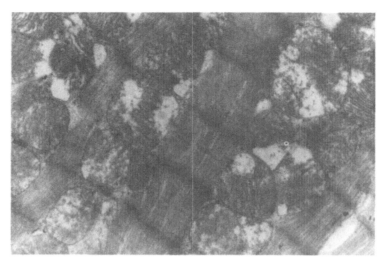

Figure 8. Electron microscopical findings. Swollen and scattered cristae of the mitochondria in the cardiac myocyte of 3 months-old WBN/Kob.

Cathecholamine concentrations

The catecholamine concentrations in the cardiac tissue tended to be low from 3 to 18 months in WBN/Kob rats. Although in WBN/Kob rats at 18 months, serum catecholamine level was low, mild hypertension existed in these animals. On the other hand, morphological features of the cardiac myocyte necrosis resembled those of the experimental low dose catecholamine myocarditis. From these results, the cause of the cardiac involvement was difficult to explain, but it is suggested that abnormalities in the sensitivities to catecholamine exist in this rat and that these abnormalities may induce Ca^{++} overload and myocardial cell death.

Comparison with human diabetic heart

Compared with human diabetic heart disease without vascular involvements, the lesion of the heart in WBN/Kob rats showed similarity in following points: focal myocytic necrosis and replacement fibrosis as well as hypertrophy and dilatation of the left ventricular wall in advanced stage. Similar findings were recognized in the human diabetic heart with hypertension. We think that WBN/Kob rat is useful as an animal model of the diabetic heart with hypertension.

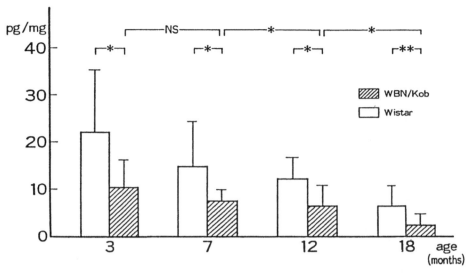

Figure 9. Epinephrine concentrations in cardiac tissue of WBN/Kob and control rats.

Summary

In this study we have revealed focal myocytic necrosis and replacement fibrosis of the myocardium, and hypertrophy and dilatation in the left ventricle in advanced stage in WBN/Kob rats. The catecholamine concentration in cardiac tissue and serum was low in these rats. These findings might suggest that abnormalities in sensitivity to catecholamines may exist in WBN/Kob rats.

References

1. Hamby RI, Zoneraich S and Sherman L. Diabetic cardiomyopathy. JAMA 1974;299:1749-1745.
2. Seneviratne BIB. Diabetic cardiomyopathy: The preclinical pahse. Br Med J 1977:1444-1446.
3. Shapiro LM, Leatherdale BA, Makkinon J, and Fletcher RF. Left vetricular function in diabetes mellitus. II: Relation between clinical features and left ventricular function. Br Heart J 1981;45:129-132.
4. Allison TB, Bruttig SP, Crass MF, Eliot RS and Shipp JC. Reduced high-energy phosphate levels in rat heart. I Effect of alloxan diabetes. Am

J Physiol 1976;230:1744-1750.
5. Penpargkul S. Abnormal Ca^{++}-transport by cardiac myocyte in the diabetic rat. Circ 1979;60(Suppl. II):147-151.
6. Dillmann WH. Diabetes mellitus induced changes in cardiac myosin of the rat. Diabetes 1980;29:579-582.
7. Heylinger CE, Pierce GN, Beamish RE and Dhalla NS. Cardiac α- and ß-adrenergic receptor alternations in diabetic cardiomyopathy. Basic Res Cardiol 1982;77:610-618.
8. Factor SM, Okun EM and Minase T. Capillary microaneurysms in the human diabetic heart. N Engl J Med 1980;302:384-388.
9. Ditzel J and Rooth G. The micro-angiopathy in diabetes mellitus. A concept regarding the mechanism of its origin. Diabetes 1955;4:474-480.
10. Fischer VW. Myocardial structure and capillary basal laminar thickness in experimentally diabetic rat. Exper and Mol Pathol 1981;35:244-251.

Biochemical and Morphologic Alterations in Cardiac Myocytes in Streptozotocin-Induced Diabetic Rats

T. Katagiri, Y. Umezawa, Y. Suwa, E. Geshi, T. Yanagishita, M. Yaida

The Third Department of Internal Medicine, Showa University School of Medicine, Tokyo, JAPAN.

Introduction

Complication of congestive heart failure in patients with diabetes mellitus has well been known in clinical practice. Impairment of cardiac function was recognized in the absence of arteriosclerotic changes in diabetics, and the concept of "diabetic cardiomyopathy" has been proposed as the diabetes specific myocardial disorder (1,2). In the clinical practice, diabetes mellitus occurs in the mature to elder age and complication of coronary arterio- or athero-sclerosis is usual. Therefore, influence of ischemia could not be excluded in clinical cases. To elucidate effect of hyperglycemic state on cardiac myocytes without vascular changes, experimental diabetes was induced in relatively young rats by single intravenous injection of streptozotocin (STZ), and the effects of abrupt and long-standing severe hyperglycemia on the cardiac micro organs such as the sarcoplasmic reticulum (SR) and the structural proteins were investigated in comparison with the fine structures of cardiac myocytes.

Materials and Methods

Experimental diabetes mellitus; One hundred and fifty male Wistar rats, weighing 180 to 200 g, were made diabetic by single injection of STZ at 65 mg/kg body weight into the tail vein under ether anesthesia. They were fed solid feed for rats in an air conditioned room and sacrificed at 1, 2, 4, 8, 12 and 16 weeks after STZ injection under ether anesthesia in the same manner as STZ was injected (DM group). To age-matched control rats same amount of physiologic saline solution was given (C group). In a part of DM group, lente insulin was injected daily for a period of 2 and 4 weeks subcutaneously from the third day, so that fasting blood glucose level was around 120 mg/dl. In some 12 weeks diabetic rats, insulin treatment was started at the beginning of the 10th week (DM+I group).

Preparation of cardiac sarcoplasmic reticulum; Cardiac SR was prepared by ultracentrifugation method as the light microsome fraction of myocardial homogenate, and Ca^{++}-stimulated ATPase activity was measured. And SR-composing proteins were fractionated by SDS polyacrylamide gel electrophoresis according to the modified method of Laemmli (cited in 3). SR constituting phospholipids were extracted by the modified method of Folch according to Yanagishita (4), and separated by two dimensional thin layer chromatography. Phospholipid fatty acids were further analysed by gas chromatography.

Preparation of total structural proteins; Crude fraction containing total structural proteins was extracted by the method of Katagiri (5), and actomyosin ATPase activity was measured in the presence of 2×10^{-5} M Ca^{++}. They were analysed by SDS-polyacrylamide gel electrophoresis in a similar manner as for the analysis of SR proteins.

Electron microscopic cytochemical ATPase study; Cytochemical ATPase reaction was carried out for electron microscopic study by the method described previously (6). Briefly, chopped heart muscle was prefixed in 2% glutaraldehyde, 5% sucrose and 0.1 M Na cacodylate (pH 7.4) at 4°C for 15 min, and cut to 40 um sections by a cryostat. ATPase reaction was carried out at 37°C in 0.01 M $CaCl_2$, 0.01 M $MgCl_2$, 0.72 mM $Pb(NO_3)_2$, 5 mM ATP, and 0.05 M trismaleate (pH 7.4) for 15 min. The section was rinsed in 0.05 M trismaleate (pH 7.4), postfixed in 1% OsO_4, ultra-thin sectioned and observed with a Hitachi H-300 electron microscope.

Results

General profiles of STZ-induced diabetic rats; Rats of DM group exhibited fasting blood glucose level of higher than 400 mg/dl (458±26) from one to sixteen weeks after STZ injection. Blood glucose of C group was maintained 100 to 110 mg/dl overall period. Increases in body and heart weights were inhibited in DM group, as shown in Figure 1, however, heart/body weight ratio increased from the 4th week, indicating development of cardiac hypertrophy in the diabetic state. In DM+I group, the fasting blood glucose level was maintained to 130 to 150 mg/dl, and body and heart weights increased at the same extent as those of C group did.

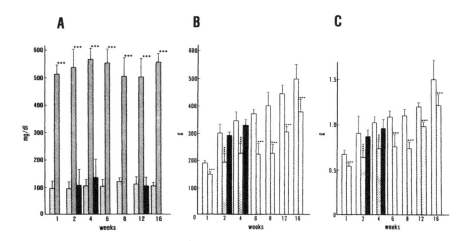

Figure 1. General profiles of STZ-induced diabetic rats. A: Fasting blood glucose (FBG), B: body weight, and C: heart weight. Dotted bars; of the C group, bars with slunting lines; of the DM group, and closed bars; of the DM+I group. Development of both of body and heart weights were inhibited in the DM group, but were prevented by insulin injection. FBG was over 400 mg/dl in the DM group. ***$p<0.001$ vs values of the C group.

Alterations in cardiac SR; Figure 2 shows Ca^{++}-stimulated ATPase activity of cardiac SR. SR from C group exhibited the activity of 3.72±0.22 umoles Pi/mg SR protein /hr at 37°C at 1 week, and the activity was not changed up to 16 weeks. But the ATPase activity of SR from DM group diminished significantly from the 1st week to about 57% of that of C group. The reduced activity remained lower until at 16 weeks after STZ injection as low as 38% on the average. In DM+I group for 2 and 4 weeks, Ca^{++}-dependent ATPase activity of cardiac SR was in the similar level to that of the control rats as shown in Figure 2.

Figure 3 shows gel electrophoresis of SR composing proteins from the rat heart muscle. SR proteins were separated to the major ATPase protein (110,000 dalton), several bands of acidic proteins (70,000-50,000) and proteolipids (-22,000). The pattern of these SR proteins was the same as that of the canine heart muscle (7). In the DM group, a marked increase in the 100,000 dalton protein suggesting the major ATPase was observed from the 4th week, and remained in the increased state until at 16 weeks. Other bands except the

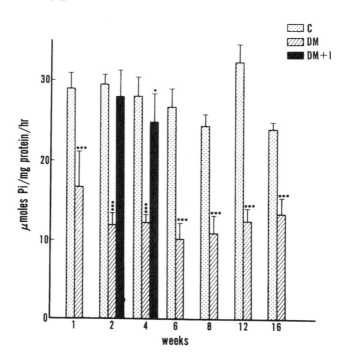

Figure 2. Ca^{++}-stimulated ATPase activity of cardiac SR from STZ-induced diabetic rats. Dotted bars; of the C group, bars with slunting line; of the DM group, and closed bars; of the DM+I group. ***p<0.001 vs values of the C group. Depression of ATPase activity in the DM group was prevented by insulin treatment.

100,000 dalton protein did not change. Compositions of cardiac SR proteins calculated from densitometric curves were shown in Table 1. In SR of the C group, the major ATPase protein occupied 25 to 30% of total SR proteins and this value was similar to that of the canine heart (7). In the DM group, the content of the major ATPase protein increased to about 150% of that of the C group notwithstanding the marked reduction in Ca^{++}-dependent ATPase activity. This evidence was the most marked in the pathophysiology of the diabetic rat heart.

Composition of SR membrane phospholipids is shown in Figure 4. Because of the limitation of the amount of specimens, data were presented collectively in relatively early, i.e. 4 to 7 and relatively chronic, i.e. 8 to 12 weeks of diabetes. In the DM group of 8 to 12 weeks, total phospholipid content

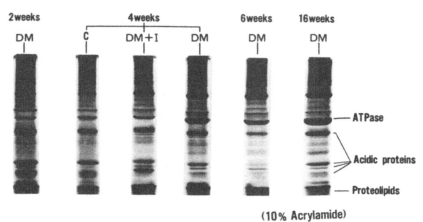

Figure 3. SDS gel electrophoresis of the cardiac SR from STZ-induced diabetic rats. Note an increase in the bands corresponding the major ATPase protein at 4 to 16 weeks in the DM group. This was prevented by insulin treatment.

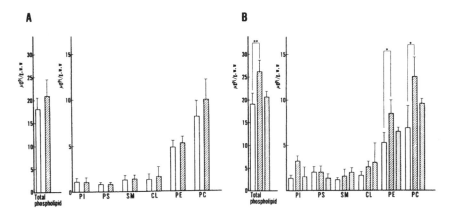

Figure 4. Compositions of SR membrane constituting phospholipids from the STZ-induced diabetic rat heart.
A: 4 to 7 weeks, and B: 8 to 12 weeks of the diabetic state. In the chronic stage, significant increases in total phospholipid content, phosphatidylcholine, and phosphatidylethanolamine. Treatment with insulin from 10th week prevented these increases. *$p<0.05$, and **$p<0.01$ vs values of the C group.

Table 1. Compositions of major ATPase protein in cardiac SR proteins from diabetic rats.

	Control	Diabetic	DM+Insulin
1 week	0.253 ± 0.062	0.246 ± 0.061	
2 weeks	0.243 ± 0.036	0.239 ± 0.021	0.240 ± 0.032
4 weeks	0.295 ± 0.025	0.452 ± 0.067***	0.303 ± 0.022
6 weeks	0.248 ± 0.023	0.392 ± 0.011***	
8 weeks	0.221 ± 0.017	0.397 ± 0.019***	
12 weeks	0.274 ± 0.020	0.483 ± 0.025***	
16 weeks	0.253 ± 0.009	0.369 ± 0.035***	

Values are expressed as mean ± S.D.   *** $p<0.001$ vs values of control rats.

increased significantly. Among the SR phospholipids, phosphatidylcholine (PC) and phosphatidylethanolamine (PE) increased significantly, and as shown in Figure 4-B; compositions of phospholipids from the DM+I group exhibited values similar to those of the C group.

Figure 5 shows fatty acid compositions of membrane phospholipids. Membrane fatty acids were separated to C16:0 (palmitic acid), C18:0 (stearic acid), C18:1 (oleic acid), C20:4 (arachidonic acid) and C22:4 (docosahexaenoic acid). In the DM group, none of new peaks of fatty acids appeared on gas chromatogram, but a significant reduction in arachidonic acid and an increase in docosahexaenoic acid were recognized in 8 to 12 weeks after STZ injection.

Alterations in the cardiac structural proteins; Ca^{++}-dependent actomyosin ATPase activity of the total structural proteins was at the level similar to that of the C group (33.4±1.8 uM Pi/mg protein/hr at 25°C) in the early period, until at 2 weeks (29.6±2.9 uM, n.s.), but it diminished significantly after 4 to 6 weeks (at 6 weeks 20.6±5.0 uM) as shown in Figure 6. But the compositions of the structural proteins did not change throughout the diabetic course up to 16 weeks in SDS gel electrophoresis.

Fine structural observation of cardiac myocytes with cytochemical ATPase activity; Figure 7 shows electron micrographs of cardiac myocytes with

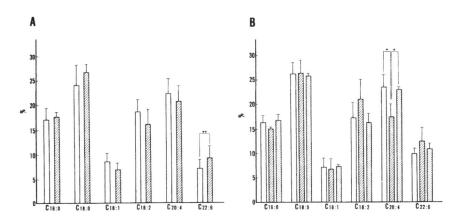

Figure 5. Compositions of phospholipid fatty acids of cardiac SR from STZ-induced diabetic rats.
A: 4 to 7 weeks, and B: 8 to 12 weeks after STZ injection. In DM+I group a decrease in arachidonic acid in the DM group was protected. **$p<0.01$ vs values of the C group.

cytochemical ATPase reaction. In a myocardial cell of the C group, fine structures were well retained, and abnormal findings were rarely observed (Fig. 7-A). Fine structures of cardiac myocytes from the DM group were relatively well-preserved in the early diabetes, i.e. 2 to 4 weeks after the administration of STZ. But in the chronic stage, i.e. 8 to 12 weeks, marked increases in secondary lysosomes and lipid droplets were recognized in number with mild coarseness of myofilaments and assemblage of mitochondria (Fig. 7-B). But such findings as contraction band and intramitochondrial dense deposits, which are usually observable in the ischemic myocardium, were seldom observed. In addition, no such abnormal findings as arteriosclerosis were rarely found in coronary arteries until at 12 weeks.

In a myocardial cell of the C group, ATPase reaction product was recognized most intensely in the terminal cisternae (TC), subsarcolemmal cisternae and longitudinal tubules (LT) of SR, and moderately on myofilaments (Fig. 7-A). In cells of the DM group, however, reduction in ATPase reaction product was noticed. It began to decrease in SR as early as 2 to 4 weeks after the administration of STZ, and decreased markedly in the chronic period,

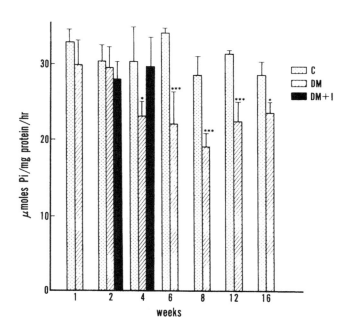

Figure 6. Ca^{++}-stimulated actomyosin-ATPase activity of the total structural proteins of STZ-induced diabetic rat heart.
Dotted bars; of the C group, bars with slunting line; of the DM group and closed bars; of the DM+I group. Diminution of ATPase activity was significant in the DM group from 4 weeks of diabetes, and protected by insulin treatment.

i.e. 8 to 12 weeks. And that on myofilament also diminished in the chronic stage. These fine structural alterations and intensity and localization of ATPase activity were summarized in Table 2.

Discussion

Congestive heart failure has often been recognized in patients with diabetes mellitus in the absence of coronary sclerotic changes (1,2), and a concept such as diabetic cardiomyopathy being characterized by cardiomegaly, cardiac dysfunction and congestive heart failure has been proposed by some investigators (1,8-12). Such abnormalities in the diabetic heart have been suggested to be caused by microangiopathy (1,8,11), which results from primary metabolic disorders in severe hyperglycemia (9,10,12); however, the cause of cardiac dysfunction in diabetic has still been unelucidated. In the diabetic heart, slowing of relaxation and depression of peak development of contraction

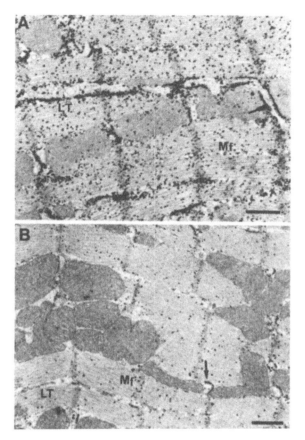

Figure 7. Electron micrographs of cardiac myocytes from STZ-induced diabetic rats. A: C group, and B: DM group at 12 weeks of diabetes. Note the marked decrease in ATPase reaction product in SR and on myofilament with increased numbers of lysosomes and assemblage of mitochondria in B. Bars indicate 1 uM. Arrows; terminal cisternae, LT; longitudinal tubules, Mf; myofibrils.

were recognized in hemodynamic study without arteriosclerotic changes (13). To eliminate the influence of vascular alterations, diabetes was induced in relatively young rats by selective destruction of pancreatic beta cells by the single administration of STZ.

Among the results obtained in the present study, the most striking

Table 2. Fine structural changes and localization and intensity of ATPase activity in streptozotocin diabetic cardiac myocytes.

	Lipid droplets	secondary lysosomes	other fine structural changes	ATPase activity TC	LT	Mf
Control	-	-	-	+++	+++	++
2 weeks	-	-	-	+++	+++	++
4 weeks	+	+	+	+++	+++	++
8 weeks	+	+	+	++	++	++
12 weeks	++	++	+	+	±	±
16 weeks	++	++	++	±	±	±

TC; terminal cisternae, LT; longitudinal tubules of SR, and Mf; myofibrils.

phenomenon was the depression of Ca^{++}-ATPase activity of SR. It began to decrease as early as within 1 week after the initiation of diabetes before the fine structural alterations in cardiac myocytes appeared, and this evidence was also confirmed by an ultrastructural study with cytochemical ATPase reaction. Depression of Ca^{++}-ATPase activity should be related to the reduction in Ca^{++}-uptake activity of SR. Similar results were also recognized by Penpargkul (14) and Ganguly (15), and also in sarcolemma (16). Interestingly, the content of the protein corresponding to the major ATPase on SDS gel electrophoresis increased notwithstanding depression of ATPase activity. Similar evidence was noticed in the phospholipid fraction of SR. Total content of inorganic phosphate in the phospholipid fraction of SR increased together with increases in the major constituents, PC and PE, even though the appearance time of increase was different.

These evidences indicate that in the diabetic heart, the function of SR is severely damaged, which results in a decrease of Ca^{++}-uptake by SR and an increase in free Ca^{++} in the cytosole. This can be seen to explain the slow relaxation and impaired peak contraction of the diabetic heart. Moreover, alterations in cardiac membrane phospholipid and fatty acid components may lead to the altered property of membrane such as fluidity.

The increase in 100,000 dalton protein suggesting the major ATPase and total phospholipid content of SR might be a suggestion of an increase in SR membrane components for the compensation of impaired SR function. There seems to be a sequential process in the pathophysiologic alterations in the diabetic myocardium. Impairment of Ca^{++}-ATPase activity was noticed earliest, i.e. within 1 week after the initiation of diabetes, and then increases in the protein suggesting the major ATPase and phospholipid content followed in the relatively chronic period. At the same time, activity of Ca^{++}-dependent actomyosin-ATPase activity significantly diminished without detectable compositional changes in electrophoresis (3). These alterations in the diabetic myocardium were completely suppressed by daily treatment with insulin, and this indicates they are diabetes specific.

With respect to the compositions of phospholipid fatty acids, decrease in arachidonic acid is of great interest. Decrease in arachidonic acid in diabetes mellitus was recognized widely in the liver, kidney, heart and serum (17,18) and was attributed to impairment of the activation of 5-desaturase, which is essential for the synthesis of arachidonic acid (17). This evidence also is related to the alterations in membrane fluidity.

In contrast to biochemical changes, fine structural alterations in cardiac myocytes were relatively mild. In disregard of reduced Ca^{++}-stimulated ATPase activity in 1 week after the onset of diabetes, fine structures of diabetic myocardial cells were almost intact. Slight ultrastructural changes such as increments of secondary lysosomes and lipid droplets were found at around 2 to 4 weeks (19-21). These changes became more intense in the chronic diabetic heart muscle with slight myofibrillar coarseness and assemblage of mitochondria. And such changes as contraction band or mitochondrial dense deposits, which are usually observable in the acute ischemic cardiac myocytes and were recognized by Jackson et al (22) in the diabetic cardiomyocytes, were not observed at all. ATPase reaction product decreased markedly in the chronic stage without severe, necrotic fine structural alterations. Reduction in actomyosin-ATPase activity was recognized by Fein et al (13), Dillmann (23) and Yaida et al (3) in the relatively chronic period of the experimental diabetic heart with change in myosin isoenzyme (23). Reduction in cytochemical ATPase activity corresponds to the diminution of ATPase activity of SR and the structural proteins. Marked diminution of Ca^{++}-ATPase activity of SR was noticed in the acute ischemic myocardial cells (6). Extent of reduction in ATPase activity of SR from diabetic heart was similar to that from the acute ischemic myocardium.

But in the acute ischemic myocardium, reduction in ATPase activity accompanies the degradation of the major ATPase protein and therefore indicate the degeneration of the membrane system (7). On the contrary, the protein corresponding with the major ATPase increased inversely in the diabetic heart. This difference indicates that the pathogenesis of metabolic impairment is quite different in ischemia and in diabetes. That is, in the diabetic heart, influence of ischemia is completely the secondary phenomenon. Similar difference is notable in the phospholipid contents and compositions. In acute myocardial ischemia degradation of phospholipids such as PC and PE were recognized in SR membrane (4), but in the diabetic heart these were increased. As the cause of diabetic myocardial impairment, participation of ischemia including the disturbance of microcirculation has been proposed by several reports (1,8,11), however, the evidence described in this paper suggests strongly that the pathogenesis is different from ischemia and is specific for diabetes mellitus. Complete prevention of these changes by insulin treatment, and the absence of coronary arterial sclerotic changes also support the diabetes specific alterations.

Summary

We studied myocardial alterations in diabetic rats induced by streptozotocin (STZ) by biochemical analyses of cardiac sarcoplasmic reticulum (SR) and structural proteins in combination with electron microscopic cytochemical studies on ATPase activity of cardiac myocytes from 1 to 16 weeks with fasting blood glucose over 400 mg/ml. Ca^{++}-dependent ATPase activity of extracted cardiac SR decreased markedly to about 40% of that of the control rat from 1 week, and reduced further until 16 weeks. But 100,000 dalton protein band corresponding major ATPase protein increased from 4 weeks. Total phospholipid content also increased in a relatively chronic period, at 8 to 12 weeks, with increases in phosphatidylcholine and phosphatidylethanolamine. Arachidonic acid decreased among phospholipid constituting fatty acids with relative increase in docosahexaenoic acid. Ca^{++}-stimulated actomyosin ATPase activity reduced gradually 18 TO 36% from 4 to 16 weeks without changes in subunit compositions in gel electrophoresis. These biochemical alterations were prevented by insulin treatment. In contrast to biochemical alterations, fine structural changes were not so severe. At 8 to 12 weeks of diabetes increases in secondary lysosomes and lipid droplets were recognized plentifully with coarseness of myofibrils and assemblage of mitochondria under morphologically intact coronary arteries. But ATPase activity decreased markedly in terminal cisternae and longitudinal tubules of SR, and those on myofilamet reduced in the chronic period, i.e. 8 to 12 weeks. Such findings as dense deposits in mitochondria or contraction band, seen in ischemic injury, were not noted. Myocardial impairment occurs in diabetic heart as early as within 1 week without vascular obstruction, and biochemical alterations in SR are more prominent that those in morphologic changes. From the evidence that these changes were prevented by insulin treatment, we conclude that these are diabetes specific myocardial disorders.

Acknowledgements

The authors wish to express sincere thanks to Professor Yasumitsu Nakai of the Department of Anatomy for his encouragement for this work. And they are also deeply indebted to Drs. Shuji Mukae, Kazuhiko Umetsu, Mamoru Mochizuki, and Noburu Konno of the Third Department of Internal Medicine, Showa University School of Medicine, for their collaboration.

References

1. Rubler S, Dlugash J, Yuceoglu YZ, Kumral T, Branwood AW, Grishman A. New type of cardiomyopathy associated with diabetic glomerulosclerosis. Am J Cardiol 1972; 30: 595-602.
2. Kannel WB, Hjortland M, Castelli WP. Role of diabetes in congestive heart failure: The Framingham Study. Am J Cardiol 1974; 34: 29-34.
3. Yaida M, Umezawa Y, Konno N, Katagiri T. Alterations in cardiac sarcoplasmic reticulum and structural proteins in streptozotocin induced diabetic rats. J Showa Med Assoc 1988; 48: 175-183.
4. Yanagishita T, Konno N, Geshi E, Katagiri T. Alterations in phopholipids in acute ischemic myocardium. Jpn Circ J 1987; 51: 41-50.
5. Katagiri T. Changes of cardiac structural proteins in myocardial infarction. Jpn Heart J 1977: 18: 711-721.
6. Ozawa K, Takeyama Y, Katagiri T. Electron microscopic studies on the ATPase activity in myocardial infarction. Jpn Circ J 1982; 46: 725-733.
7. Konno N, Yanagishita T, Geshi E, Katagiri T. Degradation of the cardiac sarcoplasmic reticulum in acute myocardial ischemia. Jpn Circ J 1987; 51: 411-420.
8. Hamby RI, Zonerai S, Sherman L. Diabetic cardiomyopathy. JAMA 1974; 229: 1749-1754.

9. Regan TJ, Ettinger PO, Khan MI, Jesrani MU, Lyons MM, Oldewurtel HA, Weber M. Altered myocardial function and metabolism in chronic diabetes mellitus without ischemia in dogs. Circ Res 1974; 35: 222-237.
10. Ahmed SS, Jaferi GA, Narang RM, Regan TJ. Preclinical abnormality of left ventricular function in diabetes mellitus. Am Heart J 1975; 89: 153-158.
11. Ledet T. Diabetic cardiopathy. Acta Path Microbiol Scand A 1976; 84: 421-428.
12. Seneviratne BIB. Diabetic cardiomyopathy: The preclinical phase. Brit Med J 1977; 1: 1444-1446.
13. Fein FS, Kornstein LB, Strobeck JE, Capasso JM, Sonnenblick EH. Altered myocardial mechanics in diabetic rats. Circ Res 1980; 47: 922-933.
14. Penpargkul S, Fein F, Sonnenblick EH, Scheuer J. Depressed cardiac sarcoplasmic reticular function from diabetic rats. J Mol Cell Cardiol 1981; 13: 303-309.
15. Ganguly PK, Pierce GN, Dhalla KS, Dhalla NS. Defective sarcoplasmic reticular calcium transport in diabetic cardiomyopathy. Am J Physiol 1983; 244: E528-E535.
16. Pierce GN, Dhalla NS. Sarcolemmal Na^+-K^+-ATPase activity in diabetic rat heart. Am J Physiol 1983; 245: C241-C247.
17. Holman RT, Johnson SB, Gerrard JM, Mauer SM, Kupcho-Sandberg S, Brown DM. Arachidonic acid deficiency in streptozotocin-induced diabetes. Proc Nat Acad Sci USA 1983; 80: 2375-2379.
18. Huang YS, Horrobin DF, Manku MS, Mitchell J, Ryan MA. Tissue phopholipid fatty acid composition in the diabetic rat. Lipids 1984; 19: 367-370.
19. Tarach JS. Electron microscopic cytochemical studies on lysosomes and peroxisomes of a rat cardiac muscle in the experimental alloxan diabetes. Acta Histochem 1978; 62: 32-43.
20. Factor SM, Minase T, Bhan R, Wolinsky H. Hypertensive cardiomyopathy in the rat: Ultrastructural features. Virchows's Arch Anat 1983; 398: 305-317.
21. Seager MJ, Singal PK, Orchard R, Pierce GN, Dhalla NS. Cardiac cell damage: A primary myocardial disease by streptozotocin-induced chronic diabetes. Br J Exp Pathol 1984; 65: 613-623.

22. Jackson CV, McGrath GM, Tahiliani AG, Vadlamudi RVSV, McNeill JH. A functional and ultrastructural analysis of experimental diabetic rat myocardium. Diabetes 1985;34:876-883.
23. Dillmann WH. Diabetes mellitus induces changes in cardiac myosin of the rat. Diabetes 1980;29:579-582.

Diabetes Prolongs the Action Potential Duration in Rat Ventricular Muscle Probably Via Enhanced Calcium Current

Seiki Nobe, Masahiro Aomine, Makoto Arita, Sukenobu Ito*, Ryosaburo Takaki*

The Department of Physiology, and the Department of Medicine,
Medical College of Oita, Oita 879-56, JAPAN*

Introduction

Diabetic cardiomyopathy arises in patients suffering from diabetes mellitus for relatively long periods, and it is not secondary to hypertension, coronary artery disease, or valvular disease (1-4). A number of studies using diabetic rats as an experimental model, disclosed mechanical, biochemical and morphological changes in the heart (5,6). Fein et al. (7) found a marked slowing of relaxation and a substantial decrease of shortening velocity in the ventricular papillary muscles obtained from streptozotocin-induced diabetic rats, in which prolongation of action potential duration (APD) was also shown (8).

The present study was undertaken to investigate possible alteration of ionic mechanism(s) which may underlie the action potential changes in diabetic heart muscles.

Methods

Male Wistar rats (200-250 g) were made diabetic by injecting streptozotocin (STZ, Sigma Chemicals, USA) (65 mg·kg^{-1}) into the tail vein. The STZ was dissolved in citrate buffer (0.05 M, 0.8 ml·kg^{-1}, pH 4.5) just before use. Control rats were given comparable volumes of vehicle (citrate buffer). Control and diabetic rats were used 30 - 40 weeks after vehicle-or STZ-injection. Nonfasting plasma glucose concentrations of both control and diabetic rats were measured in a glucose analyzer (Fuji Film, Fujichem 1000, Japan) immediately before the animals were killed for subsequent *in vitro* study.

After the animals were anesthetized with ethyl ether, heart was rapidly

Nagano, M., Mochizuki, S., Dhalla, N.S. (eds.), CARDIOVASCULAR DISEASE IN DIABETES. Copyright © 1992. Kluwer Academic Publishers, Boston. All rights reserved.

removed and the papillary muscles were excised from the left ventricle. The muscle was mounted in a tissue bath (about 1.5 ml volume) and superfused continuously with oxygenated Tyrode's solution at a constant flow rate of 5 ml·min^{-1}. The tendinous end of the muscle was connected to a force transducer (Nihon Kohden, TB-612T, Japan) via a fine silk thread to record isometric tension. The muscle was stretched to the length at which the developed tension reached maximum (L_{max}). The Tyrode's solution contained (in mM): NaCl 136.7, KCl 5.4, $CaCl_2$ 1.8, $MgCl_2$ 1.05, NaH_2PO_4 0.4, and glucose 10.0. The pH of the Tyrode's solution was 7.4 after bubbling with a 95% O_2 - 5% CO_2 gas mixture. The bath temperature was maintained at 36 ± 0.5°C. The preparations were equilibrated with the solution for at least 2 hours before starting the study.

The preparations were always stimulated at 0.2 Hz with rectangular pulses of 1 ms duration at two times the threshold, through bipolar silver wire electrodes attached to the base of the preparation. Transmembrane potentials at the distal region of the papillary muscles were recorded using conventional glass microelectrodes filled with 3 M KCl and having a tip resistance of 10 to 30 megohm. A d.c. preamplifier (Nihon Kohden, MEZ-7101) with capacitance compensation was used to record the transmembrane potential. The maximum upstroke velocity of the action potential ($\dot{V}_{max}$) was obtained by using an electronic differentiator with linear amplification from 0 to 600 V·s^{-1}. The transmembrane potential, the $\dot{V}_{max}$, and the contractile tension were displayed simultaneously on an oscilloscope (Nihon Kohden, VC-9), and photographed using a long recording camera (Nihon Kohden, RLG-6101) or a pen-chart recorder (Nihon Kohden RJG-4004). The following membrane potential variables were measured: action potential amplitude (APA); resting membrane potential (RMP); $\dot{V}_{max}$; action potential duration (APD) at the levels of 25% (APD_{25}), 50% (APD_{50}), 75% (APD_{75}) and 90% (APD_{90}) repolarization. Only data for which the microelectrode was maintained within the same cell throughout the entire experimental period were used for analysis. The following twitch tension parameters were measured: resting tension (RT); peak developed tension (DT); time to peak developed tension (TPT); time to 1/2 relaxation (T1/2R). The length and diameter of the muscle fibers were measured with the aid of a miniature scale placed under the microscope.

4-Aminopyridine, $CoCl_2$ and ryanodine were purchased from Wako Pure

Table 1. Comparison of size of preparation and contraction parameters in control and diabetic papillary muscles

	L (mm)	CSA (mm^2)	RT (mN/mm^2)	DT (mN/mm^2)	TPT (ms)	T1/2R (ms)
Control (n = 11)	5.35±0.03	0.96±0.07	5.84±0.68	6.33±0.71	70.1±1.2	35.7±1.4
Diabetic (N = 13)	5.42±0.04	0.97±0.05	6.70±0.70	6.70±0.54	81.0±2.3*	45.3±1.6*

L, muscle length; CSA, cross sectional area of muscle; RT, resting tension; DT, developed tension; TPT, time to peak tension; T1/2R, time to 1/2 relaxation. Data presented as mean±SEM. n, number of preparations.
*: p < 0.05, significant difference from control.

Chemical Industries (Japan), and were dissolved in distilled water to produce stock solution which was diluted immediately before use.

All data are expressed as mean ± SEM. Statistical analysis was performed by Student's t test, and the difference is considered significant at p < 0.05, and marked with an asterisk (*) in the figures.

Results

General aspects of experimental animals

The treatment with STZ made the rats diabetic and significantly increased the blood glucose concentration from 156 ± 7 mg/dl (n=15, control rats) to 517 ± 17 mg/dl (n=14, diabetic rats); the body weight of diabetics (351 ± 13 g) was significantly less than that of controls (573 ± 25 g).

Contractile properties

The size of preparation and mechanical data from both control and diabetic rats (stimulated at 0.2 Hz) are summarized in Table 1. The resting tension (RT) and peak developed tension (DT) were similar, but time to peak developed tension (TPT) and time to 1/2 relaxation (T1/2R) of diabetic group

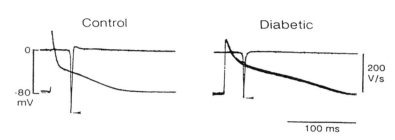

Figure 1: Representative action potentials recorded from ventricular papillary muscles of control (left panel) and diabetic (right panel) rats, stimulated at 0.2 Hz. In each panel; lower trace, action potential; upper trace, first derivative of action potential. Arrow indicates peak of the maximum upstroke velocity ($\dot{V}_{max}$) of action potential.

were significantly longer than those in control group.

Action potential characteristics

The rat ventricular action potential has a unique repolarization phase, referred to as the early phase (with brief duration) and the late phase (with long duration) (9-11). In our measurements, the APD_{25} and APD_{50} refer to the early phase; and the APD_{75} and APD_{90}, to the late phase. The early phase is determined by a combination of the decaying calcium inward current (I_{Ca}) and the increasing transient outward current (I_{to}) (11), and the late phase is primarily attributed to the inward current arising from electrogenic Na^+-Ca^{2+} exchange ($I_{Na/Ca}$) (10,12).

Figure 1 shows typical examples of the action potential of papillary muscles from control (left) and diabetic (right) rats, stimulated at 0.2 Hz. These records highlight major difference in the action potentials between the two groups; the APD was apparently longer in muscles from the diabetics than from the controls. Several features of the action potential from control and diabetic muscles are summarized in Table 2. In the diabetic muscles, the APDs (APD_{25}, APD_{50}, APD_{75} and APD_{90}) were significantly longer than those of the controls, with no significant difference in the RMP or APA. The $\dot{V}_{max}$ was significantly smaller in the diabetics than in the controls (Fig 1 and Table 2).

Effects of $CoCl_2$

Application of $CoCl_2$ (3 mM), a Ca^{2+} channel blocker, shortened the

Table 2. Action potential parameters of control and diabetic rat ventricular muscles

	RMP (-mV)	APA (mV)	$\dot{V}_{max}$ (V/s)	APD_{25} (ms)	APD_{50} (ms)	APD_{75} (ms)	APD_{90} (ms)
control (n=18)	77.1±1.0	100.7±2.0	253.4±20.4	5.2±0.4	12.0±0.8	59.1±3.8	95.0±3.7
diabetic (n=21)	77.5±0.8	97.5±1.5	178.1±12.0*	8.1±0.8*	23.4±2.8*	88.6±6.8*	134.6±7.1*

Stimulation frequency, 0.2 Hz. n, number of preparations. RMP, resting membrane potential; APA, action potential amplitude; $\dot{V}_{max}$, maximum upstroke velocity of action potential; APD_{25}, APD_{50}, APD_{75} and APD_{90}, action potential duration at repolarization levels of 25, 50, 75 and 90%, respectively. Data presented as mean±SEM. *: p < 0.05, significant difference from control.

APD in both muscle types (Fig 2A), and abolished contraction within 25 - 30 min. Figure 2B summarizes the effects of $CoCl_2$ on APDs at 4 different levels in control (open symbols) and diabetic muscles (filled symbols). $CoCl_2$ shortened the APD in both groups, but the effect seemed to be greater in the diabetic group. This became evident after subtraction of the APDs in the absence of $CoCl_2$ from the APDs in the presence of $CoCl_2$ to show Co^{2+}-induced shortening of the APDs (Fig 2C, as negative values). The Co^{2+}-induced shortening of the APD was significantly greater in the diabetics than in the controls at all levels of APD. This means that the APD of diabetic muscle tends to become close to that of control muscle in the presence of $CoCl_2$ (compare traces #2 in Fig 2A), thereby suggesting that Co^{2+}-sensitive current component prevails more in the diabetic muscles than in the control muscles.

Effects of ryanodine in absence and presence of $CoCl_2$

We observed that diabetic muscles had a more Co^{2+}-sensitive current component in the action potential than the controls (Fig 2C). The Co^{2+}-sensitive component is supposed to be composed of a Ca^{2+} inward current (I_{Ca}) and an inward current arising from electrogenic Na^+-Ca^{2+} exchange ($I_{Na/Ca}$), the operation of which is secondary to the increase in $[Ca^{2+}]_i$

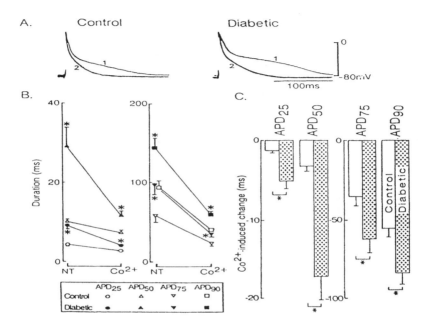

Figure 2: Effects of $CoCl_2$ (3 mM) on action potentials of control (CM) and diabetic muscles (DM), stimulated at 0.2 Hz. Preparation was superfused with 3 mM $CoCl_2$ for 30 min. A: Representative superimposed traces recorded in normal tyrode's solution (1) and with $CoCl_2$ (2). B: Summarized effects of $CoCl_2$ on the APDs from 11 CM and 11 DM, the symbols of which are shown in the inset. NT, normal Tyrode's solution; Co^{2+}, $CoCl_2$-containing solution. C: Co^{2+}-induced changes in APDs of CM (open column) and DM (stippled) obtained by subtraction of APD in the absence of $CoCl_2$ form APD in the presence of this compound.

(see discussion) (10,14).

To investigate the contribution of the increase in $[Ca^{2+}]_i$, due to the release of Ca^{2+} from the sarcoplasmic reticulum (SR), to the prolongation of APDs of the diabetic muscles, we used ryanodine, the most specific inhibitor of Ca^{2+}-release from SR (15-17). The effect of ryanodine (2 uM) appeared within 2 - 5 min after exposure, and reached steady state within 20 - 25 min, in our preparations. Figure 3A shows typical examples of ryanodine effects (traces #2) and subsequent addition of $CoCl_2$ (traces #3) on action potentials recorded from both muscle types. Figure 3B summarizes the effect of ryanodine and subsequent application of $CoCl_2$ on the APDs. The ryanodine-induced alteration in APDs, and the $CoCl_2$-induced shortening of APDs in the presence of ryanodine, were obtained from data shown in Fig 3B by subtraction, and presented in Fig 3C. In control muscles, ryanodine slightly lengthened the APDs in the early phase (APD_{25} and APD_{50}), and shortened the APDs in the late phase (APD_{75} and APD_{90}). This principle held also true, in qualitative manner, for diabetic muscles. However, the prolongation of early phase (APD_{25} and APD_{50}) was tremendous in the latter case, albeit the effect on the late phase (shortening of APD_{75} and APD_{90}) remained much the same as in the control muscles (Fig 3A and C, left).

It is noteworthy that, in the presence of ryanodine, the developed tension of control muscles virtually disappeared, leaving only 1.4 ± 0.3% of the control (ryanodine-free) tension (6.33 ± 0.71 mN/mm^2 or 100%, Table 2). By contrast, although the developed tension of diabetic muscles was also suppressed by ryanodine, the degree of suppression was significantly less ($p < 0.05$), and left a tension of as much as 4.9 ± 1.1% of the control tension (6.70 ± 0.54 mN/mm^2, Table 2). Since the release of Ca^{2+} from SR is blocked in the presence of ryanodine, this "ryanodine-resistant component of tension" is considered to be due to the direct activation of contractile protein by Ca^{2+} flowing through the Ca^{2+} channel (18,19). The finding lends support to the idea that I_{Ca} during action potential is larger in diabetic than in control muscles.

In the presence of ryanodine, application of $CoCl_2$ (3 mM) shortened the APD in both groups (Fig 3A, traces #3). However, the Co^{2+}-induced shortening of the APDs was greater in diabetics than in controls, thereby making the APDs of diabetic muscles comparable to those of controls (compare traces #3 in Fig 3A). As shown in Fig 3C (right), at all levels of APDs, Co^{2+}-sensitive component of APD was much greater in diabetics than in controls, thereby suggesting that I_{Ca} of diabetic muscles exceeds, perhaps in terms of both its amplitude and duration, that of controls in the presence of ryanodine, as was the case in the absence of ryanodine (Fig 2C).

Effects of 4-aminopyridine in absence and presence of $CoCl_2$

It is possible that the APD-prolongation in diabetic muscles would be

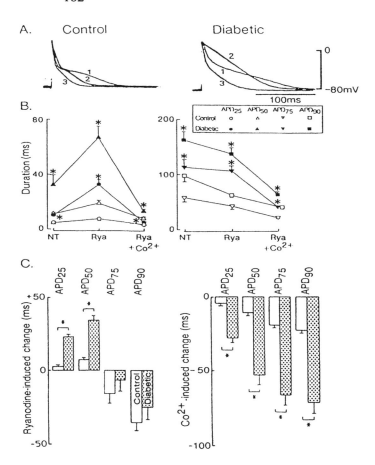

Figure 3: Effects of ryanodine (2 uM) and of ryanodine (2 uM) plus $CoCl_2$ (3 mM) on action potential of control (CM) and diabetic muscles (DM), stimulated at 0.2 Hz. A: the action potential in normal Tyrode's solution (1) superimposed on those at 30 min after application of ryanodine (2) and 30 min after application of $CoCl_2$ in presence of ryanodine (3). B: Summarized effects of ryanodine and of ryanodine plus $CoCl_2$ on the APDs from 6 CM and 6DM, the symbols of which are shown in the inset. NT, normal Tyrode's solution; Rya, ryanodine; Rya + Co^{2+}, ryanodine plus $CoCl_2$. C: Changes of APD induced by $CoCl_2$ in the presence of ryanodine ("Co^{2+}-induced change", right part) in both muscle types.

due to some dysfunction of the ionic channels that carry the transient outward current (I_{to}) which is responsible for the early phase of repolarization of the rat ventricle (11,13). Suppose this is the case, the difference in the APD between the two groups should be eliminated when the I_{to} of both preparations was sufficiently blocked by application of 4-aminopyridine (4-AP), a potent blocker of I_{to} in rat ventricular muscle (11,13). However this did not happen. As shown in Fig 4A, 4-AP (1 mM) produced approximately the same prolongation of APDs at the early Phase (APD_{25} and APD_{50}) in both preparations, and yet leaving unequivocal difference of the APDs between the groups. This is quantitatively shown in Fig 4B, in which the effects of 4-AP on the different levels of APD are summarized. Figure 4C shows 4-AP-induced lengthening of APDs, in that the APDs in the absence of 4-AP were subtracted from the APDs in the presence of 4-AP. There was no significant difference between the controls and diabetics with regard to the 4-AP-induced lengthening of the APDs.

Figure 5 shows the effects of $CoCl_2$ (3 mM) and subsequent application of 4-AP (5 mM) on the action potential. These concentrations of $CoCl_2$ and 4-AP are, respectively, considered sufficient to block the I_{Ca} and I_{to} of rat ventricular muscles (11,13,14). Even after the blockade of I_{Ca} with $CoCl_2$, the subsequent application of 4-AP lengthened the APDs to the same extent in both muscle types (Fig 5A and B). Figure 5C shows the 4-AP-induced prolongation of APDs in the presence of $CoCl_2$; 4-AP lengthened all the APDs to the same extent in both muscle types, a result comparable to the effect of 4-AP in the absence of $CoCl_2$ (Fig 4C). This again lends support to the idea that the I_{to} system is yet operating normally in diabetic muscle.

Finally, the treatment with 4-aminopyridine, $CoCl_2$ or ryanodine did not affect the RMP and APA, in both preparations.

Discussion

Electrophysiological studies of cardiac muscles from hearts subjected to chronic diabetes mellitus are relatively few (8,20). Fein et al. (8) first reported prolongation of the APD and reduction of the V_{max}, RMP and APA in the ventricular muscle from diabetic rats, albeit the underlying ionic mechanism(s) remained unexplained. The present study confirmed much of what was previously reported, except for the change in RMP (Table 2). They found depolarization of approximately 10 mV, whereas we found no depolarization.

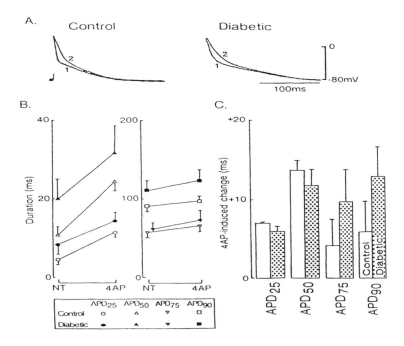

Figure 4: Effects of 4-aminopyridine (4-AP, 1 mM) on action potentials of control (CM) and diabetic muscles (DM), stimulated at 0.2 Hz. A: Action potential in normal Tyrode's solution (1) superimposed on that of 20 min after application of 4-AP (2). B: Summarized effects of 4-AP on the APDs from 4 CM and 4 DM, the symbols of which are shown in the inset. NT, normal Tyrode's solution; 4AP, 4-aminopyridine. C: 4-AP-induced changes of APDs in both muscle types.

Thus, the decrease in V_{max} (by about 27 - 42%) cannot be attributed to depolarization of the RMP, and indicates some impairment of the Rapid Na^+ current system in diabetic muscles. In single ventricular cells from diabetic rats, the action potential in about 1/4 of the myocytes tested was prolonged, with no change in RMP or APA (20). In agreement with above findings, some prolongation of corrected QT interval in electrocardiograms was reported for

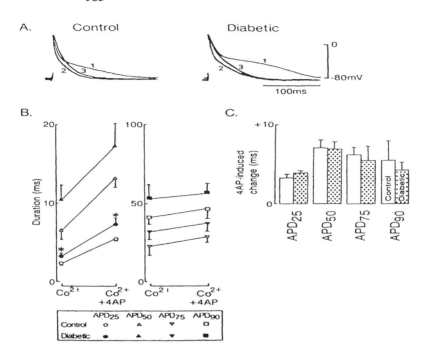

Figure 5: Effects of 4-AP (5 mM) in the presence of $CoCl_2$ (3 mM) on action potentials of control (CM) and diabetic muscles (DM), stimulated at 0.2 Hz. A: Action potential in normal Tyrode's solution (1) superimposed on those at 30 min after application of $CoCl_2$ (2) and 20 min after application of 4-AP in presence of $CoCl_2$ (3). B: Summarized effects of 4-AP on the APDs from 5 CM and 5 DM in presence of $CoCl_2$, the symbols of which are shown in the inset. Co^{2+}, $CoCl_2$; Co^{2+} + 4AP, $CoCl_2$ plus 4-aminopyridine. C: 4-AP-induced changes of APDs in the presence of $CoCl_2$ in both muscle types.

patients suffering from long-term diabetes mellitus (21).

What then is the mechanism of prolongation of APDs in diabetic muscle? So far, several ionic current components have been proposed for the build-up of repolarizing phase of rat ventricular action potentials. Among these included are: 1) A prominent transient outward current (I_{to}) contributing to early repolarization of the action potential, that is 4-AP sensitive and should therefore be a kind of K^+ current (11,13). In voltage clamp experiments, rat ventricular I_{to} was recorded even in the presence of

Co^{2+}, indicating that the current activation has nothing to do with transient increase of $[Ca^{2+}]_i$ that was proposed for sheep Purkinje fibres (I_{bo}) (22) and rabbit ventricular muscles ($I_{K,Ca}$) (23). The I_{to} of rat ventricular muscle was rapidly activated (~ 10 ms), and inactivated with a single component of current decay (τ = 30 - 40 ms). The repriming time was fairly short (~ 25 ms) (13). 2) A Ca^{2+} current (I_{Ca}), which may oppose the outward I_{to} and tend to lengthen the APD (11,14,24). 3) An inward current arising from electrogenic Na^+-Ca^{2+} exchange ($I_{Na/Ca}$), that is enhanced by an increase in intracellular Ca^{2+} concentration ($[Ca^{2+}]_i$), most of which is derived from Ca^{2+} released from the SR, and which is sensitive to, and effectively blocked by ryanodine (10,12,19). This electrogenic (inward) $I_{Na/Ca}$ is particularly important in producing the late phase of the rat ventricular action potential (10,12). The time course of $I_{Na/Ca}$ was similar to that of the intracellular Ca^{2+} transient monitored by aequorin and proportional to the time course of the developed tension (18,25). 4) A time-dependent K^+ current (I_{K1}) and Na^+,K^+-pump current may also contribute to the APD shortening because they are all outwardly directed. A time-dependent (delayed) K^+ current (I_K) was omitted from consideration (9, 26), because a voltage-clamp experiment using single cells from rat ventricles revealed no appreciable I_K activation (14,27).

From all these current components responsible for the formation of repolarization phase of rat ventricular muscles, we excluded a significant role of I_{K1} in alteration of APDs in diabetic muscle since the RMP was found not to be decreased in the present study (Table 2). Eventually, we focus our attention on alterations of two inward currents (I_{Ca} and $I_{Na/Ca}$) and one outward current (I_{to}) as candidates for the prolongation of APD. Among these currents, I_{to} does not seem to be important for the prolongation of the early phase of action potentials, because 4-AP, a potent inhibitor of this current, lengthened the early phase of repolarization to the same extent in both muscle types, either in the absence (Fig 4), or in the presence (Fig 5) of $CoCl_2$, indicating that I_{to} channels of diabetic muscles may be intact.

We then examined the possibility that I_{Ca} and/or $I_{Na/Ca}$ are involved in the prolongation of APDs. Application of $CoCl_2$ markedly shortened all levels of APDs in both control and diabetic muscles, with much greater effects on the latter (Fig 2). At the same time, the developed tension (DT) was totally abolished in both muscle types, indicating the key role of I_{Ca} for activation of contraction. The amplitude of DT of rat ventricular muscle depends mostly on the amount of cytosolic Ca^{2+} released from SR (10,15,19,28), and this Ca^{2+}, via acceleration of Na^+-Ca^{2+} exchange, produces $I_{Na/Ca}$, an inward current, which is subsequently responsible for the maintenance of late phase of action potential (APD_{75} and APD_{90}) (10,12). Prolongation of the time to peak tension (TPT) and time to half relaxation (T1/2R) of contraction in the diabetic muscle (Table 2) may be, at least in part, related to this prolongation of APD and suggests prolonged increase in cytosolic free Ca^{2+} concentration after depolarization.

It has been demonstrated that the Ca^{2+} uptake by SR is impaired in diabetic animals (29). Thus, we speculated that the APD of diabetic muscle is longer because of sustained increases in $[Ca^{2+}]_i$ (and hence persistent $I_{Na/Ca}$), due to retarded Ca^{2+} uptake in the SR. However this speculation does not fit with the present results we obtained in the presence of ryanodine (Fig 3). In other words, if the APD difference between the control and diabetic muscles is simply derived from the difference in $I_{Na/Ca}$ or the difference in APD should disappear in the presence of ryanodine, because this agent totally inhibits the Ca^{2+} release from SR in both control and diabetic muscles (15-17). Actually this was not the case (cf. traces #2 in Fig 3A). On the contrary, if the difference in APD depends on the difference in the I_{Ca}, the APD difference, especially in the early phase (APD_{25} and APD_{50}), would remain unchanged or become more pronounced in the presence of ryanodine, because SR-derived increase in $[Ca^{2+}]_i$, a factor facilitating inactivation of Ca^{2+} channels (19,30,31), does not occur in this situation, thereby disclosing inherent abnormality of Ca^+ channels existing in diabetic muscles. Indeed, ryanodine did not eliminate the difference in APD_{25} and APD_{50} but rather enhanced it (Fig 3), a finding in keeping with the latter hypothesis, that is, enhanced I_{Ca} is perhaps involved in the lengthening of APDs in diabetic muscle. This idea reconciles with the finding that ryanodine-resistant component of twitch contraction, that is directly (not via released Ca^{2+} from SR) activated by transsarcolemmal Ca^{2+} influx (18,19), was significantly larger in diabetic muscles than in the controls, and that, in the presence of ryanodine, blockage of I_{Ca} by $CoCl_2$ had much greater shortening effects on APD_{25} and APD_{50} in diabetic muscles (Fig 3C, right).

If the APD-prolongation observed in diabetic muscles is due exclusively to altered I_{Ca}, the difference in APD between both muscle types should disappear when the I_{Ca} was totally blocked. However, there still remained slight but significant difference in the APDs in the presence of $CoCl_2$ (Fig 2A and B). We attribute this residual APD-difference to: 1) insufficient blockade of I_{Ca}, or 2) contribution of the other still unknown current component(s), for prolongation of the APDs. Final conclusion must await further study.

Summary

The effects of chronic diabetes on electromechanical properties of isolated ventricular papillary muscles were studied, using rats made diabetic by single intravenous injection of streptozotocin (65 mg·kg^{-1}), for 30 - 40 weeks. Conventional glass microelectrodes and tension-recording techniques were used. We found: 1) The maximum upstroke velocity of the action potential of diabetic muscles (DM) was significantly decreased compared to control muscles (CM), with no difference in the resting potential. 2) The action potential duration (APD) of DM was significantly longer than that of CM. 3) A Ca^{2+} channel blocker, $CoCl_2$, shortened all levels of APDs, with much greater effect on DM. 4) Ryanodine lengthened the early phase of APDs while shortened the late phase of APDs in both groups, and did not diminish the APD difference in the early phase recognized between the groups, but rather enhanced it. 5) Developed tension in the presence of ryanodine (ryanodine-resistant tension component) was significantly greater in DM than in CM. 6) A blocker of transient outward current, 4-aminopyridine, lengthened the early phase of APDs in both groups, the same amount. All these findings taken together suggest that altered Ca^{2+} current, unlike altered Na^+-Ca^{2+} exchange current and altered transient outward current, is responsible for the prolongation of APDs in the diabetic rat ventricular muscle.

Acknowledgments

We thank K. Takahashi and K. Goto for help in preparing diabetic rats, and M. Makino for the measurement of plasma glucose concentration.

References

1. Hamby RI, Zoneraich S, Sherman S. Diabetic cardiomyopathy. J Am Med Assoc 1974;229:1749-1754.

2. Kannel WB, Hjortland M, Castelli WP. Role of diabetes in congestive heart failure: the Framingham Study. Am J Cardiol 1974;34:29-35.
3. Regan TJ, Lyons MM, Ahmed SS, Levinson GE, Oldewurtel HA, Ahmed MR, Haider B. Evidence for cardiomyopathy in familial diabetes mellitus. J Clin Invest 1977;60:885-899.
4. Rubler S, Dlugash J, Yuceoglu YZ, Kumral T, Branwood AW, Grishman A. New type of cardiomyopathy associated with diabetic glomerulosclerosis. Am J Cardiol 1972;30:595-602.
5. Gotzsche O. Myocardial cell dysfunction in diabetes mellitus. A review of clinical and experimental studies. Diabetes 1986;35:1158-1162.
6. Tahiliani AG, McNeill JH. Diabetes-induced abnormalities in the myocardium. Life Sci 1986;38:959-974.
7. Fein FS, Kornstein LB, Strobeck JE, Capasso JM, Sonnenblick EH. Altered myocardial mechanics in diabetic rats. Circ Res 1980;47:922-933.
8. Fein FS, Aronson RS, Nordin C, Miller-Green B, Sonnenblick EH. Altered myocardial response to ouabain in diabetic rats: mechanics and electrophysiology. J Mol Cell Cardiol 1983;15:769-784.
9. Watanabe T, Delbridge LM, Bustamante JO, McDonald TF. Heterogeneity of the action potential in isolated rat ventricular myocytes and tissue. Circ. Res 1983;52:280-290.
10. Mitchell MR, Powell T, Terrar DA, Twist VW. The effects of ryanodine, EGTA and low-sodium on action potentials in rat and guinea-pig ventricular myocytes: evidence for two inward currents during the plateau. Br J Pharmac 1984;81:543-550.
11. Mitchell MR, Powell T, Terrar DA, Twist VW. Strontium, nifedipine and 4-aminopyridine modify the time course of the action potential in cells from rat ventricular muscle. Br J Pharmac 1984;81:551-556.
12. Noble D. Experimental and theoretical work on excitation and excitation-contraction coupling in the heart. Experientia 1987;43:1146-1150.
13. Josephson IR, Sanchez-Chapula J, Brown AM. Early outward current in rat single ventricular cells. Circ Res 1984;54:157-162.
14. Josephson IR, Sanchez-Chapula J, Brown AM. A comparison of calcium currents in rat and guinea pig single ventricular cells. Circ Res 1984;54:144-156.

15. Sutko JL, Willerson JT. Ryanodine alteration of the contractile state of rat ventricular myocardium. Comparison with dog, cat, and rabbit ventricular tissues. Circ Res 1980;46:332-343.
16. Sutko, JL, Kenyon JL. Ryanodine modification of cardiac muscle responses to potassium free solutions: Evidence for inhibition of sarcoplasmic reticulum calcium release. J Gen Physiol 1983;82:385-404.
17. Rousseau E, Smith JS, Meissner G. Ryanodine modifies conductance and gating behavior of single Ca^{2+} release channel. Am J Physiol 1987;253:C364-C368.
18. Marban E, Wier WG. Ryanodine as a tool to determine the contributions of calcium entry and calcium release to the calcium transient and contraction of cardiac Purkinje fibers. Circ Res 1985;56:133-138.
19. Callewaert G, Cleemann L, Morad M. Epinephrine enhances Ca^{2+} current-regulated Ca^{2+} release and Ca^{2+} reuptake in rat ventricular myocytes. Proc natl Acad Sci USA 1988;85:2009-2013.
20. Horackova M, Murphy MG. Effects of chronic diabetes mellitus on the electrical and contractile activities, $^{45}Ca^{2+}$ transport, fatty acid profiles and ultrastructure of isolated rat ventricular myocytes. Pflugers Arch 1988;411:564-572.
21. Kahn JK, Sisson JC, Vinik AI. QT interval prolongation and sudden cardiac death in diabetic autonomic neuropathy. J Clin Endocrinol Metab 1987;64:751-754.
22. Coraboeuf E, Carmeliet E. Existance of two transient outward currents in sheep cardiac Purkinje fibers. Pflugers Arch 1982;392:352-359.
23. Hiraoka M, Kawano S. Calcium-sensitive and insensitive transient outward current in rabbit ventricular myocytes. J Physiol(Lond) 1989;410:187-212.
24. Mainwood GW, McGuigan JAS. Evidence for inward calcium current in the absence of external sodium in rat myocardium. Experientia 1975;31:67-69.
25. Mitchell MR, Powell T, Terrar DA, Twist VW. Calcium-activated inward current and contraction in rat and guinea-pig ventricular myocytes. J Physiol(Lond) 1987;391:545-560.
26. Hilgemann DW, Noble D. Excitation-contraction coupling and extracellular calcium transients in rabbit atrium: reconstruction of basic cellular mechanisms. Proc R Soc Lond 1987;B230:163-205.

27. Yatani A, Imoto Y, Goto M. The effects of caffeine on the electrical properties of isolated, single rat ventricular cells. Jpn J Physiol 1984;34:337-349.
28. Allen DG, Eisner DA, Pirolo JS, Smith GL. The relationship between intracellular calcium and contraction in calcium-overloaded ferret papillary muscles. J Physiol(Lond) 1985;364:169-182.
29. Penpargkul S, Fein F, Sonnenblick EH, Scheuer J. Depressed cardiac sarcoplasmic reticular function from diabetic rats. J Mol Cell Cardiol 1981;13:303-309.
30. Mitchell MR, Powell T, Terrar DA, Twist VW. Ryanodine prolongs Ca-currents while suppressing contraction in rat ventricular muscle cells. Br J Pharmac 1984;81:13-15.
31. Schouten VJA. The negative correlation between action potential duration and force of contraction during restitution in rat myocardium. J Mol Cell Cardiol 1986;18:1033-1045.

Increases in Voltage-Sensitive Calcium Channel of Cardiac and Skeletal Muscle in Streptozotocin-Induced Diabetic Rats

A. Kashiwagi, Y. Nishio, T. Ogawa, S. Tanaka, M. Kodama, T. Asahina, M. Ikebuchi, Y. Shigeta

The Third Department of Medicine, Shiga University of Medical Science, Seta, Ohtsu, Shiga, JAPAN. 520-21

Introduction

Many lines of evidence including epidemiological (1), clinical (2,3) and experimental (4,5) studies have shown the existence of specific abnormalities in cardiac muscle in diabetes. Recently, it has been suggested that Ca^{2+} overload into cardiac muscle may be one of the contributing factors for cardiomyopathy (6). Furthermore, an increase in tissue Ca^{2+} level has been reported in chronic diabetic rats (7), which may be associated with cardiomyopathy in diabetes (8). Interestingly, Afzal N. et al. (9) have shown that treatment of streptozotocin-diabetic rats with verapamil, a voltage-sensitive Ca^{2+} channel blocker, improves cardiac dysfunction. These reports suggest that an excess Ca^{2+} influx through voltage-sensitive Ca^{2+} channel may induce cardiomyopathy in diabetes. However, there has been no report on voltage sensitive Ca^{2+} channel in diabetic rat heart. Therefore, in the present study, we have examined the status of Ca^{2+} channels in cardiac muscle as well as skeletal muscle membrane from control and streptozotocin-induced diabetic rats using [^{3}H]PN200-110, a dihydropyridine derivative as a ligand.

Materials and Methods

Animals; Male Sprague-Dawley rats weighing 180-200 g were randomly separated into control and experimental groups. The experimental animals were anesthetized with diethyl ether and given an injection of streptozotocin (STZ;55mg/kg, iv) in 0.05M citrate buffer (pH 4.5). These animals were maintained on laboratory chow and water *ad libitum* for 10 weeks after the induction of diabetes. The control animals received only buffer. Plasma

Table 1. Characteristics of experimental animals.

Group	Number	Body weight (g)	Ventricular weight (g)	Plasma glucose (mM)	Plasma IRI (u U/ml)
Control	18	480 ± 11	1.22 ± 0.02	8.0 ± 0.4	59 ± 6
Diabetic	28	268 ± 15*	0.77 ± 0.02*	27.7 ± 2.6*	16 ± 4*

Data are expressed at means ± SE. * $P < 0.01$ as compared with control.

Table 2. Characteristics of [^{3}H]PN200-110 binding to cardiac and skeletal muscle membrane fraction isolated from control and diabetic rats.

Group	Muscle	Number	5'-nucleotidase (n mole/min/mg prot.)	[^{3}H]PN200-110 binding (fmole/mg prot.) Bmax	Kd(pM)
Control	Heart	6	14.7 ± 0.5	62 ± 4	134 ± 14
	Skeletal	4	10.9 ± 1.0	170 ± 4	1100 ± 20
Diabetic	Heart	7	14.5 ± 0.4	100 ± 6*	129 ± 9
	Skeletal	4	13.0 ± 0.9	421 ± 17*	700 ± 90

Date are expressed as means ± SE. * $P < 0.01$ as compared with control.

insulin level was measured by radioimmunoassay (10) and plasma glucose level was measured by hexokinase method (11). The characteristics of the experimental animals are shown in Table 1.

Preparation of cardiac and skeletal muscle membrane; After the rat was killed, the heart was quickly removed and perfused with cold Krebs-Ringer phosphate buffer containing 5 mM glucose and then atrium was trimmed. Then, we prepared a crude membrane fraction from the remaining ventricular tissue following a previous method with some modifications (12). Briefly, the ventricular tissue taken from the control and diabetic rats was minced in 6 volumes of cold 50 mM Tris-HCl buffer (pH 7.4) containing 5 mM EDTA, 0.3mM PMSF (phenyl methyl sulfonyl fluoride), 50U/ml aprotinin and 10 uM benzethonium chloride and homogenized with a polytron at a half maximal speed

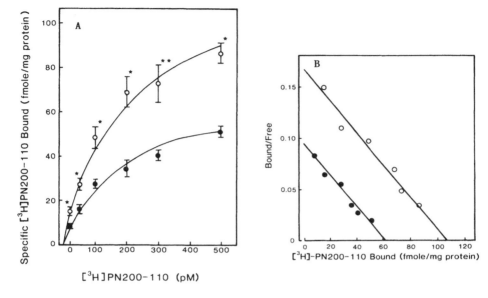

Figure 1. A: Specific [^{3}H]PN200-110 binding to cardiac membrane fraction isolated from control (closed circles) and 10-wk-diabetic (open circles) rats. Values are expressed as means ± SE (n=4) *P<0.01, **P<0.05 as compared with the control. B: Mean Scatchard plots of [^{3}H]PN200-110 binding to cardiac membrane.

for 20 sec two times. The homogenate was centrifuged at 500 x g for 10 min and the supernatant was centrifuged at 40,000 x g for 15 min. The pellet was suspended and homogenized in 10 mM histidine buffer (pH 7.5) containing 0.1 mM PMSF and used as crude cardiac membrane.

Skeletal muscle membrane was prepared from hind limb muscles according to the method of Amira K. et al. (13). Tissue was minced in 10 volumes of cold 10 mM NaHCO$_3$ buffer (pH 7.4) containing 0.25M sucrose, 5 mM NaN$_3$ and 0.1 mM PMSF and homogenized with polytron at a half maximal speed for 20 sec. After centrifugation at 1,200 x g for 10 min, the supernatant was stocked. The pellet was rehomogenized at 9,000 x g for 10 min. Finally, the supernatant was spun at 190,000 x g for 60 min. The pellet was resuspended in 50 mM Tris-HCl buffer (pH 7.5) containing 0.1 mM PMSF. The samples were frozen at -70 °C until use.

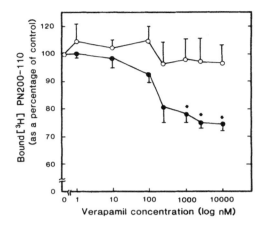

Figure 2. Effect of verapamil on specific [^{3}H]PN200-110 binding to cardiac membrane isolated from control (closed circles) and diabetic (open circles) rats. Data are expressed as means ± SE (n=3). *P<0.05 compared with the diabetic rats.

Protein concentration was measured by the method dscribed by Lowry et al. (14) with bovine serum albumin as a standard. 5'-nucleotidase activity was measured according to the method described by Newby et al. (15).

Calcium channel binding assay; Dihydropyridine-sensitive Ca^{2+} channel in membrane fraction was measured according to the previous method with some modifications (16). Two hundred ug of membrane protein was incubated at 37 °C for 15 min in the presence of 1 ml of 50 mM Tris-HCl (pH 7.5) and 0.1 mM PMSF containing 20-500 pM [^{3}H]PN200-110 (isopropyl 4-(2,1,3-benzoxadiazol 4-yl)-1,4-dihydro-2,6-dimethyl-5-methoxycarbonyl-pyridine-3-carboxylate) for cardiac membrane and 200 5000pM [^{3}H]PN200-110 for skeletal muscle membrane, respectively. The incubation was terminated by an addition of 10 ml of cold 10 mM Tris-HCl (pH 7.4) buffer and kept a 4 °C for 30 min. Applying this procedure, the non-specific binding decreased by 30% without a significant decrease in the specific binding. Membrane bound [^{3}H]PN200-110 was separated from free [^{3}H]PN200-110 by vacuum filtration through the Whatman GF/B glass fiber filter (Clifton, NJ). The filter was washed with a 4ml of 10 mM Tris-HCl buffer for 5 times before counting. Following this procedure, the specific binding was saturated after 15 min-incubation at 37° C and was kept constant for a further 15 min. The non-specific binding was

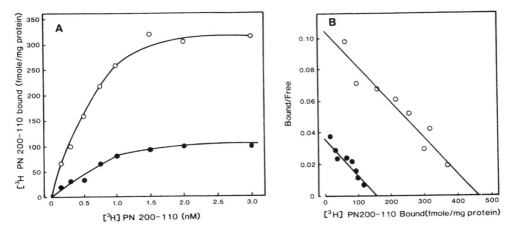

Figure 3. A: A representative [^{3}H]PN200-110 binding to skeletal muscle membrane fraction isolated from control (closed circles) and diabetic (open circles) rats. B: Scatchard plots of [^{3}H]PN200-110 binding shown in Fig 4A. Data are expressed as means of the duplicate measurements.

determined in the presence of 2 uM nitrendipine (less than 30% of the total binding in the presence of the highest ligand concentration). Allosteric inhibition of [^{3}H]PN200-110 binding to cardiac membrane by verapamil was measured by incubating 200 ug protein of cardiac membrane in the presence of 200 pM [^{3}H] PN200-110 in the absence or presence of 1-10000 nM verapamil. The binding study was performed under dim light.

Chemicals; [^{3}H]PN200-110 (2597.4 GBq/mmol) and [^{14}C]AMP were purchased from New England Nuclear (Boston, MA). Nitrendipine was a gift from Yoshitomi Pharmaceutical Co. (Osaka, Japan) and streptozocin was generously provided from Upjohn Co. (Kalamazoo, MI). All other chemicals were reagent-grade products obtained from commercial sources.

Statistical analysis; The equilibrium dissociation constant (Kd) and the maximum binding sites (B_{max}) for [^{3}H]PN200-110 were calculated from Scatchard analysis with linear regression. Differences were evaluated by Student's t-test with P<0.05 indicating significance.

Results

STZ-induced diabetic rats showed significantly higher plasma glucose level (P<0.01) and lower plasma insulin level (P<0.01) than those of the control (Table 1). STZ-induced diabetic rats showed an impairment of increases in both body weight and ventricular weight (P<0.01).

As shown in Fig. 1A, the [^{3}H]PN200-110 binding to cardiac membrane isolated from the 10-wk-diabetic rats significantly (p<0.01) increased at all [^{3}H]PN200-110 concentrations compared with those of the 10-wk-control rats. Fig. 1B showed linear scatchard plots of the binding indicating the difference in B_{max} without any difference in Kd between the two groups. As summarized in Table 2, only binding site (B_{max}) in the diabetic group (100 ± 6 fmol/mg protein) increased significantly (P < 0.05) in comparison to that (62 ± 4 fmol/mg protein) in control rats. As shown in Fig. 2, [^{3}H]PN200-110 binding to cardiac membrane isolated from control rats was significantly (P<0.05) inhibited by verapamil, a phenylalkylamine Ca^{2+} channel antagonist. In contrast, the binding to cardiac membrane isolated from diabetic rats showed no inhibition in the presence of verapamil. Furthermore, the specific [^{3}H]PN200-110 binding to skeletal muscle membrane isolated from the diabetic rats also showed more binding sites (B_{max}) than those of normal rats without a significant difference in Kd between the two groups (Fig. 3A and 3B). As summarized in Table 2, the maximum binding sites (B_{max}) of [^{3}H]PN200-110 to skeletal muscle membrane isolated from diabetic rats was 2.5 fold greater (P<0.01) than those of the control without a significant difference in Kd. 5'-Nucleotidase activity in cardiac and skeletal muscle membrane fraction was similar between the control and diabetic rats, respectively.

Discussion

In the present study, we found a 61% increase in the maximum [^{3}H]PN200-110 binding sites (B_{max}) in cardiac membrane isolated from diabetic rats compared with that of the control rats without any difference in Kd. [^{3}H]PN200-110, a voltage-sensitive Ca^{2+} channel antagonist, can label alpha$_1$-subunit of the L-type (dihydropyridine class) of Ca^{2+} channel. An L-type Ca^{2+} channel is also present in skeletal muscle, although the property of skeletal muscle L-type Ca^{2+} channels is somewhat different from that present in cardiac muscle (17). In the present study, skeletal muscle membrane isolated from the 10-week-diabetic rats showed the marked (2.5 fold) increase in the B_{max} compared with the control skeletal muscle. Both cardiac and skeletal muscle membrane fractions isolated from control and diabetic rats showed similar 5'-nucleotidase activities. Thus it is evident that there occurs a change in voltage-sensitive Ca^{2+} channel of cardiac and skeletal muscle membrane isolated from diabetic rats.

As previously described (18), [^{3}H]PN200-110 binding to control cardiac membrane was allosterically inhibited in the presence of verapamil, a phenylalkylamine Ca^{2+} antagonist. However, the [^{3}H]PN200-110 binding to cardiac membrane isolated from diabetic rats was not inhibited by verapamil, suggesting that an abnormality in subunit interactions of the receptor in diabetic cardiac membrane. In the present study, we have no further explanation for this qualitative change of dihydropyridine Ca^{2+} channel in diabetic cardiac muscle.

It can be argued that the increased number of the voltage-sensitive Ca^{2+} channel is secondary to insulin deficiency or cardiac dysfunction in STZ-diabetic rats (4,19), or toxicity of the drug on cardiac tissue. At least the latter possibility may be unlikely by the fact that B_{max} of [^{3}H]PN200-110 in cardiac membrane isolated from obese diabetic rats (Wistar fa/fa rats) increased by 34% (P<0.01) compared with that of the lean littermate (data not shown). Furthermore, in a preliminary study, we could prevent the significant increase in the [^{3}H]PN200-110 binding to cardiac membrane in streptozotocin-induced diabetic rats by a 8-week-insulin treatment (data not shown). Therefore, although the exact mechanism of this phenomena remains unsolved in the present study, the increases in voltage sensitive calcium channel of cardiac muscle may be associated with the metabolic abnormalities in diabetes.

It is well known that Ca^{2+} movement through voltage-sensitive Ca^{2+} channel is essential in excitation-contraction coupling in cardiac muscle (20). In the present study, we did not measure the actual Ca^{2+} movement into cardiac myocytes. However, if the open probability of the channel is similar between control and diabetic rats, more Ca^{2+} might flow inside the cardiac cells during the plateau of the action potential. This is advantageous for producing a positive inotropic effect during systole. On the other hand, an increase in voltage-sensitive Ca^{2+} channel may also suggest excessive accumulation of Ca^{2+} in the depolarized state, which may induce cardiomyopathy as described in Syrian cardiomyopathic hamster (6). In fact, it has been reported that the occurrence of the intracellular Ca^{2+} overload (8) and an increase in tissue Ca^{2+} content (7) are present in chronic diabetic heart. These may lead to the development of cardiomyopathy (8). Interestingly, Afzal N. et al. (9) have reported that _in vitro_ treatment of streptozotocin-induced diabetic rats with verapamil can prevent diabetes-induced functional, metabolic and ultrastructural abnormalities in cardiac muscle (9). Therefore, in terms of Ca^{2+} overload in diabetic heart, the present significant increase in voltage-sensitive Ca^{2+} channel in diabetes may contribute to an increase in Ca^{2+} influx and is compatible with the effectiveness of verapamil on diabetes-induced cardiac abnormalities. Furthermore, depression in the sarcoplasmic reticular Ca^{2+} uptake (21), the decrease in sarcolemmal Ca^{2+}-pump and Na^{+}-Ca^{2+} exchange activities (22) and reduced mitochondrial capacity to accumulate Ca^{2+} (23) have been reported in chronic diabetic rat heart. Taking together all this data including the present results, Ca^{2+} overload and a possible increase in free cytosolic Ca^{2+} concentration may be present in myocardial cells in chronic diabetes and this may lead to the development of cardiomyopathy. This possibility will be evaluated in the future study.

Summary

Voltage-sensitive Ca^{2+} channel in cardiac and skeletal muscle membrane isolated from normal and diabetic rats was measured by using [^{3}H]PN200-110, a dihydropyridine derivative as a ligand. Both cardiac and skeletal muscle [^{3}H]PN200-110 binding sites increased as compared with the control without any difference in Kd of the binding. However, the verapamil-dependent inhibition of [^{3}H]PN200-110 binding was different between the control and diabetic rats. These results indicate both quantitative and qualitative changes in cardiac muscle voltage-sensitive Ca^{2+} channel in diabetic rats as compared with control rats which may serve as a mechanism for Ca^{2+} overload in diabetic heart.

Acknowledgements

This study was supported in part by a research grant-in-aid from the Ministry of Education, Science, and Culture, Japan.

References

1. Kannel WB, Hjoltland M, and Castelli WP. Role of diabetes in congestive heart failure: The Framingham study. Am J Cardiol 1974;34:29-34.
2. Factor M, Minase T and Sonnenblick EH. Clinical and morphological features of human hypertensive diabetic cardiomyopathy. Am Heart J 1980;99:446-58.

3. Hamby RI, Zoneraich S and Sherman S. Diabetic cardiomyopathy. J Am Med Assoc 1979;229:1749-54.
4. Fein FS, Strobeck JE, Malhotra A, Scheuer J and Sonnenblick EH. Reversibility of diabetic cardiomyopathy with insulin in rats. Circ Res 1981;49:1251-61.
5. Regan TJ, Ettinger PO, Khan MI, Jesuani MV, Lyon MM, Oldewurtel, HA and Weber M. Altered myocardial function and metabolism in chronic diabetes mellitus without ischemia in dogs. Cir Res 1974;35:222-37.
6. Wagner JA, Reynolds, IJ, Weisman HF, Dudeck P, Weisfeldt ML and Snyder SH. Calcium antagonist receptors in cardiomyopathic hamster: Selective Increase in Heart, Muscle, Brain. Science 1986;25:515-18.
7. Nagase N, Tamura Y, Kobayashi S, Saito K, Saito M, Niki T, Chikamori K and Mori H. Myocardial disorders of hereditarily diabetic KK mice. J Mol Cell Cardiol 1981;13(Suppl. 2):70.
8. Dhalla NS, Pierce GN, Innes IR and Beamish RE, Pathogenesis of cardiac dysfunction in diabetes mellitus. Can J Cardiol 1985;1:263-84.
9. Afzal N, Ganguly PK, Dhalla KS, Pierce GN, Singal PK and Dhalla NS. Beneficial effects of verapamil in diabetic cardiomyopathy. Diabetes 1988;37:936-42.
10. Hoffman WS. A rapid photometric method for the determination of glucose in blood and urine. J Biol Chem 1973;248:12051-55.
11. Hales C and Randle P. Immunoassay of insulin with insulin anti-body precipitate. Biochem J 1963;88:137-146.
12. Jones JR, Besch HR Jr., Fleming JW, MaConnauhey MM and Watanabe AM. Separation of vesicles of cardiac sarcolemma from vesicles of cardiac sarcoplasmic reticulum. J Biol Chem 1979;254:530-539.
13. Amira K, Ramlal T, Young DA and Holloszy JO. Insulin-induced translocation of glucose transporters in rat hindlimb muscles. FEBS Letters 1987;224:224-230.
14. Lowry OH, Rosebrough HJ, Farr AL and Randall RJ. Protein measurement with the Folin phenol reagent. J Biol Chem 1951;193:265-275.
15. Newby AC, Luzio JP and Hales CN. The properties and extracellular location of 5'-nucleotidase of the rat fat cell plasma membrane. Biochem J 1975;146:625-633.
16. Goll A, Ferry DR and Glossmann H. Target size analysis of skeletal muscle Ca^{2+} channels. Positive allosteric heterotropic regulation by

d-cis-diltiazem is associated with apparent channel oligomer dissociation. FEBS Letters 1983;157:63-67.
17. Chang FC and Hosey MM. Dihydropyridine and phenylalkylamine receptors associated with cardiac and skeletal muscle calcium channels are structurally different. J Biol Chem 1988;263:18929-37.
18. Ehlert FJ, Roeske WR, Itoga E and Yamamura HI. The binding of [^{3}H]nitrendipine receptors for calcium channel antagonists in the heart, cerebral cortex, and ileum of rats. Life Sci 1982;30:2191-2202.
19. Vadlamudi RVSV and McNeill JH. Effect of experimental diabetes on isolated rat heart responsiveness to isoproterenol. Can J Physiol Pharmacol 1984;62:124-31.
20. Fleckenstein A. Specific pharmacology of calcium in myocardium, cardiac pacemaker, and vascular smooth muscle. Ann Rev Pharmacol Toxicol 1977;17:149-66.
21. Penpargul S, Fein F, Sonnenblick EH and Scheuer J. Depressed cardiac sarcoplasmic reticular function from diabetic rats. J Mol Cell Cardiol 1981;13:303-309.
22. Makino N, Dhalla KS, Elimban V and Dhalla NS. Sarcolemmal calcium transport in streptozocin-induced diabetic cardiomyopathy in rats. Am J Physiol 1987;253:E202-207.
23. Pierce GN and Dhalla NS. Mitochondrial abnormalities in diabetic cardiomyopathy. Can J Cardiol 1985;1:48-54.

Changes in Cell Morphology, $[Ca^{2+}]_i$ and pH_i During Metabolic Inhibition in Isolated Myocytes of Diabetic Rats Using Dual-Loading of Fura-2 and BCECF

H. Hayashi, N. Noda, H. Miyata, S. Suzuki, A. Kobayashi, M. Hirano#,
T. Kawai#, T. Hayashi* and N. Yamazaki.

Third Department of Internal Medicine, Hamamatsu University School of Medicine, Hamamatsu, JAPAN. #Hamamatsu Photonics K.K., Hamamatsu, JAPAN. *Medical Photonics, Hamamatsu University School of Medicine, Hamamatsu, JAPAN.

Introduction

Diabetes Mellitus (DM) has been shown to be associated with heart failure in the absence of atherosclerosis (1,2), suggesting a diabetic cardiomyopathy (3,4). The mechanism of heart failure due to the diabetic cardiomyopathy remains to be elucidated. The small vessel disease (5) and the abnormalities of subcellular mechanisms such as myosin ATPase (6) and myosin isoenzymes (7), have been reported in DM myocardium. Recently, abnormalities of Ca^{2+} metabolism have been reported in DM myocardium, which showed decreased Ca^{2+}-ATPase of sarcoplasmic reticulum (SR) (8,9) and sarcolemma (10). It has also been reported that the activity of Na^+/Ca^{2+}-exchange was lower in DM myocardium (11). Previous reports have suggested the possibility of the Ca^{2+} overload in diabetic cardiomyopathy (11).

Mortality in DM patients after acute myocardial infarction has been reported to be high comparing with that of non-diabetic patients (12). Experimental studies have also suggested that DM myocardium was more sensitive to ischemia/reperfusion (13,14). The Ca^{2+} overload is supposed to be the final common pathway of cell necrosis in ischemia/reperfusion (15). However, the time course and magnitude of the rise in $[Ca^{2+}]_i$ were highly variable in previous experiments (16-18), and there has been little study to determine whether the rise in $[Ca^{2+}]_i$ contributes to cellular damage.

It is also possible that other metabolic alterations, including impaired energy metabolism (19), lactate accumulation and acidosis (20) may be

Nagano, M., Mochizuki, S., Dhalla, N.S. (eds.), CARDIOVASCULAR DISEASE IN DIABETES. Copyright © 1992. Kluwer Academic Publishers, Boston. All rights reserved.

important in the pathogenesis of irreversible cell injury, with Ca^{2+} accumulation simply representing a secondary consequence. Accelerated anaerobic pathway during hypoxia produces lactate, causing the decrease in pH_i (21,22). Recent studies indicate that an increase in $[Ca^{2+}]_i$ in cardiac muscle cells is associated with a decrease in pH_i and vice versa (23,24), and that $[Ca^{2+}]_i$ in myocytes is influenced by pH_i (25).

In this study, $[Ca^{2+}]_i$ and pH_i were measured simultaneously in isolated rat ventricular myocytes using, respectively, the fluorescent indicators fura-2 and BCECF (26). The first purpose of this study was to measure $[Ca^{2+}]_i$ and pH_i of streptozotocin-induced DM rat myocytes. The second was to investigate whether DM myocytes were more sensitive to metabolic inhibition caused by sodium cyanide (NaCN) than those of control rats, and to investigate the relation between cell injury, $[Ca^{2+}]_i$ and pH_i.

Materials and Methods

Animals: Male Wistar rats of 200-220 g in the diabetic group received 45 mg/kg streptozotocin in citrate buffer (0.1 M citric acid and 0.1 M sodium citrate, pH 4.5) intravenously, while control rats in the age-matched group were treated with citrate buffer alone. The rats in the two groups were allowed free access to food and water, kept for 8 weeks. Blood glucose was measured every 2 weeks after the injection of streptozotocin using the glucose oxidase method. Diabetic rats with blood glucose less than 500 mg/dl were not used.

Isolation of rat ventricular myocytes: Ventricular myocytes were isolated from rats following the method described by Hayashi et al. (27). The hearts were excised, attached to the bottom of a Langendorff column (60 cm height), and perfused with solutions gassed with 95% O_2 - 5% CO_2 and maintained at 36 ± 0.5 °C and pH 7.4. The first perfusate was Ca^{2+}-free Krebs solution to wash out the blood remaining in the heart cavities and coronary arteries. After 3-4 min of the initial perfusion, 50 ml of low $CaCl_2$ (50 uM) Krebs solution containing enzymes (500 U/ml collagenase type V and 200 U/ml trypsin Type III, Sigma Chemical Co.) were added to the column and perfused for 3-5 min. Finally, Ca^{2+}-free Krebs solution was introduced to wash out the residual enzyme solution in the heart. The ventricles were cut into small fragments with iris scissors, and myocytes were dispersed by gentle agitation in oxygenated Ca^{2+}-free Krebs solution. Finally, the

Ca^{2+} concentration in the cell suspension was raised to 2.45 mM by the addition of $CaCl_2$.

Dual-loading of fura-2 and BCECF (Figure 1); The cells were loaded with 5 uM fura-2/AM and 0.5 uM BCECF/AM for 40 min at 37 °C. The cells were washed three times with modified Krebs solution before study, and was placed in an experimental chamber, which was mounted on the stage of a Nikon TMD inverted microscope and a Nikon Fluor 20 x, (N.A. :0.75) objective. The myocytes were superfused with modified Krebs solution (mM): NaCl 113.1, KCl 4.6, $CaCl_2$ 2.45, $MgCl_2$ 1.2, $NaHPO_4$ 3.5, $NaHCO_3$ 21.9, and glucose 5, equilibrated with 95% O_2-5% CO_2 (pH 7.4). Excitation light was provided by 300 W Xenon lamp and passed through an interference and neutral density filter to select wavelength and intensity. A low-light, intensified silicon target (SIT) camera (Hamamatsu Photonics K.K.) collected fluorescent images that were fed to a computer (ARGUS: Hamamatsu Photonics K.K.). All filters had half-band widths of 10 nm. After passing the filters, the exciting light was reflected by a dichroic mirror. This had a half-pass wavelength of 400 nm for fura-2 and 510 nm for BCECF, which was changed manually. Changes in cell shaper were monitored with a video analytical technique. In measurement of $[Ca^{2+}]_i$, fura-2 fluorescence elicited the cells at 340 nm and 380 nm was measured at 500 nm (emission: bandpass 20 nm). Fluorescence ratios were obtained by dividing pixel by pixel, the 340 nm image after background subtraction by the 380 nm image after background subtraction. In mesurement of pHi, the fluorescent signal was obtained with excitation wavelengths at 490 nm and 450 nm, and emission wavelength at 505-560 nm. Fluorescent ratios were also obtained by dividing pixel by pixel, the 490 nm image after background subtraction by the 450 nm image after background subtraction (26).

Calibration of fura-2 and BCECF fluorescences; We used in vivo calibration according to the method described by Li et al. (28). Briefly, the cells were loaded with fluorescent probes, and were then superfused with a glucose-free buffer containing carbonyl cyanide m-chlorophenylhydrazone (CCCP: 5.0 uM: an inhibitor of oxidative phosphorylation) and amytal (3.3 mM: an inhibitor of NADH dehydrogenase) for 15-20 min to deplete intracellular ATP stores. R_{max} was determined by adding the Ca^{2+} ionomycin (10 uM) and $CaCl_2$ (5 mM). R_{min} was determined by adding the Ca^{2+} ionomycin (10 uM) and 10 mM EGTA to the external solution. $[Ca^{2+}]i$ is related to the ratio of measured fluorescence signals elicited at two excitation wavelengths according

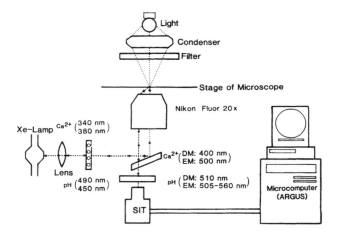

Figure 1. Schematic diagram of dual-loading using fura-2 and BCECF.

to the following equation (29). $[Ca^{2+}]_i = Kd \times \beta \times (R - R_{min}) / (R_{max} - R)$. The measured ratios of the cell could be converted directly to $[Ca^{2+}]_i$ with this equation.

The in vivo calibration curve was generated in BCECF-loaded, and dual-loaded myocytes by the addition of 10 /ml nigericin, a K^+/H^+ ionophore, in 130 mM KCl, 1 mM $MgCl_2$, 15 mM MES (2-[N-Morpholino] ethnesulfonic acid), 15 mM Hepes buffer at 37 °C. The pH was adjusted appropriately with KOH. The BCECF or dual-loaded cells were incubated with the solution for at least 5-10 min to allow complete equilibration before recording the data.

Sodium cyanide (NaCN) was purchased from Sigma, and pH of the solution was adjusted with HCl to 7.4. Data are presented as mean ± S.E. Differences between control and DM groups were analyzed by Student's t-test or analysis of variance. The p values less than 0.05 were considered significant.

Results
1) Effects of dual-loading of fura-2 and BCECF on calibration curve:

Figure 2A shows in vivo calibration curve of fura-2 fluorescence using fura-2-loaded and dual-loaded cells. Agreement between fura-2 and dual-loading was quite acceptable. Figure 2 B shows in vivo calibration curves generated in BCECF-loaded, and dual-loaded myocytes. Fluorescence ratios were

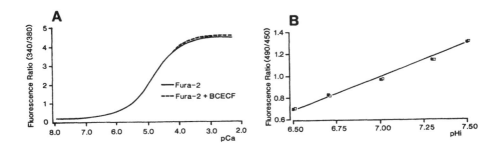

Figure 2. Effects of dual-loading on the in vivo calibration curves of fura-2 and BCECF fluorescence. A: Fura-2 fluorescence ratio and pCa_i. B: BCECF fluorescence ratio and pH_i. (open circles: BCECF-loaded cells; closed circles: dual-loaded cells).

linearly related to pH from 6.5 to 7.5, and there was no statistical difference between BCECF-loaded and dual-loaded cells.

Using the dual-loading method, we could measure $[Ca^{2+}]_i$ and pH_i in rat myocytes simultaneously. This represents a substantial advantage to investigate the interaction of $[Ca^{2+}]_i$ and pH_i in a cell.

2) General Characteristics of Animals;

As shown in Table 1, the heart-to-body weight ratio was significantly higher in DM rats than the age-matched control rats. Though ketonuria was occasionally seen in DM rats at 1 week after the injection of streptozotocin, there was no ketonuria from 2 to 8 weeks after the injection.

3) $[Ca^{2+}]_i$ and pH_i of DM myocytes;

After the isolation procedure, 20-40% of all cells were rod-shaped cells with clear striae. There was no difference in the % of rod-shaped cells between control and DM rats. $[Ca^{2+}]_i$ and pH_i of isolated ventricular myocytes during the control perfusion with oxygenated Krebs' solution are also shown in Table 1. The mean value of $[Ca^{2+}]_i$ of DM rats (53±3 nM) was significantly lower than that of the control rats (75±5 nM, p<0.01). There was no difference in pH_i between control and DM rats.

Table 1. General characteristics, $[Ca^{2+}]_i$ and pH_i of control and DM rats.

	Control	(n)	DM	(n)
Body wt. (g)	341 ± 8	(13)	183 ± 6*	(16)
Heart wt. (g)	1.02 ± 0.04	(13)	0.81 ± 0.03*	(16)
Heart wt./Body wt. (mg/g)	3.00 ± 0.10	(13)	4.46 ± 0.12*	(16)
Blood glucose (mg/dl)	164 ± 5	(13)	559 ± 7*	(16)
$[Ca^{2+}]_i$ (nM)	75 ± 5	(36)	53 ± 3*	(61)
pH_i	7.06 ± 0.02	(36)	7.07 ± 0.02	(61)

Values are mean±S.E. *Significantly different (p<0.01) from the control rats.

4) Effects of Sodium Cyanide on $[Ca^{2+}]_i$ and pH_i:

The cells were superfused with substrate-free Krebs' solution which contained 2 mM NaCN for 30 min. Figure 3 is a typical example of a diabetic myocyte during the NaCN perfusion. The upper column shows $[Ca^{2+}]_i$ and the lower column shows pH_i. The ratios were expressed as the density changes, and the upper in the right bar indicates that $[Ca^{2+}]_i$ and pH_i are high. As the cell was shortened (middle) and rounded (right) during the NaCN perfusion, $[Ca^{2+}]_i$ increased while pH_i decreased.

Figure 4 A shows the relationship between cell morphology and $[Ca^{2+}]_i$ in control and DM rats during the perfusion with glucose-free NaCN solution. When the cells were shortened, $[Ca^{2+}]_i$ increased to 150±22 nM (p<0.05 vs rod-shaped cells before NaCN) in control rats, and to 112±29 nM in DM rats. When the cells were rounded, $[Ca^{2+}]_i$ increased significantly in both control and DM rats (421±106 and 172±21 nM, respectively). The mean value of $[Ca^{2+}]_i$ in control rats when cells were rounded, was significantly higher than that of DM rats (p<0.05). Figure 4 B shows the relationship between cell morphology and pH_i. When cells were rounded, pHi decreased significantly in both control and DM rats. (6.87±0.10 in control rats, p<0.05; 6.91±0.05 in DM rats, p<0.05). There was no difference between pH_i of two groups.

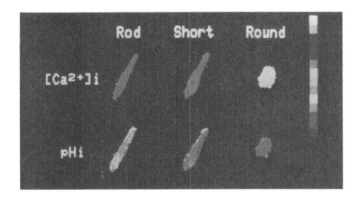

Figure 3. An example of the effect of NaCN (2 mM) on $[Ca^{2+}]_i$ (upper column), and pH_i (lower column). The upper density of the right bar shows the higher $[Ca^{2+}]_i$ or pH_i.

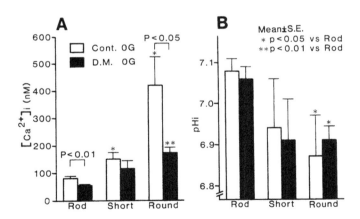

Figure 4. The relation between cell morphology, $[Ca^{2+}]_i$ and pH_i during the perfusion of substrate-free solution which contained 2 mM NaCN. A: Cell morphology and $[Ca^{2+}]_i$. B: Cell morphology and pH_i. Cont: control rats, n=23. DM: n=36. *Significantly different from rod-shaped control cells.

Table 2. Effects of NaCN on the % of rod-shaped cells, $[Ca^{2+}]i$ and pHi in the absence or the presence of glucose.

	Time (min)	0	10	20	30
Cont. 0G	% rod-shaped cells	100	83	57	30
(n=23)	$[Ca^{2+}]_i$	82 ± 8	125 ± 30	243 ± 85	480 ± 151
	pH_i	7.08 ± 0.03	7.07 ± 0.04	7.01 ± 0.05	6.96 ± 0.05
Cont. 50G	% rod-shaped cells	100	95	90*	90*
(n=20)	$[Ca^{2+}]_i$	76 ± 8	115 ± 15	166 ± 53	194 ± 93
	pH_i	7.08 ± 0.02	7.03 ± 0.04	6.99 ± 0.03	6.92 ± 0.04
DM 0G	% rod-shaped cells	100	94	64	47
(n=36)	$[Ca^{2+}]_i$	56 ± 4	104 ± 12	135 ± 21	281 ± 54
	pH_i	7.06 ± 0.03	7.08 ± 0.04	6.99 ± 0.04	6.95 ± 0.03
DM 50G	% rod-shaped cells	100	95	84	42
(n=19)	$[Ca^{2+}]_i$	53 ± 5	105 ± 12	122 ± 15	243 ± 72
	pH_i	7.09 ± 0.04	7.07 ± 0.04	6.94 ± 0.05	6.90 ± 0.05

Values are mean ± S.E. $[Ca^{2+}]_i$ and pH_i are means of all cells. Cont.: Control rats. DM: Diabetic rats. NaCN (2 mM) was applied in the absence (0G) or the presence (50G) of 50 mM glucose. *Significantly different (p<0.01) from control 0G group.

5) Effects of glucose;

Table 2 shows the % of rod-shaped cells, $[Ca^{2+}]_i$ and pH_i during the NaCN perfusion in the absence or presence of glucose in control and DM rats. After 30 min perfusion of NaCN, there was no difference in the % of rod-shaped cells (30% in the control group, and 47% in DM group). When 50 mM glucose was present in the perfusion media, the % of rod-shaped cells was significantly higher in the control group (90% after 30 min in 50 mM glucose, p<0.01). The % of rod-shaped cells was, however, 42% at 30 min in DM group when 50 mM glucose was present in the perfusion media, which was not different from that of glucose-free perfusion.

The effects of NaCN on $[Ca^{2+}]_i$ and pH_i of all cells from 4 groups are also shown in Table 2. $[Ca^{2+}]_i$ increased gradually in all four groups. Though the increase in $[Ca^{2+}]_i$ was larger in the control-0 mM glucose group, the differences were not significant (analysis of variance).

There were no difference in pH_i.

6) Effects of insulin in DM rats;

Regular insulin (25 mU/ml) was, then, added to the NaCN solution in the presence of glucose (15 mM). The % of rod-shaped cells after 30 min was 88%, which was significantly higher than that (47%) during the substrate-free perfusion (p<0.01). When insulin and glucose was present, $[Ca^{2+}]_i$ was 92 ± 24 nM at 30 min, and was significantly lower than that during the glucose-free NaCN solution (p<0.01). The % of rod-shaped cells during the perfusion with NaCN which contained only insulin was 50% at 30 min, which was not different from that in the control solution.

Discussion

Dual-loading of fura-2 and BCECF; It is difficult to calibrate the fluorescence changes produced by fura-2 added as the AM ester in cardiac muscle. This is because: (a) compartmentation of fura-2 (30) and (b) incomplete de-esterification of fura-2/AM (31). Therefore we used in vivo calibration, and have developed a new method for measuring the fura-2 and BCECF fluorescence signals in rat myocytes simultaneously (26). This technique should be applicable to other cell types, and $[Ca^{2+}]_i$ and pH_i could be measured under comparable condition. This represents a substantial advantage to investigate the interaction of $[Ca^{2+}]_i$ and pH_i in a cell. There are, however, several possibilities that might distort the present $[Ca^{2+}]_i$ measurement. These include: (a) photobleaching of fura-2 (32) and (b) buffering of intracellular Ca^{2+} by the intracellular fura-2 (33).

$[Ca^{2+}]_i$ in DM myocytes; Though Ca^{2+} overload has been implicated in the diabetic cardiomyopathy, pathological studies have not shown the abnormal Ca^{2+} deposit in diabetic myocardium (34). This study showed that $[Ca^{2+}]_i$ in DM rat myocytes was significantly lower than that of control rats. Horackova et al. (35) have recently reported that the Ca^{2+} content was decreased in DM rat myocytes using the radioisotope method. Bergh et al. (36) have recently shown that Ca^{2+} net flux was significantly reduced in both acute (4 days) and chronic (8 weeks) DM rat myocardium. It has been also reported that Ca^{2+} uptake stimulated by ß-adrenergic agonist, was decreased in DM rat hearts (37). The low Ca^{2+} uptake might explain the low $[Ca^{2+}]_i$ of DM myocytes in this study.

There are two other possible reasons of the lower $[Ca^{2+}]_i$ in DM myocytes. One is the duration of diabetic state as we have used animals of 8 weeks after the injection of streptozotocin. Since it has been reported that positive and negative dp/dt of left ventricle were reduced in DM rats more than 30 days after the injection of streptozotocin (38), the contractile activity and/or $[Ca^{2+}]_i$ may be different according to the duration of diabetic state. Another possible reason is related to the isolated myocytes used in this study. If there were heterogeneous progression in diabetic cardiomyopathy, rod-shaped myocytes might have been obtained from the intact part of DM myocardium. There was, however, no difference in the % of rod-shaped cells after the cell isolation between the control and DM rats (35).

Effects of NaCN on cell morphology and $[Ca^{2+}]_i$; The % of rod-shaped cells of DM rats was not different from that of control rats during the NaCN perfusion without glucose. Most experimental data have suggested that DM myocardium was more sensitive to ischemia or reperfusion. However, Vogel and Apstein (39) recently reported that the severity of injury after ischemia/reperfusion is not different between DM and normal rabbit myocardium. Tani and Neely (40) have suggested that DM rat myocardium was more resistant to ischemia/reperfusion injury. Though ischemia is not the same with the substrate-free NaCN perfusion, we could study the effect of metabolic inhibition independently of vascular component or hormonal effects, by using isolated myocytes.

We have already reported that there was a positive relation between $[Ca^{2+}]_i$ and the % of cell shortening or rounding in guinea pig ventricular myocytes during the perfusion of strophanthidin (41). The value of $[Ca^{2+}]_i$ in DM rats when cells were rounded, was significantly lower than that of control rats. This could be due to the higher sensitivity of myofibrils in DM myocytes. Fein et al. (42) have reported that the changes in contractile activity caused by ouabain or increased $[Ca^{2+}]_o$ (12 mM), were greater in diabetic myocardium than control myocardium. Another possible reason is that although the elevation of $[Ca^{2+}]_i$ is the cause of irreversible cell injury, other factors such as ATP depletion (19) or low pH_i (20) may play important roles. There was, however, no difference in pH_i when cells were rounded between the normal and DM myocytes. Previous studies using aequorin have shown that $[Ca^{2+}]_i$ rose abruptly after the cell had gone into contracture during metabolic inhibition (16,17). Barry et al. (43) have recently reported using indo-1 that the early component of cell contracture during metabolic inhibition was due to increase in $[Ca^{2+}]_i$.

Effects of glucose and insulin; It has been reported that hypoxic contracture could be precipitated by the fall of ATP (44), and that the ATP content of DM rat myocardium was lower than that of control rat myocardium (45). It has also been reported that ATP content of DM rat myocardium during ischemia was lower than that of control rat myocardium (45). It is likely that the difference in the value of $[Ca^{2+}]_i$ between control and DM when cells were rounded, might be related with the difference of ATP level, since the intracellular Ca^{2+} homeostasis is regulated by ATP (46).

Though glucose increased the % of rod-shaped cells in the control groups than that in the substrate-free NaCN solution, the % of rod-shaped cells in DM was not different by the addition of glucose. It is likely that the difference was due to the disturbance of glucose utilization in DM myocardium, since DM myocardium was shown to have decreased glucose utilization (47). The increase of glucose utilization during hypoxia is lower in DM myocardium than normal myocardium. When insulin and glucose were added in the NaCN solution, the % of rod-shaped cells in DM rats was significantly higher. It has been reported that the addition of insulin during hypoxia markedly stimulated the glucose uptake even in DM myocardium (47), and the lower level of ATP was reversed by the perfusion of insulin with glucose. The effect of insulin on the sensitivity to NaCN in DM myocytes was likely to be related with the stimulation of glucose utilization.

pH_i during NaCN perfusion; The present data indicated that there was no difference in pH_i between control and DM myocytes. There was no ketonuria in DM rats which were used in this study. When oxidative phosphorylation was inhibited, glycolysis and glucose uptake are accelerated. This anaerobic pathway produces lactate, causing the decrease in pH_i (21,22).

There was a decrease in pH_i as $[Ca^{2+}]_i$ increased during the NaCN perfusion. It has been shown that an increase in $[Ca^{2+}]_i$ in cardiac muscle cells is associated with a decrease in pH_i and vice versa (23,24), and that $[Ca^{2+}]_i$ in cardiac myocytes is also influenced by pH_i (25). It has been proposed that the increase in $[Ca^{2+}]_i$ produced by intracellular acidosis is due to displacement of Ca^{2+} from common intracellular binding sites, presumably components of the mitochondria and/or SR (23). It is also, however, possible that the intracellular acidosis produced by metabolic inhibition might result directly from an increase in $[Ca^{2+}]_i$, since Allen et al. (48) have suggested that intracellular acidification caused by an elevation of $[Ca^{2+}]_i$ was due primarily to stimulated anaerobic metabolism and consequent increased production of lactate.

Summary

$[Ca^{2+}]_i$ was lower in DM rat myocytes, and it was suggested that there was disturbance in intracellular Ca^{2+} homeostasis in DM. Although $[Ca^{2+}]_i$ possibly play an important role in the irreversible cell injruy during metabolic inhibition, $[Ca^{2+}]_i$ might not be the only cause of the cell injury. Since there was a close relationship between energy metabolism and irreversible cell injury, the difference in the response to metabolic inhibition between DM and control rats was suggested to be related with the disturbance of energy metabolism in DM myocardium.

References
1. Kannel WB, Hjortland M and Castelli WP. Role of diabetes in congestive heart failure: The Framingham Study. Am J Cardiol 1974;34:29-34.
2. Regan TJ, Ettinger PO, Khan MI, Jesrani MU, Lyons MM, Oldewurtel HA and Weber M. Altered Myocardial function and metabolism in chronic diabetes mellitus without ischemia in dogs. Cir Res 1974;35:222-237.
3. Regan TJ, Lyons MM, Ahmed SS, Levinson GE, Oldewurtel HA, Ahmad MR and Haider B. Evidence for cardiomyopathy in familial diabetes mellitus. J Clin Invest 1977;60:885-899.
4. Fein FS and Sonnenblick EH. Diabetic Cardiomyopathy. Prog Cardiovasc Disease 1985;27:255-270.
5. Hamby RI, Zoneraich S and Shermann L. Diabetic cardiomyopathy. JAMA 1974;229:1749-1754.
6. Malhotra A, Penpargkul S, Fein FS, Sonnenblick EH and Scheuer J. The effect of streptozotocin-induced diabetes in rats on cardiac contractile proteins. Circ Res 1981;49:1243-1250.
7. Dillmann WH. Diabetes mellitus induces changes in cardiac myosin of the rat. Diabetes 1980;29:579-582.
8. Penpargkul S, Fein FS, Sonnenblick EH, and Scheuer J. Depressed cardiac sarcoplasmic reticular function from diabetic rats. J Mol Cell Cardiol 1981;93:303-309.

9. Lopaschuk GD, Tahiliani AG, Vadlamudi RVSV, Katz S and McNeill JH. Cardiac sarcoplasmic reticulum function in insulin- or carnitine-treated diabetic rats. Am J Physiol 1983;245:H969-H976.
10. Heyliger CE, Prakash A and McNeill JH. Alterations in cardiac sarcolemmal Ca^{2+} pump activity during diabetes mellitus. Am J Physiol 1987;252:H540-H544.
11. Makino N, Dhalla KS, Elimban V and Dhalla NS. Sarcolemmal Ca^{2+} transport in streptozotocin-induced diabetic cardiomyopathy in rats. Am J Physiol 1987;253:E202-207.
12. Gwilt DJ, Petri M, Lewis PW, Nattrass M and Pentecost BL. Myocardial infarct size and mortality in diabetic patients. Br Heart J 1985;54:466-472.
13. Feuvray D, Idell-Wenger JA and Neely JR. Effects of ischemia on rat myocardial function and metabolism in diabetes. Circ Res 1979;44:322-329.
14. Nadeau A, Tancrede G, Jobidon C, D'Amours C and Rousseau-Migneron S. Increased mortality rate in diabetic rats submitted to acute experimental myocardial infarction. Cardiovasc Res 1986;20:171-175.
15. Nayler WG and Daly MJ. Calcium and the injured cardiac myocytes. In: Physiology and Pathophysiology of the Heart, N Sperelakis (Ed.) Martinus Nijhoff Publishing, 1984;477-492.
16. Cobbold PH and Bourne PK. Aequorin measurements of free calcium in single heart cells. Nature 1984;312:444-446.
17. Allen DG and Orchard CH. Intracellular calcium concentration during hypoxia and metabolic inhibition in mammalian ventricular muscle. J Physiol (Lond) 1983;339:107-122.
18. Smith GL and Allen DG. Effects of metabolic blockade on intracellular calcium concentration in isolated ferret ventricular muscle. Circ Res 1988;62:1223-1236.
19. Jennings RB and Reimer KA. Lethal myocardial ischemic injury. Am J Pathol 1981;102:241-255.
20. Neely JR and Grotyohann LW. Role of glycolytic products in damage to ischemic myocardium. Dissociation of adenosine triphosphate levels and recovery of function of reperfused ischemic hearts. Circ Res 1984;55:816-824.
21. Ellis D and Noireaud J. Intracellular pH in sheep Purkinje fibres and

ferret papillary muscles during hypoxia and recovery. J Physiol (Lond) 1987;383:125-141.
22. Eisner DA, Nichols CG, O'Neill SC, Smith GL and Valdeolmillos M. The effects of metabolic inhibition on intracellular calcium and pH in isolated rat ventricular cells. J Physiol (Lond) 1989;411:393-418.
23. Vaughan-Jones RD, Lederer WJ and Eisner DA. Ca^{2+} ions can affect intracellular pH in mammalian cardiac muscle. 1983;301:522-524.
24. Kim D, Cragoe Jr, EJ and Smith TW. Relations among sodium pump inhibition, Na-Ca and Na-H exchange activities, and Ca-H interaction in cultured chick heart cells. Circ Res 1987;60:185-193.
25. Bers DM and Ellis D. Intracellular calcium and sodium activity in sheep heart Purkinje fibres. Effect of changes of external sodium and intracellular pH. Pfluegers Arch 1982;393:171-178.
26. Miyata H, Hayashi H, Suzuki S, Noda N, Kobayashi A, Fujiwake H, Hirano M and Yamazaki N. Dual loading of the fluorescent indicator fura-2 and 2,7-biscarboxyethyl-5(6)-carboxyfluorescein (BCECF) in isolated myocytes. Biochem Biophys Res Commun 1989;163:500-505.
27. Hayashi H, Ponnambalam C, McDonald TF. Arrhythmic activity in reoxygenated guinea pig papillary muscles and ventricular cells. Circ Res 1987;61:124-133.
28. Li Q, Altschuld RA and Stokes BT. Quantitation of intracellular free calcium in single adult cardiomyocytes by fura-2 fluorescence microscopy: Calibration of fura-2 ratios. Biochem Biophys Res Commun 1987;147:120-126.
29. Grynkiewicz G, Poenie M and Tsien RY. A new generation of Ca^{2+} indicators with greatly improved fluorescence properties. J Biol Chem 1985;260:3440-3450.
30. Highsmith S, Bloebaum P and Snowdowne KW. Sarcoplasmic reticulum interacts with the Ca^{2+} indicator precursor fura-2-AM. Biochem Biophys Res Commum 1986;138:1153-1162.
31. Scanlon M, Williams DA and Fay FS. A Ca^{2+}-insensitive form of fura-2 associated with polymorphonuclear leukocytes. Assessment and accurate Ca^{2+} measurement. J Biol Chem 1987;262:6308-6312.
32. Becker PB and Fay FS. Photobleaching of fura-2 and its effect on determination of calcium concentrations. Am J Physiol 1987;253:C613-C618.

33. Timmerman MP and Ashley CC. Fura-2 diffusion and its use as an indicator of transient free calcium changes in single striated muscle cells. FEBS Lett 1986;209:1-8.
34. Jacson CV, McGrath GM, Tahiliani AG, Vadlamudi RVS, and McNeill JH. A functional and ultrastructural analysis of experimental diabetic rat myocardium. Manifestation of a cardiomyopathy. Diabetes 1985;34:876-883.
35. Horackova M and Murphy MG. Effects of chronic diabetes mellitus on the electrical and contractile activities, $^{45}Ca^{2+}$ transport, fatty acid profiles and ultrastructure of isolated rat ventricular myocytes. Pflugers Arch 1988;411:564-572.
36. Bergh CH, Hjalmarson A, Sjogren KG and Jacobsson B. The effect of diabetes on phosphatidylinositol and calcium influx. Horm Metabol Res 1988;20:381-386.
37. Gotzsche O. Decreased myocardial calcium uptake after isoproterenol in streptozotocin-induced diabetic rats. Studies in the in vitro perfused heart. Lab Invest 1983;48:156-161.
38. Vadlamudi RVSV, Rodgers RL and McNeill JH. The effect of chronic alloxan and streptozotocin-induced diabetes on isolated rat heart performance. Can J Physiol Pharmacol 1982;60:902-911.
39. Vogel WM and Apstein CS. Effects of alloxan-induced diabetes on ischemia-reperfusion injury in rabbit hearts. Circ Res 1988;62:975-982.
40. Tani M and Neely JR. Hearts from diabetic rats are more resistant to in vivo ischemia: Possible role of altered Ca^{2+} metabolism. Circ Res 1988;62:931-940.
41. Miyata H, Hayashi H, Kobayashi A and Yamazaki N. Effects of strophanthidin on intracellular Ca^{2+} concentration and cellular morphology of guinea pig myocytes. Cardiovasc Res 1989;23:378-384.
42. Fein FS, Aronson RS, Nordin C, Miller-Green B and Sonnenblick EH. Altered myocardial response to ouabain in diabetic rats: Mechanism and electrophysiology. J Mol Cell Cardiol 1983;15:769-784.
43. Barry WH, Peeters GA, Rasmussen Jr CAF and Cunningham MJ. Role of changes in $[Ca^{2+}]_i$ in energy deprivation contracture. Circ Res 1987;61:726-734.
44. Allen DG, Morris PG, Orchard CH and Pirolo JS. A nuclear magnetic resonance study of metabolism in the ferret heart during hypoxia and inhibition of glycolysis. J Physiol (Lond) 1985;361:185-204.

45. Bhimji S, Godin DV and McNeill JH. Coronary artery ligation and reperfusion in rabbits made diabetic with alloxan. J Endocr 1987;112:43-49.
46. Carafoli E. The homeostasis of calcium in heart cells. J Mol Cell Cardiol 1985;17:203-212.
47. Morgan HE, Cadenas E, Regen DM and Park CR. Regulation of glucose uptake in muscle. 2. Rate-limitiing steps and effects of insulin and anoxia in heart muscle from diabetic rats. J Biol Chem 1961;236:262-268.
48. Allen DG, Eisner DA, Morris PG, Porolo JS and Smith GL. Metabolic consequences of increasing intracellular calcium and force production in perfused ferret hearts. J Physiol (Lond) 1986;376:121-141.

Abnormal Phosphorylation: Cause of Reduced Responsiveness to Isoproterenol in Diabetic Heart

S.W. Schaffer, S. Allo and G. Wilson

Departments of Pharmacology and Anatomy, University of South Alabama School of Medicine, Mobile, AL 36688, USA

Introduction

One of the major complications of both insulin-dependent and noninsulin-dependent diabetes is the development of a cardiomyopathy (1-4). In animal models which resemble insulin-dependent diabetes, this condition is associated with defects in both the rate of contractile development and relaxation (1-4). Also abnormal in these animals is the inotropic and chronotropic responses to different pharmacologic agents. For example, ouabain and ß-adrenergic receptor-mediated positive inotropic responses are significantly depressed (5,6), while hyperresponses to milrinone and alpha-adrenergic agents have been reported (7,8).

Like insulin-dependent diabetic animals, noninsulin-dependent diabetic rats also exhibit defects in the rate of contractile development and relaxation and in the response to ß-adrenergic agents (9,10). They also undergo changes in myosin isozyme content and alterations in calcium homeostasis similar to those reported in insulin-dependent diabetes (9). However, some important fundamental differences in both contractile function and cardiac metabolism exist between the insulin-dependent and noninsulin-dependent diabetic cardiomyopathies. While the mobilization of fatty acids and the accumulation of toxic lipid amphiphiles appear to play an important role in the development of the insulin-dependent diabetic cardiomyopathy, these factors play no apparent role in the noninsulin-dependent diabetic disease (11). Similarly, reduced diastolic compliance plays a significant role in the depression of contractile function only in the noninsulin-dependent diabetic heart (9). Also different between the two types of

Nagano, M., Mochizuki, S., Dhalla, N.S. (eds.), CARDIOVASCULAR DISEASE IN DIABETES. Copyright © 1992. Kluwer Academic Publishers, Boston. All rights reserved.

diabetes is the basis for abnormal responses to various inotropic agents.

Recently it has been observed that ß-adrenergic receptor number and affinity remain unchanged in the noninsulin-dependent diabetic heart (10). Moreover, isoproterenol-mediated stimulation of adenylate cyclase is unaffected in the noninsulin-dependent diabetic (10). Since defects in the response to ß-adrenergic agonists have been attributed to alterations in receptor number and stimulation of adenylate cyclase in the insulin-dependent diabetic (12,13), the mechanism underlying the defect in ß-adrenergic responsiveness must be different in the two types of diabetes. These differences are explored further in this report.

Methods

The chemically-induced noninsulin-dependent diabetic condition was produced as described previously (14). These animals exhibited the characteristic pattern of noninsulin-dependent diabetes. Their fasting and nonfasting blood glucose levels were only slightly elevated; fasting levels were 132 ± 4 and 114 ± 3 mg/dl for noninsulin-dependent diabetic and nondiabetic, respectively. One hour following a glucose challenge of 2 g/kg i.p., blood glucose levels typically rose to values from 500-600 mg/dl in the diabetic rats, but only 200-300 mg/dl in the control rats. At the same time, plasma insulin levels increased to a value of 20 ± 4 and 9 ± 2 ng/ml in the noninsulin-dependent diabetic and nondiabetic, respectively. However, characteristic of noninsulin-dependent diabetes, plasma insulin levels in the diabetic group began to decrease at a time when glucose levels continued to rise. All animals were studied after 10 - 12 months of age.

The sarcolemma preparation was isolated from nondiabetic and noninsulin-dependent diabetic hearts using a slight modification of the method of Pitts (15). Membrane yield was similar in the two groups. Both preparations contained approximately 30% leaky, 35% inside-out and 35% right-side out vesicles. Sarcolemmal markers adenylate cyclase and Na^+,K^+ ATPase were concentrated approximately 9-13 fold relative to the homogenate in both preparations. By comparison, the purity factor for cytochrome c oxidase was 0.3-0.4 for the two preparations, indicating minimal mitochondrial contamination of the sarcolemma preparation. Based on the low rates of oxalate-facilitated and P-nitrophenylphosphate supported calcium accumulation, sarcoplasmic reticular contamination was also minimal in both preparations.

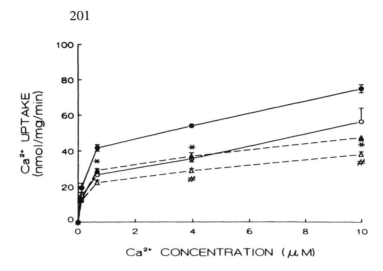

Figure 1. Effect of noninsulin-dependent diabetes on sarcolemmal ATP-dependent calcium transport. Sarcolemma was prepared from nondiabetic (●,○), and noninsulin-dependent diabetic (▲,△) rats using the method of Pitts (15). The membrane was either incubated in the presence (●,▲) or absence (○, △) of 150 units of cAMP-dependent protein kinase catalytic subunit prior to assaying ATP-dependent calcium uptake. The rate of ATP-dependent calcium transport was determined over a free calcium concentration range of 0.06 - 10 uM. Values shown represent the means ± S.E.M. of 5 preparations. * and # denote significant differences (p < 0.05) between diabetic and nondiabetic sarcolemma incubated in the presence and absence of cAMP-dependent protein kinase, respectively.

Membrane phosphorylation was determined according to the method of Caroni and Carafoli (16). Sarcolemma (20 ug protein) were preincubated for 5 minutes at 37°C in 20 mM MOPS buffer (pH 7.0) containing 160 mM KCl, 5 mM $MgCl_2$ and 0.1 mM EGTA in the presence and absence of 150 units cAMP-dependent protein kinase catalytic subunit. The phosphorylation reaction was initiated by addition of 50 uM [γ-^{32}P]-ATP and terminated at the appropriate time by addition of 3 ml of 20 mM MOPS buffer (pH 7.0) containing 160 mM KCl, 1.0 mM ATP and 40 mM K_2HPO_4 and by rapidly filtering the reaction mixture over Whatman GF/B filters. The filters were washed twice with 3 ml of the 20 mM MOPS buffer and then counted for radioactivity.

During the analysis of individual sarcolemmal protein bands by gel electrophoresis, the phosphorylation reaction was allowed to proceed for 30 seconds, at which time it was terminated by the adition of 10 ul of a 0.125 M

Tris (pH 6.8) stop solution containing 20% glycerol, 7 mM ß-mercaptoethanol and 5% SDS and then heated for 3 minutes at 80°C. The samples were then subjected to SDS gel electrophoresis using a 10% polyacrylamide slab gel. Following the run, the gels were dried and exposed to Kodak X-AR5 X-ray film using intensifying screens.

The method of Ingebritsen et al (17) was used to mesure the activities of individual protein phosphatases. In this reaction, the substrate denatured, ^{32}P-sarcolemma was prepared according to the procedure of Sulakhe et al (18).

Results

Several investigators (19,20) have reported that sarcolemmal calcium pump activity is depressed in hearts isolated from rats with insulin-dependent diabetes. Figure 1 reveals that this defect is not only observed in insulin-dependent diabetes, but also using sarcolemma prepared from noninsulin-dependent diabetic rats. The defect in noninsulin-dependent diabetic hearts was apparent at medium calcium concentrations greater than 1 uM, where ATP-dependent calcium uptake was significantly reduced.

Larger differences in calcium transport between noninsulin-dependent diabetic and age-matched control sarcolemma were observed upon treatment of the membranes with the catalytic subunit of cAMP-dependent protein kinase. This occurred because protein kinase-mediated stimulation of calcium transport was greater in the nondiabetic. For example, in a medium calcium concentration of 0.06 uM, calcium uptake of nondiabetic and diabetic preparations increased 57% and 14%, respectively. Although not as pronounced, similar diabetes-linked differences in the amount of stimulation were also noted at other calcium concentrations. On the average (over the entire calcium concentration range of 0.06 to 10 uM), protein kinase caused a 46% (range 33 to 57%) increase in calcium transport in the control group, but only half that amount (22%, range 8 to 31%) in the diabetic group.

It has generally been accepted that stimulation of calcium transport by cAMP-dependent protein kinase involves the phosphorylation of a specific sarcolemma-associated protein (21,22), which upon phosphorylation promotes either directly or indirectly the activation of the calcium pump. While the identity of this protein has not been established, it seems reasonable to expect that changes in the phosphorylation state of the membrane would alter its activity. Therefore, with the aim of clarifying the basis underlying the

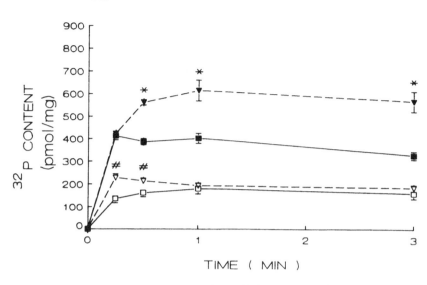

Figure 2. Effect of noninsulin-dependent diabetes on membrane phosphorylation. Sarcolemma from nondiabetic (□,■) and noninsulin-dependent diabetic (▽,▼) rats were prepared according to the method of Pitts (15). The rate of radioactive phosphate incorporation into membrane proteins was determined using sarcolemma incubated in medium containing (■,▼) or lacking (□,▽) 150 units cAMP-dependent protein kinase catalytic subunit. Values shown represent the means ± S.E.M. of 4 preparations. * and # denote significant differences ($p < 0.05$) between diabetic and control sarcolemma incubated in the presence and absence of cAMP-dependent protein kinase, respectively.

reduced response of diabetic sarcolemma to the effects of cAMP-dependent protein kinase, the phosphorylation properties of isolated nondiabetic and diabetic sarcolemma were evaluated. Figure 2 reveals that the levels of ^{32}P incorporation into isolated sarcolemma were significantly greater in noninsulin-dependent diabetic preparations.

In the absence of added protein kinase, the initial rate of membrane phosphorylation was elevated in the diabetic, although the maximal extent of phosphorylation was virtually identical in the two groups. Incubation of the membranes with extrinsic cAMP-dependent protein kinase increased the extent of phosphorylation in both preparations, although maximal levels reached were greater in the diabetic. Significantly, these differences in the phosphorylation properties of the two groups disappeared upon inclusion of a protein phosphatase inhibitor, such as 10 mM NaF, in the incubation medium,

Table 1. Effect of noninsulin-dependent diabetes on sarcolemma-associated protein phosphatase activity.

Enzyme	Activity (pmol/mg/hr)	
	Nondiabetic	Diabetic
Protein phosphatase 1	36.8 ± 4.0	16.4 ± 3.6*
Protein phosphatase 2A	60.0 ± 12.8	48.8 ± 9.2
Protein phosphatase 2B	ND	ND
Protein phosphatase 2C	4.8 ± 3.2	5.6 ± 2.4

Sarcolemma from nondiabetic and noninsulin-dependent diabetic rats was prepared according to the method of Pitts (15). The activities of the protein phosphatases were assayed according to the method of Ingebritsen et al (17) using denatured, phosphate labeled sarcolemma as substrate. Values shown represent the means ± S.E.M. of four preparations. ND signifies no detectable activity. * represents significant difference between the diabetic and nondiabetic groups ($p < 0.05$).

suggesting that diabetes may affect the levels of the protein phosphatases associated with the membrane (data not shown).

The identity of the protein phosphatase altered by noninsulin-dependent diabetes was determined by assaying the activity of each of the protein phosphatases in the cell membrane. Using labelled, denatured cell membrane as a substrate, it was found that more than 90% of the protein phosphatase activity of nondiabetic and noninsulin-dependent diabetic sarcolemma was either protein phosphatase 1 or 2A (Table 1). The only phosphatase affected by diabetes was protein phosphatase 1, which was reduced approximately 50%.

While decreased protein phosphatase 1 activity provides an adequate explanation for the increase in total membrane phosphorylation, it is less able to account for the effect of cAMP-dependent protein kinase on sarcolemmal ATP-dependent calcium transport. Therefore, the possibility that noninsulin-dependent diabetes affects the phosphorylation of a specific sarcolemmal protein was considered. To examine this point, sarcolemma from diabetic and nondiabetic rats were phosphorylated with cAMP-dependent protein kinase and individual membrane phosphoproteins were then separated from each other by SDS polyacrylamide gel electrophoresis. In the absence of both a phosphatase

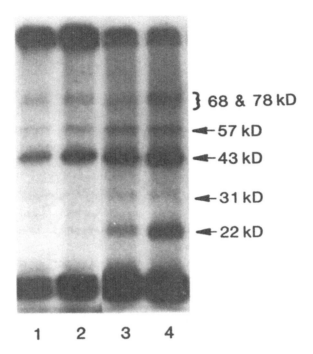

Figure 3. Effect of noninsulin-dependent diabetes on sarcolemmal protein phosphorylation pattern. Sarcolemma was isolated from nondiabetic and noninsulin-dependent diabetic hearts using the method of Pitts (15). The isolated membranes were phosphorylated in medium containing radioactive ATP in the presence or absence of 150 units cAMP-dependent protein kinase catalytic subunit. After termination of the reaction, the solubilized membrane proteins were subjected to polyacrylamide gel electrophoresis, followed by autoradiography. Shown is an autoradiogram of nondiabetic (Lanes 1 and 3) and diabetic (Lanes 2 and 4) samples incubated in the presence (Lanes 3 and 4) or absence (Lanes 1 and 2) of cAMP-dependent protein kinase.

inhibitor and extrinsic protein kianse, the dominant proteins phosphorylated by the intrinsic protein kinases exhibited molecular weights of 9 kD, 43 kD, 57 kD and 68 kD; the extent of phosphorylation of each protein was greater in the diabetic (Figure 3).

Preincubation of membranes with 150 units cAMP-dependent protein kianse appeared to potentiate the differences between the diabetic and nondiabetic phosphorylation pattern by causing further phosphorylation of proteins with molecular weights of 9 kD, 31 kD, 43 kD, 49 kD, 57 kD, 68 kD and 78 kD. However, inclusion of the phosphatase inhibitor NaF in the reaction medium eliminated many of the observed differences. A few bands exhibited either a higher or lesser degree of membrane phosphorylation under these conditions, presumably because diabetes directly affects either the amount or the phosphorylation properties of these proteins (data not shown).

Discussion

One of the characteristic features of the noninsulin-dependent diabetic cardiomyopathy is decreased diastolic compliance, resulting in impaired myocardial filling and cardiac output. This defect appears to develop in part because the heart loses its ability to regulate calcium homeostasis, particularly during diastole (9). Since one of the most important transport systems controlling calcium homeostasis during diastole is the sarcolemmal calcium pump (16), it follows that ventricular stiffness may be the direct consequence of the diabetes-mediated decrease in sarcolemmal calcium pump activity.

The mechanism by which diabetes affects the activity of the sarcolemmal calcium pump is a matter of speculation. Makino et al (19) have argued that changes in the phospholipid composition of diabetic sarcolemma might affect the microenvironment of the Ca^{2+} stimulated ATPase, thereby reducing its activity. Our data open up a new possibility; that is, the defect may reside in one or more of the factors (cAMP-dependent phosphorylation, calmodulin, potassium and pH) which regulate the calcium pump (21,22). Clearly, the effectiveness of one of these regulators, cAMP-dependent phosphorylation, is dramatically blunted in membrane derived from diabetic hearts.

The basis for decreased responsiveness to cAMP-dependent stimulation of calcium transport in diabetic sarcolemma is presently unknown. This is not surprising because very little is known about the mechanism underlying the regulation of the calcium pump by protein kinase. While some studies have implicated the phospholamban-like protein as the substrate of protein kinase which upon being phosphorylated modulates calcium pump activity (22), not all investigators support this view (23). Although this study does not provide any new information regarding the identity of the phosphoprotein modulator, it is interesting that the phosphorylation state of the phospholamban-like protein is increased in diabetes. If the assumption were made that this protein is the modulator responsible for the regulation of the calcium pump, it follows that the decrease in calcium pump activity must be independent of the phosphorylation event. This could occur if the regulation of the calcium pump by its modulator were uncoupled. Further studies using rapid kinetics will be required to test this hypothesis.

Changes in calcium pump activity represent only one process affected by phosphorylation. Sperelakis and coworkers (24) have provided convincing evidence that the calcium channel is fully activated only after membrane phosphorylation. There is also some evidence that the sarcolemmal sodium-calcium exchanger is affected by membrane phosphorylation (25). It would be reasonable to expect that these reactions also would be altered as a result of the diabetes-mediated alterations in membrane phosphorylation.

Also affected by membrane phosphorylation is insulin responsiveness (26). It is now generally accepted that full expression of insulin action depends upon activation of the insulin receptor tyrosine kinase. The activity of this kinase has been found recently to be decreased by the phosphorylation of the insulin receptor by cAMP-dependent protein kinase (27). The diabetes-linked decrease in phosphatase 1 activity would presumably have a similar effect because it would help maintain the insulin receptor in a more phosphorylated state, thereby contributing to the loss in insulin responsiveness. This reaction may be very significant in light of the observation that insulin resistance is a characteristic feature of noninsulin-dependent diabetes.

Summary

Noninsulin-dependent diabetes is associated with a decrease in sarcolemmal ATP-dependent calcium uptake. This effect was potentiated upon incubation of the membranes with cAMP-dependent protein kinase, raising the possibility that certain diabetes-linked defects in calcium transport are caused by abnormalities in the regulation of the calcium transporters by cAMP-dependent phosphorylation. This idea was reinforced upon examination of the phosphorylation properties of nondiabetic and diabetic sarcolemma. As a result of the diabetes-linked decrease in protein phosphatase 1 activity, ^{32}P incorporation into sarcolemmal proteins was enhanced in the diabetic. Analysis of individual sarcolemmal phosphoproteins by SDS polyacrylamide gel electrophoresis indicated that diabetes was associated with an elevation in membrane phosphorylation of some proteins, but a decrease in the phosphorylation state of other phosphoproteins. The possibility that the dramatic change in membrane phosphorylation contributes to defective sarcolemmal calcium transport is discussed.

Acknowledgements

This research was supported by a grant from the National Institutes of Health (DK 36440).

References

1. Fein FS and Sonnenblick EH. Diabetic cardiomyopathy. Prog Cardiovasc Dis 1985;27:255-270.
2. Regan TJ. Congestive heart failure in the diabetic. Ann Rev Med 1983;34:161-168.
3. Schaffer SW, Artman MF and Wilson GL. Properties of insulin-dependent and noninsulin-dependent diabetic cardiomyopathies. In: Pathogenesis of Myocarditis and Cardiomyopathy (edited by Kawai C and Abelmann WH), University of Tokyo Press, Tokyo, 1987, pp. 149-162.
4. Tahiliani AG and McNeill JH. Diabetes-induced abnormalities in the myocardium. Life Sci 1986;38:959-974.
5. Fein FS, Aronson RS, Nordin C, Miller-Green B and Sonnenblick EH. Altered myocardial response to ouabain in diabetic rats: Mechanics and electrophysiology. J Mol Cell Cardiol 1983;15:769-784.
6. Vadlamudi RVSV and McNeill JH. Effect of experimental diabetes on isolated rat heart responsiveness to isoproterenol. Can J Physiol Pharmacol 1984;62:124-131.
7. Goyal RK and McNeill JH. Effects of chronic streptozotocin-induced diabetes on the cardiac responses to milrinone. Can J Physiol Pharmacol 1985;63:1620-1623.
8. Jackson CV, McGrath GM and McNeill JH. Alterations in alpha-adrenoceptor stimulation of isolated atria from experimental diabetic rats. Can J Physiol Pharmacol 1986;64:145-151.
9. Schaffer SW, Mozaffari MS, Artman M and Wilson GL. Basis for myocardial mechanical defects associated with noninsulin dependent diabetes. Am J Physiol 1989;256:E25-E30.
10. Allo SN, Lincoln TM and Schaffer SW. Reduced cardiac response to isoproterenol in noninsulin-depedent diabetes. The Pharmacologist 1989;31:185.
11. Schaffer SW, Mozaffari MS, Cutcliff CR and Wilson GL. Postreceptor myocardial metabolic defect in a rat model of noninsulin-dependent diabetes mellitus. Diabetes 1986;35:593-597.

12. Nishio Y, Kashiwagi KA, Kida Y, Kodama M, Abe N, Saeki Y anmd Shigeta Y. Deficiency of cardiac ß-adrenergic receptor in streptozotocin-induced diabetic rats. Diabetes 1988;37:1181-1187.
13. Gotzsche O. The adrenergic ß-receptor adenylate cyclase system in heart and lymphocytes from streptozotocin-diabetic rats. Diabetes 1983;32:1110-1116.
14. Schaffer SW, Tan BH and Wilson GL. Development of a cardiomyopathy in a model of noninsulin-dependent diabetes. Am J Physiol 1985;248:H179-H185.
15. Pitts BJR. Stoichiometry of sodium-calcium exchange in cardiac sarcolemmal vesicles. J Biol Chem 1979;254:6232-6235.
16. Caroni P and Carafoli E. Regulation of calcium-pumping ATPase of heart sarcolemma by a phosphorylation-dephosphorylation process. J Biol Chem 1981;256:9371-9373.
17. Ingebritsen TS, Stewart AA and Cohen P. The protein phosphatases involved in cellular regulation. Eur J Biochem 1983;132:297-307.
18. Sulakhe PV and Drummond GI. Protein kinase-catalyzed phosphorylation of muscle sarcolemma. Arch Biochem Biophys 1974;161:448-455.
19. Makino N, Dhalla KS, Elimban V and Dhalla NS. Sarcolemmal calcium transport in streptozotocin-induced diabetic cardiomyopathy in rats. Am J Physiol 1987;253:E202-E207.
20. Heyliger CE, Prakash A and McNeill JH. Alterations in cardiac sarcolemmal calcium pump activity during diabetes mellitus. Am J Physiol 1987;252:H540-H544.
21. Caroni P, Zurini M, Clark A and Carafoli E. Further characterization and reconstitution of the purified calcium-pumping ATPase of heart sarcolemma. J Biol Chem 1983;258:7305-7310.
22. Lamers JMJ. Calcium transport systems in cardiac sarcolemma and their regulation by the second messengers cyclic AMP and calcium-calmodulin. Gen Physiol Biophys 1985;4:143-154.
23. Presti CF, Jones LR and Lindemann JP. Isoproterenol-induced phosphorylation of a 15 kilodalton sarcolemmal protein in intact myocardium. J Biol Chem 1985;260:3860-3867.
24. Sperelakis N. Regulation of calcium slow channels of cardiac muscle by cyclic nucleotides and phosphorylation. J Mol Cell Cardiol 1988;20(Suppl II):75-105.

25. Caroni P and Carafoli E. The regulation of the sodium-calcium exchanger of heart sarcolemma. Eur J Biochem 1983;132:451-460.
26. Zick Y. The insulin receptor: Structure and function. Critical Rev Biochem Mol Biol 1989;24:217-269.
27. Roth RA and Beaudin J. Phosphorylation of purified insulin receptor by cAMP kinase. Diabetes 1987;36:123-126.

Electron Microscopic Cytochemical Studies on ATPase and Acid Phosphatase Activities of Cardiac Myocytes in Streptozotocin Induced Diabetic Rats

Y. Suwa, Y. Umezawa, M. Yaida, Y. Takeyama and T. Katagiri

*Third Department of Internal Medicine, Showa University School of Medicine,
Tokyo 142, JAPAN*

Introduction

It has often been reported that a crisis of congestive heart failure is frequently observed in patients with diabetes mellitus independent of coronary artery disease or hypertension (1). In this respect, a contraction/relaxation disorder of the cardiac muscle has also been noted in animal experiments. The dysfunction of the heart observed in diabetes is known as so-called diabetic cardiomyopathy (2). However for its causes, while complex factors such as intramyocardial microangiopathy and myocardial metabolic disorder caused by diabetes are suspected, a definitive conclusion has not yet been drawn.

ATPase is one of the essential enzymes in myocardial energy metabolism and is well known to be closely related to myocardial metabolism. And, acid phosphatase (AcPase), one of the lysosomal enzymes, is also known to participate in certain forms of damage or pathologic change of cells and organs. There have been many previous reports that mentioned ultrastructural changes in the cardiac muscles of experimental diabetic animals, but histocytochemical studies on enzymatic activities such as ATPase, AcPase activities, etc., in comparison with morphologic changes are few (3-13). Therefore, we studied cytochemical alterations in ATPase and AcPase activities of streptozotocin (STZ)-induced diabetic rats from early to chronic stages with an electron microscopy.

Materials and Methods

Animal experiments

Male Wistar rats weighing 180 to 200 g were made diabetic with a single intravenous injection of STZ at 65 mg/kg to the tail vein (14). Age-matched

Nagano, M., Mochizuki, S., Dhalla, N.S. (eds.), CARDIOVASCULAR DISEASE IN DIABETES. Copyright © 1992. Kluwer Academic Publishers, Boston. All rights reserved.

normal control rats were used for comparison. Rats showing fasting blood glucose levels of over 400 mg/dl at 2, 4, 6, 8, 12 and 16 weeks after STZ injection were selected for the diabetic group. Body weight and blood glucose level were measured once a week and before sacrifice. The beating heart was removed immediately after thoracotomy performed under anesthesia with ether, myocardial wet weight was measured, and the removed myocardial tissue was used for the following experiments.

Cytochemical procedures

The myocardial tissue was cut into small blocks with a razor blade. Specimens were immediately prefixed with 0.25% glutaraldehyde and 2% paraformaldehyde in 0.1 M sodium cacodylate (pH 7.4) at 4°C for 20 min, rinsed in 0.1 M sodium cacodylate (pH 7.4) thrice and cut into 40 um thick frozen sections at -20°C with a cryostat. The thin sections were rinsed in 0.1 M tris-maleate (pH 7.4) and incubated in the modified solutions of Wachstein and Meisel for ATPase reaction or of Gomori for AcPase activity at 37°C for 60 min (15-18). After incubation, the sections were rinsed briefly in 0.1 M cacodylate, postfixed in 1% OsO_4 at 4°C for 60 min, and embedded in Epon 812 after dehydration through a graded series of ethanol and propylene oxide. Ultrathin sections were cut on an ultramicrotome, double-stained with uranyl acetate and lead citrate, and examined with a Hitachi H-300 electron microscope. In some experiments, the sections were observed without double staining to examine the reaction product for ATPase or acid phosphatase. As a control experiment, the reaction was done in a medium without ATP or ß-glycerophosphate. As a control experiment for ATPase activity, the reaction was also carried out in a reaction media with the addition of 1 mM L-bromotetramisole as an inhibitor of non-specific alkaline phosphatase, or with the addition of 0.1 mM ouabain as an inhibitor of Na^+-K^+-ATPase.

Results

1) General profile

The diabetic rats showed fasting blood glucose over 400 mg/dl at the time of sacrifice, and these values were significanly higher than those found in the control rats (Fig. 1). Both heart and body weights decreased significantly in the diabetic rats compared with those in the control rats

(Figs. 2, 3). Heart/body weight ratios tended to increase significantly in the diabetic rats in comparison with those in the control rats (Fig. 4).

2) Ultrastructural findings

The ultrastructural features of the myofilaments, mitochondria, sarcoplasmic reticulum and other organelles in the diabetic left ventricular cells appeared not to be so severe in comparison with those of age-matched control tissues (Figs. 5-11). In the diabetic myocardial cells, however, from the early stage (about 4 weeks after STZ injection), a number of lipid droplets and lysosomes were observed to be increased (Figs. 9-11). In addition, slight dilatation of the sarcoplasmic reticulum-transverse tubular system and slight loss of myofilaments were seen in the diabetic rats about 12-16 weeks after STZ injection (Figs. 7, 11).

3) Cytochemical activities

The chronological changes in the intensity and the localization of ATPase and AcPase activities in the diabetic myocardial cells were summarized in Table 1.

In the control rats, the reaction product of ATPase activity was observed intensely in the terminal cisternae of the sarcoplasmic reticulum (SR), and moderately on the myofilaments and in the longitudinal tubules of SR in myocardial cells. However, no reaction products were found in the nuclei, sarcolemma or lysosomes (Fig. 5). In control experiments in which ATP-free media were used, almost no reaction product was found. In other control experiments in which an incubation medium with L-bromotetramisole or ouabain was used, the reaction product was noted as intense as that with the original incubation medium.

In the diabetic rats of the early stage (about 4 weeks after STZ injection), ATPase activity was seen to be slightly decreased in the terminal cisternae and the longitudinal tubules of SR and on the myofilaments when compared with that of control (Fig. 6).

In the chronic stage (about 12 - 16 weeks after STZ injection), ATPase reaction product on the myofilaments in the terminal cisternae and the longitudinal tubules of SR appeared to be markedly decreased (Fig. 7).

On the other hand, dense acid phosphatase reaction product was found in the terminal cisternae and the longitudinal tubules of SR and in the primary

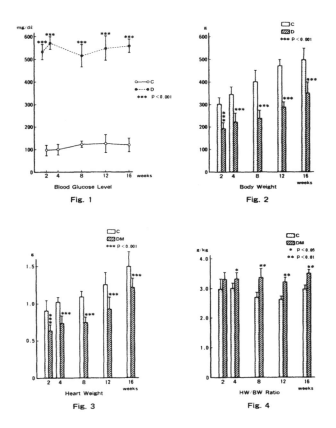

Figure 1. Blood glucose level. C: age matched controls, DM: STZ-induced diabetic rats. Values are expressed as means ± SD. *** P < 0.001 against control value.

Figure 2. Body weight.

Figure 3. Heart weight.

Figure 4. Heart/body weight ratio.

Bars indicate mean S ± SD
* P < 0.05, ** p < 0.01, *** p < 0.001 against control value.

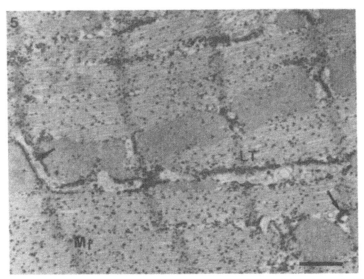

Figure 5. Electron micrograph of ultrastructural localization of ATPase reaction product in the myocardial cells of 16 weeks control rat. A bar indicates 1 um. ATPase activity was intensely observed in TC of SC and moderately of Mf and in LT of SR.

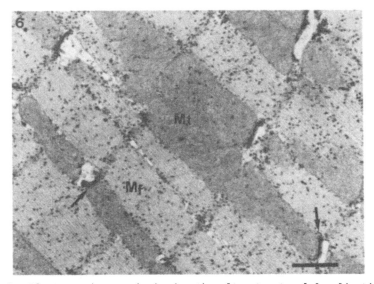

Figure 6. Electron micrograph showing the ultrastructural localization of ATPase activity in myocardial cells of 4 weeks diabetic rat. A bar indicates 1 um. ATPase activity was seen to be slightly decreased in TC (arrows) and LT of SR and on Mf.

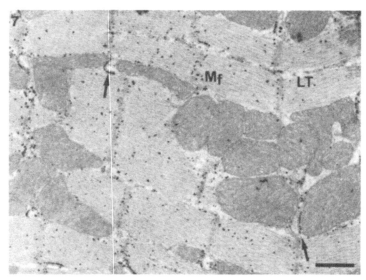

Figure 7. Electron micrograph showing ATPase activity in the myocardial cells of 16 weeks diabetic rat. A bar indicates 1 um. ATPase activity was evidently decreased in TC (arrows) of SR and on Mf. In LT of SR, ATPase activity decreased markedly.

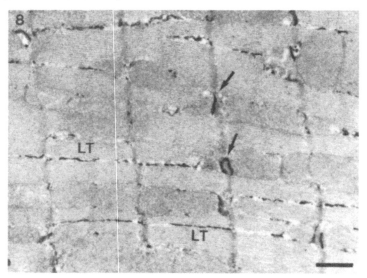

Figure 8. Electron micrograph of ultrastructural localization of AcPase reaction product in the myocardial cells of 16 weeks control rat. A bar indicates 1 um. Note the intense acid phosphatase reaction product in TC and LT of SR.

Table 1. Distribution and intensity of ATPase and acid phosphatase activities in the diabetic myocardial cells of STZ-induced diabetic rats.

			Cont	4w	8w	12w	16w
ATPase activity	SR	TC	+++	++	++	+	+
		LT	+++	++	++	±	±
	Mf		+++	++	++	+	+
AcPase activity	SR	TC	+++	++	++	+	+
		LT	+++	++	++	+	+
	Ly		+++	+++	+++	+++	+++
Fine structural change			-	-	-	+	+

+++ = markedly intense; ++ = intense; + = moderate; ± = faint; - = none

Abbreviations in Figures and Table 1 are used as follows:
LT, longitudinal tubules; Lp: lipid droplet; Ly, lysosome; Mf, myofilament; Mt, mitochondria; SR, sarcoplasmic reticulum; TC, terminal cisternae.

lysosomes in the control rats. Number of lysosomes and residual bodies were small in the normal myocardial cells (Fig. 8). The reaction product was not found in the myocardial cells incubated in the medium without the substrate.

In the diabetic rats of the early stage (about 4 weeks after STZ injection), localization of AcPase activity was also similar in diabetic rat myocardial cell to that of control (Fig. 9). In the chronic stage (about 8 - 12 weeks after STZ injection), the intensity of the AcPase activities of terminal cisternae and longitudinal tubules of SR in the diabetic rat myocytes also decreased (Figs. 10, 11).

Discussion

The ultrastructural changes in diabetic cardiac myocyte are characterized by an increase in lipid droplets and enlargement in the number and size of the lysosomes. The increase in lipid droplets is reported by many

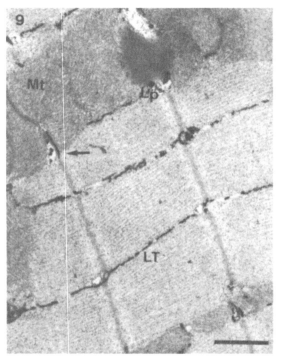

Figure 9. Electron micrograph showing AcPase activity in the myocardial cells of 4 weeks diabetic rat. AcPase activity was similar in comparison with that of control. Lipid droplets increased in DM.

morphological studies (3-13). In the cardiac muscle of diabetic patients and experimental diabetic animals, it is thought that energy production in the heart muscle becomes lipid-dependent owing to the decreased utilization of glucose, then the oxidation of fatty acids is accelerated and the intramyocardial lipids are increased. Tarach (3) also reported an enlargement in the number and size of the lysosomes. Vtynrin (19) described how an increase in the lysosomes shows an impairment of the fundamental activity of the cell. Hyperglycemia, caused by hypoinsulinemia which is induced by the destruction of Langerhans' B cell with streptozotocin, brings about various impairments. As diabetes is a disease based on insulin deficiency, this induces various metabolic changes. Consequently, myocardial cells may be

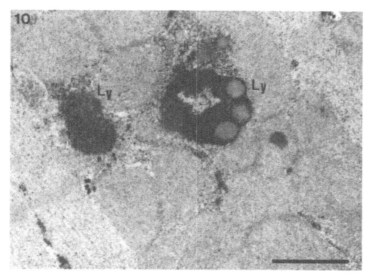

Figure 10. Electron micrograph showing AcPase activity in the myocardial cells of 16 weeks diabetic rat. Slightly mitochondrial swelling and an increase in the number of size and lysosomes are apparent.

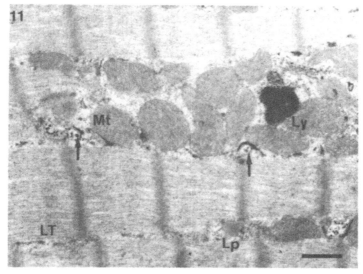

Figure 11. Electron micrograph showing AcPase activity in the myocardial cells of 16 weeks diabetic rat. AcPase activity decreased distinctly in TC (arrows) and LT of SR compared with those of control.

impaired and enlargement in the number and size of the lysosomes may be observed. In patients with diabetes mellitus, complication of cardiac hypertrophy is often reported (2,20,21). In this study, the ratio between heart and body weights in the diabetic rats was greater than that of the control group, and this suggests the presence of cardiac hypertrophy. It is likely that compensatory mechanism induces cardiac hypertrophy by the increasing load on the heart under imbalance of carbohydrates and lipids and diabetic situations such as polyposia. In diabetics, the frequency of heart failure is higher than that in the non-diabetic cases (1), and after an autoptic report of Rubler (2), the presence of cardiac impairment was shown even in cases without coronary sclerosis in many studies. Ultrastructural studies have also been reported (3-13). Decreases in contractile proteins, the swelling and destruction of mitochondria, the formation of a contraction band were observed about 12-24 weeks after STZ injection (4). On the contrary, it was stated that the above morphological changes were not noted but only the swelling of mitochondria and the increase of lipid droplets were recognized at 12 weeks after STZ injection (8). Thus, morphological changes in the ultrastructure of the myocardial cell in the diabetic heart varies in each report both in man and in experimental diabetic animals. Such differences in the results are presumed to be due to the differences in animal species, dose of streptozotocin, and the affected period of diabetes or in the tissue fixation method.

For the diabetic cardiac muscle, the formation of contraction bands and the expansion of the intercalated disc are also reported (4,6,11) and intracellular Ca^{++} overload was speculated to attribute to such diabetic cardiomyopathy accompanying the impairment of cardiac dysfunction or ultrastructural alterations (22-24). Afzal et al described how the morphological changes in the myocardial cells in STZ diabetic rats could be improved by the administration of Ca^{++} antagonist and this might support the above supposition (12). Intramyocardial microangiopathy has been noticed as a cause of diabetic cardiomyopathy (2,20). In the reports of Rubler (2) and Hamby (20), morphologic changes in the intramyocardial small vessels and interstitium are described, and the relationship to diabetic cardiomyopathy was speculated. Ledet reported similar results, but no special findings about the changes on the capillary level were made (25). But hypertrophy was also observed in the basement membranes of the intramyocardial capillaries of diabetics (5) and the presence of capillary microaneurysms was detected in the cardiac muscles (26). From these reports, it seems likely that microangiopathy is closely related to the myocardial effects of diabetes. On the contrary, it was reported that differences in ultrastructural changes between diabetic and normal rat myocardium were not significant until 6 weeks (4). It was also stated that fibrosis in the interstitium and small blood vessel walls of diabetic rats at 8 weeks after STZ injection was not different from that in normal rats (7).

Therefore, the final conclusion about the cause of diabetic cardiomyopathy has not yet been drawn. In general, Ca^{++} overload has been pointed out as a mechanism of the development of myocardial impairment. But intracellular Ca^{++} concentration and kinetics are regulated by various functions, such as sarcolemma, sarcoplasmic reticulum and mitochondria. Yaida and coworkers (14) and Dhalla and associates (27) reported, in STZ DM rats, reduced Ca^{++} ATPase activity of SR, which is considered to have an important role in the relaxation of the cardiac muscle. There are suggestions about the abnormality of the structural proteins of the cardiac muscle by some reports, of which one, by using isolated papillary muscles from experimental diabetics, noted decreased contraction ability, delayed relaxation time, and reduced actomyocin ATPase activity (28,29), and one found an abnormality of the myosin isozyme and reduced myosin ATPase activity (30). On the other hand, in the case of the diabetic heart, it is said that when a decrease in elasticity of the cardiac muscle and a stiffening of the ventricular wall occur, then a decrease in the compliance and the distensibility of the whole heart appear (29); however, there is a report that the hypofunction of the heart in diabetic rats appears more rapidly than a manifestation of ultrastructural changes (4).

In this study, both ATPase and AcPase activities decreased more markedly in SR though no severe changes in the ultrastructures were recognized. From these findings, it is suggested that because of the abnormal metabolism of the cardiac muscle in diabetics, functional abnormality of the intracellular small organs such as SR occurs firstly and then diabetic cardiomyopathy develops because of this abnormality which acts as a trigger.

Summary

We studied cytochemical alterations in ATPase and acid phosphatase (AcPase) activities in cardiac myocytes of streptozotocin (STZ)-induced diabetic rats from 2 to 16 weeks. Male Wistar rats were made diabetic with a single STZ I.V. at 65 mg/kg. Myocardial specimens were prefixed, and reacted by modified methods of Wachstein and Meisel and of Gomori for ATPase and AcPase, and examined with an electron microscope. Diabetic rats (DM) showed fasting blood glucose of over 400 mg/dl at the time of sacrifice after 4 to 16 weeks after STZ injection. Body and heart wet weights were significantly decreased in DM. Lipid droplets and lysosomes increased in myocardial cells in DM but ultrastructural changes were not so severe through the course of DM up to 16 weeks. ATPase activities were recognized intensely in sarcoplasmic reticulum (SR) and on myofilaments, and those of AcPase in SR and lysosomes. Both ATPase and AcPase activities decreased progressively after 8-12 weeks in DM. Among them, ATPase activities in SR decreased markedly. These findings suggest that decreases in ATPase and AcPase activities in diabetic myocardial cells may be closely related to cardiac dysfunction though the ultrastructural changes were not so severe.

Acknowledgements

The authors wish to express their sincere thanks to Professor Yasumitsu Nakai of Showa University for his guidance and encouragement to this work. We are also greatly indebted to Drs. Hitoshi Kanaya, Shigeo Hasegawa and Shuji Mukae of Showa University for their collaboration.

References

1. Kannel WB, Hjortland M and Castelli WP. Role of diabetes in congestive heart failure: The Framingham study. Am J Cardiol 1974;34:29-34.
2. Rubler S, Dlugash J, Yuceoglu YZ, Kumal T, Branwood AW and Grishman A. New type of cardiomyopathy associated with diabetic glomerulosclerosis. Am J Cardiol 1972;30:595-602.
3. Tarach JS. Electron microscopic cytochemical studies on lysosomes and peroxisomes of rat cardiac muscle in the experimental alloxan diabetes. Acta Histochem Bd 1978;62:32-43.
4. Jackson CV, McGrath GM, Tahiliani AG, Vadlamudi RS and McNeill JH. A functional and ultrastructural analysis of experimental diabetic rat myocardium. Diabetes 1985;34:876-883.
5. Fischer VW, Leskiw ML and Barner HB. Myocardial structure and capillary basal laminar thickness in experimentally diabetic rats. Exp Mol Pathol 1981;35:244-256.

6. Seager MJ, Singal PK, Orchard R, Pierce GN and Dhalla NS. Cardiac cell damage: A primary myocardial disease in streptozotocin-induced chronic diabetes. Br J Exp Path 1984;65:613-623.
7. Factor SM, Minase T, Bhan R, Wolinsky H and Sonnenblick EH. Hypertensive diabetic cardiomyopathy in the rat: Ultrastructural features. Pathol Anat 1983;398:305-317.
8. McGrath GM and McNeill JH. Cardiac ultrastructural changes in streptozotocin-induced diabetic rats: Effects of insulin treatment. Can J Cardiol 1986;2:164-169.
9. Koltai MZS, Balogh I, Wagner M and Pogatsa G. Diabetic myocardial alterations in ultrastructure and function. Exp Path 1984;25:215-221.
10. Bhimji S, Godin DV and McNeill JH. Myocardial ultrastructural changes in alloxan-induced diabetes in rabbits. Acta Anat 1986;125:195-200.
11. Hisao Y, Suzuki K, Abe H and Toyota T. Ultrastructural alterations in cardiac muscle of diabetic BB Wistar rats. Pathol Anat 1987;411:45-52.
12. Afzal N, Ganguly PK, Dhalla KS, Pierce GN, Singal PK and Dhalla NS. Beneficial effects of verapamil in diabetic cardiomyopathy. Diabetes 1988;37:936-942.
13. Giacomelli F and Wiener J. Primary myocardial disease in the diabetic mouse. Lab Invest 1979;40:460-473.
14. Yaida M, Umezawa Y, Konno N and Katagiri T. Alterations in cardiac sarcoplasmic reticulum and structural proteins in streptozotocin-induced diabetic rats. J Showa Med 1988;48(2):175-182.
15. Wachstein M and Meisel E. Histochemistry of hepatic phosphatases at a physiolosic pH, with special reference to the demonstration of bile canaliculi. Am J Clin Pathol 1957;27:13-23.
16. Gomori G. An improved histochemical technique for acid phosphatase. Stain Tech 1950;25:81-85.
17. Kanaya H, Akiyama K, Kitsu T, Takeyama Y and Katagiri T. Studies on ultrastructure and cytochemical ATPase activity in human cardiac myocytes from biopsies from patients with various heart diseases. Jpn Circ J 1987;51:1241-1249.
18. Nakamura N, Sasai Y, Takeyama Y and Katagiri T. Electron microscopic cytochemical studies on acid phosphatase activity in acute myocardial ischemia. Jpn Circ J 1983;24:595-606.
19. Vtyurin BV. Concerning the structure and function of lysosomes. Arkh Pathol 1968;30:51-56.

20. Hamby RI, Zoneraich S and Sherman L. Diabetic cardiomyopathy. JAMA 1974;229:1749-1754.
21. Regan TJ, Ettinger PO, Khan MI, Jesrani MU, Lyons MM, Oldewurtel HA and Weber M. Altered myocardial function and metabolism in chronic diabetes mellitus without ischemia in dogs. Circ Res 1974;35:222-237.
22. Pierce GN and Dhalla NS. Sarcolemmal Na^+-K^+-ATPase activity in diabetic rat heart. Am J Physiol 1983;245:C241-C247.
23. Pierce GN, Kutyrk MJB and Dhalla NS. Alterations in Ca^{2+} binding and composition of the cardiac sarcolemmal membrane in chronic diabetes. Proc Natl Acad Sci 1983;80:5412-5416.
24. Penpargkul S, Fein F, Sonnenblick EH and Scheuer J. Depressed cardiac sarcoplasmic reticular function from diabetic rats. J Mol Cell Cardiol 1981;13:303-309.
25. Ledet T. Diabetic cardiomyopathy. Quantitative histological studies of the heart from young juvenile diabetics. Acta Pathol Microbiol Scand Sect A 1976;84:421-428.
26. Factor SM, Okun EM and Minase T. Capillary microaneurysms in the human diabetic heart. N Engl J Med 1980;307:384-388.
27. Ganguly PK, Pierce GN, Dhalla KS and Dhalla NS. Defective sarcoplasmic reticular calcium transport in diabetic cardiomyopathy. Am J Cardiol 1983;244:E528-E535.
28. Horackova M and Murphy MG. Effects of chronic diabetes mellitus on the electrical and contractile activities, $^{45}Ca^{2+}$ transport, fatty acid profiles and ultrastructure of isolated rat ventricular myocytes. Pflugers Arch 1988;411:564-572.
29. Fein FS, Kornstein LB, Strobeck JE, Capasso JM and Sonnenblick EH. Altered myocardial mechanics in diabetic rats. Circ Res 1980;47:922-933.
30. Dillmann WH. Diabetes mellitus induces changes in cardiac myosin of the rat. Diabetes 1980;29:579-582.

Myocardial Isoenzyme Distribution in Chronic Diabetes: Comparison with Isoproterenol-Induced Chronic Myocardial Damage

H. Hashimoto, Y. Awaji, Y. Matsui, K. Kawaguchi,
N. Akiyama, K. Okumura, T. Ito, T. Satake

The Second Department of Internal Medicine, Nagoya University School of Medicine, Nagoya 466, JAPAN.

Introduction

In the chronically diabetic heart, it has been reported that the activity of several enzymes bound to cell structures, such as sarcoplasmic reticular Ca^{++} ATPase, sarcolemmal Na^+-K^+ ATPase and myosin ATPase is depressed and that the isoenzyme distribution of myosin ATPase is altered (1,2). However, the changes in the activity and isoenzyme distribution of creatine kinase (CK: EC 2.7.3.2) and lactate dehydrogenase (LD: EC 1.1.1.27) which are mainly "soluble" enzymes and clinically important markers of myocardial necrosis (3) have not been reported in the diabetic heart previously. Therefore, in this study we measured total and isoenzyme activities of myocardial CK and LD in rats with insulin dependent diabetes and compared them with control. Since intracellular calcium overload has been suggested in the pathogenesis of diabetic cardiomyopathy (1,2,4), we also measured the activity of the same (iso)enzymes in the myocardium of rats chronically injected with isoproterenol, a pure ß-adrenergic stimulant, which develop cardiomyopathy with intracellular calcium overload (5).

Methods
Animal Preparation

Insulin dependent diabetes mellitus was induced in 30 male Wistar rats weighing between 210 and 320 g by a single injection of 65 mg/kg streptozocin dissolved with 0.1 N citrate buffer into the tail vein. Rats were killed 4 (n=11) and 8 (n=19) weeks after streptozocin injection. Among 19 rats killed at 8 weeks, 9 were injected subcutaneously with 3 U protamine zinc insulin daily during the last 4 weeks before sacrifice. Sixteen control animals, age and sex matched with the diabetic rats, were injected only with 0.1 N citrate buffer and killed 4 (n=8) and 8 (n=8) weeks after the injection.

Catecholamine cardiomyopathy was produced in 20 male Wistar rats weighing between 250 and 350 g by chronic subcutaneous administration of 0.25 (n=9), 0.5 (n=6) and 1.0 (n=5) mg/kg isoproterenol, a pure β-receptor agonist (6). Rats were injected daily with isoproterenol for 3 weeks and decapitated. Eleven age-matched male rats were injected daily with saline for 3 weeks and killed as the control.

After decapitation of each animal, the heart was quickly removed, washed with ice-cooled saline and blotted. Great vessels, atria and right ventricle were dissected and left ventricle was weighed and stored at -70°C until analysis. Body weight was measured in all animals and venous blood for the determination of glucose was drawn from diabetic rats and their controls before sacrificing the animals. The use and care of the animals in this study were in accordance with Guidelines for Animal Experimentation in Nagoya University School of Medicine.

Measurements

Transmural myocardial sample weighing between 20 and 30 mg was obtained from the left ventricle. The sample was weighed, quickly immersed in 0.1 M phosphate buffer (4°C), pH 7.4, containing 1 mM ethylenediamine tetra-acetic acid and 1 mM β-mercaptoethanol, and homogenized with a glass-Teflon homogenizer for 3 min at 4°C. The homogenate was divided into two aliquots. Triton 100X was added to one aliquot to a final concentration of 0.1%, which was then stirred for 30 min at 4°C. Both aliquots were centrifuged at 16000 g for 15 min at 4°C. The supernatant with Triton 100X was used for the determination of CK, and the supernatant without Triton 100X was used for the determination of LD. Protein was determined according to the method of Lowry. Blood glucose was measured by glucose oxidase method.

Total CK activity was assayed according to the method of Rosalki (7). CK isoenzyme distribution was determined by cellulose acetate membrane electrophoresis. Separation was achieved at 200 V for 17 min at 4°C. The membrane was stained with Cardiotrac CK reagent (Corning, Palo Alto, USA), incubated at 37°C for 10 min, dried, and scanned with a fluorescent densitometer. Activity attributable to each of CK subunits (CK-M and CK-B) was considered equivalent.

Total LD activity was measured according to the method of Wroblewski and LaDue (8). LD isoenzyme distribution was determined by cellulose acetate membrane electrophoresis. Separation was achieved at 200 V for 20 min at 4°C. The membrane was stained with Titan LDH Isoenzyme Reagent (Helena), incubated at 37°C for 10 min, placed in 3% acetic acid for 15 min, and scanned with a densitometer. Activity attributable to each of LD subunits (LD-H and LD-M) was considered equivalent.

Results were expressed as the mean ± SEM. The statistical differences between the mean values were evaluated by one way analysis of variance and Duncan's multiple range test.

Results

In rats injected with streptozocin, blood glucose 4 and 8 weeks after the injection was 680±40 and 427±15 mg/dl, respectively, which was significantly higher than the controls (126±2 and 122±4 mg/dl). In diabetic rats with insulin treatment, blood glucose (138±25 mg/dl) was not statistically different from control.

Both left ventricular and body weights were significantly smaller in diabetic rats compared with control. Left ventricle/body weight ratios were significantly greater in diabetic compared with control rats because reduction in body weight exceeded that in left ventricular weight. Insulin treatment completely and partly normalized left ventricular weight and body weight, respectively, in diabetic animals. In rats injected with isoproterenol, significant increases in left ventricular weight and decreases in body weight compared with their controls were observed. Accordingly, left ventricular/body weight ratio increased in isoproterenol group dose-dependently (Fig. 1).

In diabetic rats, myocardial mean total CK activity decreased by 23 and 31% (4 and 8 weeks after injection of streptozocin, respectively) compared with control. This change resulted from reduction in all fractions of CK isoenzyme. The reduction in CK isoenzyme activity was greatest in MB (57 and 62%), followed by BB (53 and 52%), mitochondria (44 and 49%) and MM (10 and 15%) fractions (Fig. 2, Table 1). Accordingly, reduction in the activity attributable to CK subunit was greatest in B, followed by mitochondria and M subunits (Fig. 4). Insulin treatment competely restored total, MM, MB and BB CK activity and partially restored mitochondrial CK activity (Fig. 2,Table 1).

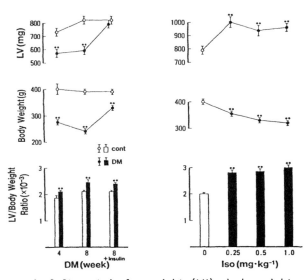

Figure 1. Changes in left ventricular weight (LV), body weight and LV/body weight ratio in diabetic rats (DM) and rats injected with isoproterenol (ISO). Each value represents mean ± SEM. Open circles and open bars indicate control animals, and solid circles and solid bars indicate diabetic rats (left panel) or rats injected with isoproterenol (right panel).
**p<0.01 compared with control.

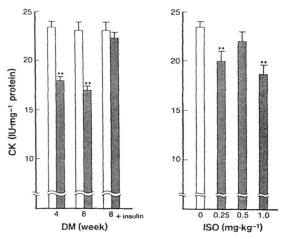

Figure 2. Changes in myocardial creatine kinase (CK) activity in diabetic rats (DM) and rats injected with isoproterenol (ISO). Each value represents mean ± SEM. Open bars indicate control animals and hatched bars indicate diabetic rats (left panel) or rats injected with isoproterenol (right panel).
**p<0.01 compared with control.

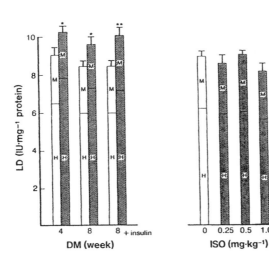

Figure 3. Changes in myocardial lactate dehydrogenase (LD) activity in diabetic rats (DM) and rats injected with isoproterenol (ISO). Each value represents mean ± SEM. Open bars indicate control animals and hatched bars indicate diabetic rats (left panel) or rats injected with isoproterenol (right panel). M and H indicate activity attributable to LD-M and LD-H subunit, respectively.
*$p<0.05$ compared with control, **$p<0.01$ compared with control.

Total LD and LD_1 activity significantly increased in the diabetic rat heart which was due to the increase in LD-H subunit. After treatment with insulin, LD-M subunit also increased as well as H subunit (Fig. 3, Table 1). Accordingly, the proportion of LD-M decreased in the diabetics, and this was normalized by insulin treatment (Table 1).

In rats injected with isoproterenol, total CK activity was significantly reduced except in 0.5 mg/kg group because of reduction in MM and mitochondrial CK activity while CK BB increased (Fig. 2, Table 1). Accordingly, activity attributable to CK-M and mitochondrial subunits decreased and CK-B subunit increased (Fig. 4). In the isoproterenol group, total LD activity was unchanged (Fig. 3). However, increase in LD-M subunit and decreases in LD-H subunit and LD_1 were observed in rats injected with larger dose (1.0 mg/kg) of isoproterenol (Fig. 4, Table 1).

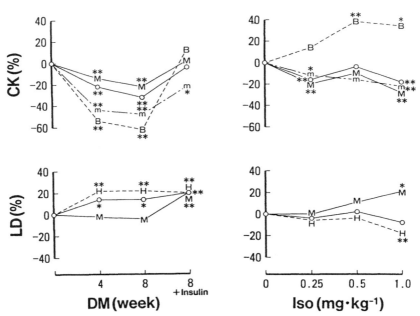

Figure 4. Changes in the activity attributable to each isoenzyme subunit of creatine kinase (CK) and lactate dehydrogenase (LD) in the heart of diabetic rats (DM) and rats injected with isoproterenol (ISO). Each point represents mean percent change compared with control (positive value = % increase, negative value = % decrease, 0 = no change compared with control). Open circle indicates total activity of CK or LD. Upper panels: M = CK-M subunit, B = CK-B subunit, m = mitochondrial CK subunit. Lower panels: H = LD-H subunit, M = LD-M subunit.
*p<0.05 compared with control, **p<0.01 compared with control.

Discussion

Time dependent changes in serum enzymes such as creatine kinase (CK) and lactate dehydrogenase (LD) and their isoenzymes have been widely used for the estimation of myocardial infarct size as well as for its diagnosis (9). Infarct size is calculated on the assumption that amount of enzyme contained in unit weight of infarcted myocardium are both constant (9). Studies have shown that total or isoenzyme activity of myocardial CK and LD changes in correlation with mechanical overload or possibly with ischemia (10,11,12,13) and that myocardial reperfusion changes the ratio of CK recovery from blood, making the interpretation of enzymatically estimated infarct size more complicated.

Table 1. Changes in myocardial isoenzyme activity of creatine kinase (CK) and lactate dehydrogenase (LD) in experimental cardiomyopathies

			CK				LD	
	n	MM	MB	BB	mito	LD$_1$	M%
4 week cont	8	15.4 (0.6)	3.0 (0.2)	0.38 (0.05)	4.3 (0.5)	2.9 (0.1)	28.0 (0.7)
DM	11	13.9 (0.4)*	1.3 (0.1)**	0.18 (0.01)**	2.4 (0.2)**	3.9 (0.2)**	23.9 (0.4)**
		-10%	-57%	-53%	-44%	+37%	-15%
DM 8 week cont	8	13.7 (0.5)	3.4 (0.2)	0.40 (0.05)	5.3 (0.5)	2.7 (0.1)	28.7 (0.4)
DM	10	11.6 (0.4)**	1.3 (0.1)**	0.19 (0.02)**	2.7 (0.2)**	3.7 (0.2)**	24.0 (0.7)**
		-15%	-62%	-52%	-49%	+39%	-16%
DM+I	9	13.9 (0.3)	3.5 (0.2)	0.45 (0.04)	4.1 (0.3)*	3.2 (0.1)*	28.3 (0.6)
		+1%	+3%	+13%	-22%	+19%	-1%
cont	11	13.3 (0.2)	3.2 (0.3)	0.52 (0.05)	6.4 (0.2)	2.6 (0.1)	30.2 (0.7)
0.25 mg/kg	9	10.2 (0.5)**	3.5 (0.2)	0.66 (0.05)	5.5 (0.3)*	2.3 (0.1)	31.3 (0.6)
		-23%	+9%	+27%	-14%	-10%	+4%
ISO 0.5 mg/kg	6	11.5 (0.7)*	4.1 (0.2)	0.90 (0.09)**	5.5 (0.3)	2.3 (0.1)	33.2 (0.9)*
		-14%	+28%	+73%	-14%	-12%	+10%
1.0 mg/kg	5	9.4 (0.6)**	3.5 (0.2)	1.02 (0.13)**	4.9 (0.4)**	1.5 (0.2)**	38.5 (1.3)**
		-29%	+9%	+96%	-23%	-41%	+27%

Unitless values represent mean (SEM) activity of isoenzymes (IU/mg protein) except M%. M% represents proportion of LD-M subunit in percentage. Values with % indicate either percent increase (positive numbers) or percent decrease (negative numbers) compared with control. cont = control animals, DM = diabetic rats, DM+I = diabetic rats treated with insulin, ISO = rats injected with isoproterenol. * p<0.05 compared with control, ** p<0.01 compared with control.

Although patients with diabetes mellitus have been shown to have a higher rate of mortality and increased incidence of congestive heart failure compared with non-diabetic patients when they develop acute myocardial infarction, infarct size estimated by CK or CK MB isoenzyme has been reported smaller in diabetic patients (14) and animals (15) compared with non-diabetic control. Diabetic heart has been shown to have molecular and cellular abnormality such as reduced activity of membrane-associated enzymes (1) and decreased myocardial contractility even in the absence of atherosclerotic coronary disease, suggesting a diabetic cardiomyopathy (2). However, changes in the activity of CK, LD, AST and their isoenzymes in the diabetic heart have not been fully investigated previously. Therefore, in this study we measured myocardial isoenzyme activity of CK and LD in rats with insulin dependent diabetes mellitus induced by streptozocin and compared it with the control. We also measured the activity of the same enzymes in the heart of the rat chronically injected with isoproterenol, a model of catecholamine-induced myocardial injury (6).

Our result showed that CK activity was decreased and LD activity was increased in the diabetic heart. The reduction in CK became greater with time after induction of diabetes (4 weeks: -23% of the control, 8 weeks: -31%). The activities of all CK isoenzymes decreased and the reduction was greater in the order of CK MB (-62% at 8 weeks), BB (-52%), mitochondria (-49%) and MM (-15%) isoenzymes. Accordingly, activity attributable to CK-B subunit decreased most (-61% at 8 weeks) followed by mitochondria (-49%) and M (-21%) subunits. Reduced CK isoenzyme activities were completely restored by the administration of insulin except the partial recovery observed in mitochondrial CK. Although total CK activity was depressed to nearly the same extent in the two types of cardiomyopathies, isoenzyme shift of CK in isoproterenol treated rats was quite different from that in diabetic animals. In isoproterenol treated rats, CK MB and BB were either increased or unchanged although CK MM was decreased as much as the diabetic heart. Thus, CK-B subunit increased significantly in isoproterenol treated rats (+33%: 1.0 mg/kg/day). Changes in myocardial LD isoenzymes in diabetic rats were also divergent from the isoproterenol group. LD_1 activity increased significantly in diabetic rats while it decreased in isoproterenol treated rats. Activity attributable to LD-H subunit significantly increased in the diabetics while it decreased in isoproterenol treated rats, thus the proportion of LD-M subunit decreased in the diabetics and increased in the isoproterenol group.

Several investigators have reported that pressure-overloaded and hypertrophied heart accumulates CK-B and LD-M subunits (10,13). It has also been suggested that CK-B is accumulated in ischemic myocardium (11) and that increased tissue LD-M content is related to the decreased oxygen availability in the tissue (12,16). These isoenzyme shifts are considered to be the molecular "adaptation" of myocardium to the mechanical stress or ischemia and possibly to serve as the compensatory mechanism in the failing heart because the affinity of CK-B to creatine phosphate is higher than CK-M (17) and LD-M favors anerobic metabolism compared with LD-H (16). Relative myocardial ischemia due to increased myocardial oxygen demand coupled with hypotension is the possible pathogenesis of the cardiomyopathy in rats treated with isoproterenol (18). On the other hand, metabolic and biochemical disorders induced by insulin deficiency is the primary cause of diabetic cardiomyopathy. Thus, increased LD-M proportion and CK-B in isoproterenol treated rats may indicate relative myocardial hypoperfusion in these animals and may serve as compensatory mechanism in the failing heart. Decreased LD-M proportion and CK-B in diabetic rats related directly to insulin deficiency and may indicate either lack of "compensation" to relative myocardial ischemia or absence of ischemia per se. Although generation and utilization of high energy phosphates are disturbed in the diabetic rat heart, energy consumption is also suppressed because of the depressed activities of myocardial ATPases and hypothyroidism associated with diabetes (2). Therefore, it is likely that energy supply and demand are balanced at lower level in the diabetic heart. However, it is possible that these isoenzyme shift may become a deleterious factor once ischemia occurs in the diabetic heart.

Although the left ventricle/body weight ratio significantly increased in diabetic rats and isoproterenol-treated rats compared with their controls, left ventricular weight was smaller than control in diabetic rats while it was larger than control in the isoproterenol group. In diabetic rats, the decrease in body weight was prominent compared with the isoproterenol group. Thus, diabetes mellitus had a little different effect on left ventricular and body weights compared with the isoproterenol-induced cardiomyopathy.

It has generally been accepted that infarct size is one of the most important predictors of prognosis and mortality in patients with acute myocardial infarction. The higher rate of mortality and increased tendency of heart failure in diabetic patients are also well known clinical investigations (14,19). However, infarct size in diabetic versus non-diabetic patients is still controversial. Experimental studies have shown that anatomical infarct size in diabetic animals is equal to that in non-diabetic animals (20). Human study has reported that infarct size estimated by QRS score of electrocardiogram in diabetic patients is larger than that in non-diabetic patients (21). On the other hand, infarct size estimated by serum CK or CK MB activity have been reported smaller in diabetic patients compared with non-diabetic patients (14,19). Infarct size estimated by plasma CK and CK MB in diabetic rats has also been suggested smaller than that in non-diabetic rats (15). The result of the present study show that both total CK and CK MB activities are decreased in the diabetic rat heart whereas further studies of CK isoenzyme analysis in the heart from diabetic humans could explain the discrepancy of infarct size as determined by enzymatic and anatomic methods in diabetes mellitus.

Summary

Myocardial isoenzyme activity of creatine kinase (CK) and lactate dehydrogenase (LD) was measured in diabetic rats (4 and 8 weeks after i.v. streptozocin, n=21) and rats injected with isoproterenol (0.25, 0.5 and 1.0 mg/kg/day, 3 weeks, n=20). Age-matched intact animals were the controls (n=8 to 11). Left ventricle/body weight ratio increased in both groups compared with the controls. Total CK and CK MM activity significantly decreased in both groups. CK MB and BB decreased by 62 and 52% in diabetic rats while they increased by 9 and 96% in isoproterenol-treated rats. Thus, CK-B subunit decreased by 61% in diabetic group and increased by 38% in isoproterenol group while CK-M subunit was decreased in both groups. Mitochondrial CK decreased in both groups. Total LD activity increased in diabetics while it was unchanged in isoproterenol group. LD-H subunit increased by 21% in diabetics and decreased by 18% in isoproterenol group. Accordingly, proportion of LD-M, and index of anerobic metabolism, decreased in diabetics and increased in isoproterenol group. Changes in CK-M and CK-B subunits and LD-M proportion in the diabetic heart were normalized by insulin treatment. Increased LD-M proportion and CK-B observed in isoproterenol group may be a metabolic "compensation" to decreased perfusion and substate. Decreased LD-M proportion and CK-B in the diabetic heart was insulin-dependent and may indicate either lack of "compensation" to myocardial ischemia or absence of ischemia per se. Decreased myocardial CK and CK MB activity possibly causes underestimation of infarct size measured by enzymatic methods in the diabetic heart.

Acknowledgement

We thank Mr. Tomoyuki Moriya of the Institute for Laboratory Animal Research for animal care and Miss Keiko Sakai for secretarial help. This study was supported in part by a Grant-in-Aid for General Scientific Research from the Ministry of Education, Science and Culture in Japan (No. 01570481).

References

1. Makino N, Dhalla KS, Elimban V, Dhalla NS. Sarcolemmal Ca^{++} transport in streptozotocin-induced diabetic cardiomyopathy in rats. Am J Physiol 1987;253:E202-7.
2. Tahiliani AG, McNeill JH. Diabetes-induced abnormalities in the myocardium. Life Sci 1986;38:959-74.
3. Witteveen SAGJ, Hemker HC, Hollaar L, Hermens WTH. Quantitation of infarct size in man by means of plasma enzyme levels. Br Heart J 1975;37:936-42.
4. Afzal N, Ganguly PK, Dhalla KS, Pierce GN, Singal PK, Dhalla NS. Beneficial effects of verapamil in diabetic cardiomyopathy. Diabetes 1988;37:936-42.
5. Fleckenstein A, Frey M, Fleckenstein-Grün G. Myocardial and vascular damage by intracellular calcium overload. Preventive actions of calcium antagonists. In: Godfraind T, Vanhoutte PM, Govoni S, Paoletti R, (eds.) Calcium Entry Blockers and Tissue Protection, New York: Raven Press, 1985:91-105.
6. Rona G, Chappel CI, Balazs T, Gaudry R. An infarct-like myocardial lesion and other toxic manifestations produced by isoproterenol in the rat. Arch Pathol 1959;67:443-55.
7. Rosalki SB. An improved procedure for serum creatine phosphokinase determination. J Lab Clin Med 1967;69:696-705.
8. Wroblewski F, LaDue JS. Lactic dehydrogenase activity in blood. Proc Soc Exp Biol Med 1955;90:210-3.
9. Roberts R, Henry PD, Sobel BE. An improved basis for enzymatic estimation of infarct size. Circulation 1975;52:743-54.

10. Ingwall JS. The hypertrophied myocardium accumulates the MB-creatine kinase isozyme. Eur Heart J 1984;5(Suppl. F):129-39.
11. Ingwall JS, Kramer MF, Fifer MA, Lorell BH, Shemin R, Grossman W, Allen PD. The creatine kinase system in normal and diseased human myocardium. N Engl J Med 1985;313:1050-4.
12. Ballo JM, Messer JV. Lactate dehydrogenase isoenzymes in human hearts having decreased oxygen supply. Biochem Biophys Res Commun 1968;33:487-91.
13. Sobel BE, Henry PD, Ehrlich BJ, Bloor CM. Altered Myocardial lactic dehydrogenase isoenzymes in experimental cardiac hypertrophy. Lab Invest 1970;22:23-7.
14. Jaffe AS, Spadaro JJ, Schechtman K, Roberts R, Geltman EM, Sobel BE. Increased congestive heart failure after myocardial infarction of modest extent in patients with diabetes mellitus. Am Heart J 1984;108:31-7.
15. Nadeau A, Tancrede G, Jobidon C, D'amours C, Rousseau-Migneron S. Increased mortality rate in diabetic rats submitted to acute experimental myocardial infarction. Cardiovasc Res 1986;20:171-5.
16. Dawson DM, Goodfriend TL, Kaplan NO. Lactic dehydrogenases: Functions of the two types. Science 1964;143:929-33.
17. Szasz G, Gruber W. Creatine kinase in serum: 4. Differences in substrate affinity among the isoenzymes. Clin Chem 1978;24:245-9.
18. Blasig IE, Zipper J, Muschick P, Modersohn D, Löwe H. Absolute and relative myocardial ischemia by isoproterenol overdosage. Biomed Biochim Acta 1985;44:1641-9.
19 Stone PH, Muller JE, Hartwell T, York BJ, Rutherford JD, Parker CB, Turi ZG, Strauss HW, Willerson JT, Robertson T, Braunwald E, Jaffe AS, the MILIS Study Group. The effect of diabetes mellitus on prognosis and serial left ventricular function after acute myocardial infarction: Contribution of both coronary disease and diastolic left ventricular dysfunction to the adverse prognosis. J Am Coll Cardiol 1989;14:49-57.
20. Vogel WM, Apstein CS. Effects of alloxan-induced diabetes on ischemia-reperfusion injury in rabbit hearts. Circ Res 1988;62:975-82.
21. Rennert G, Saltz-Rennert H, Wanderman K, Weitzman S. Size of acute myocardial infarts in patients with diabetes mellitus. Am J Cardiol 1985;55:1629-30.

In Vivo ^{31}-NMR Spectroscopic Investigation of Myocardial Energy Metabolism in Alloxan-Induced Diabetic Rabbits.

T. Misawa, Y. Kutsumi, H. Tada, S. Hayashi, H. Kato, H. Nishio, K. Toyoda, S. Kim, R. Fujiwara, T. Hayashi, T. Nakai, S. Miyabo

The Third Department of Internal Medicine, Fukui Medical School, Fukui, JAPAN.

Introduction

It is widely recognized that diabetic patients are more prone to cardiovascular disease with myocardial infarction and congestive heart failure than the general population (1). Also, it is commonly believed that the diabetic myocardium is more sensitive to ischemia than the normal myocardium. To investigate whether it is due to abnormal diabetic metabolism of high energy phosphates (HEP), we measured the change of HEP and mechanical function during regional ischemia and reperfusion of diabetic and normal rabbit hearts.

Previous studies on diabetic myocardial HEP in intact animals have been performed by obtaining biopsy tissue samples, which has obvious disadvantages for the stabililty of the animal preparation and for rapid sequential correlations with regional myocardial blood flow and function. The use of in vivo P-31 nuclear magnetic resonance spectroscopy (^{31}P-MRS) for determining myocardial HEP stores overcomes these disadvantages.

In the present study, we measured serial change of HEP during ischemia and reperfusion in alloxan-induced diabetic hearts in the open chest anesthetized rabbit model by using NMRS with surface coil, gated by respiration and LV pressure.

Methods

Animal Model: Diabetes was induced in male New Zealand rabbits (2.0~3.0kg) by slow intravenous bolus injection of 80 mg/kg alloxan (2). Rabbits were housed with ad libitum access to normal lab chow and water. Animals (n=6) were used for experiments at 6-10 weeks. Animals were included in the diabetic group if mean weekly non-fasting blood glucose was greater than 250 mg/dl. On the day of the experiment, serum acetoacetate and ß-hydroxybutyrate were measured. The normal comparison group (n=6) consisted of age-matched animals, one not given alloxan and the other with an equal number that were given alloxan but were normoglycemic (blood glucose<125 mg/dl).

Preparation: Rabbits were anesthetized with intravenous sodium pentobarbital (20 mg/kg). Anesthesia was maintained during experiment with intermittent intraperitoneal sodium pentobarbital. A 4F catheter was placed in left ventricle through the carotid artery. This catheter was connected to a Spectramed Disposable Transducer kit T4812AD-R (Spectramed Medical Products, Singapore) for continuous measurement of pressure and heart rate on Polygraph System RM6200 (Nihon Koden Kogyo, Japan). It could be used for arterial blood sampling, too. The trachea was then isolated, and animals were intubated via tracheostomy. Rabbits were then ventilated via a rodent ventilator on 100% oxygen. The animals then underwent a left lateral thoracotomy through the fifth intercostal space. The heart was suspended in a pericardial cradle. The large marginal branch of the left circumflex coronary artery, which runs subepicardially, was identified. A 5-0 suture was then placed through the myocardium underneath this artery slightly distal to the atrioventricular groove. The suture was then completed with a polyethylene tube, which served as a reversible snare occluder. To identify the anatomic region at risk, hearts were isolated and perfused with dye (Monostral blue) after ligation of the coronary artery at the previous site of occlusion.

NMR Spectroscopy: Phosphorus-31 spectra were acquired using a Otsuka Electrics 2.0 tesla nuclear magnetic resonance spectrometer (BEM 250/80). A 2.0 mm diameter, two-turn surface coil was positioned over the surface of the left ventricle. This coil was tuned with the external tuning circuit to 35.3 MHz, the phosphorus resonant frequency at this field strength. Local magnetic field homogeneity was optimized by shimming on the proton signal, yielding water line widths between 0.5 and 0.8 ppm. Phosphorus spectra were obtained using a single 90° pulse having a pulse width of 45 us and an interpulse delay of 2 seconds. To improve the signal to noise ratio, data acquisition was gated to the onset of inspiration and upslope of LV pressure. Sixty free induction decays were summed for each measurement. A hexamethyl phosphoramide (HMPA) external standard was placed in the center of the surface coil. To assess the ischemia and reperfusion-induced changes in pH_i, the chemical

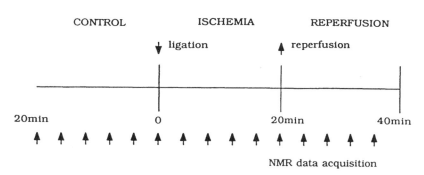

Figure 1. Experimental protocol.

shift of the pH-dependent Pi peak (∂o) relative to the pH-independent PCr peak was determined. Intracellular pHi was then calculated from the chemical shift data and Pi titration curve by the following equation:

$$pH_i = pk - \log 10(\partial o - \partial B)/(\partial A - \partial o)$$

where $\partial A = 3.290$, $\partial B = 5.805$, and $pK = 6.90(3)$.

Experimental Protocol

Figure 1 shows the protocol of experiments. Hemodynamic parameters (left ventricular pressure and heart rate) and arterial blood gases were monitored during the surgical preparation and throughout the experiment. Following acquisition of control spectra (600 spectra), the LCX was occluded for 20 minutes and reperfused for at least 20 minutes. High grade ventricular arrhythmias were treated with lidocaine (20 mg intravenously). Two control rabbits and 2 diabetic rabbits expired before the occlusion period.

Statistical Comparisons

Data are presented as mean ±95% confidence limits. Results are compared using Student's t-test. A p value <0.05 was considered significant. Statistical analysis was done by means of a commercially available statistics program on a Macintosh SE microcomputer (Apple Computer, Inc, Calif.).

Table 1. Characterization of Diabetic State in Rabbits

Variable	Normal	Diabetic
Blood glucose (mg/dl)	115 ± 7.5	415.7 ± 37.6†
Plasma acetoacetate (uM)	24.3 ± 3.8	51.1 ± 3.9†
Plasma ß-hydroxybutyrate (uM)	51.6 ± 12.6	158.0 ± 4.4†
IRI (uU.ml)	18.4 ± 4.0	6.4 ± 0.6†
Body weight (kg)	3.4 ± 0.3	2.7 ± 0.2

† Significant difference compared with normal rabbit by Student's t-test.
Values are means ± SEM.

Results

Characterization of Diabetic State: With the model of alloxan-induced diabetes used, it was possible to produce diabetes for 6-10 weeks in most of our rabbits. Overt diabetes ensued within 1-2 days after injection of alloxan, as manifested by increase in food and water uptake and increase in urine excretion associated with glycosuria. Some diabetic animals showed severe dehydration and died within one week after the onset of diabetes.

Characteristics of normal and diabetic animals used in the isolated heart experiments are shown in Table 1. The mean body weight of control and diabetic rabbits after 6-10 weeks was 3.4±0.3 and 2.7±0.2, respectively.
Blood glucose, plasma acetoacetate and ß-hydroxybutyrate were significantly elevated in the diabetic animals. By contrast, there was a decrease in serum insulin. Hemodynamic changes during ischemia followed by reperfusion in control and diabetic rabbits.

Before the onset of ischemia, left ventricular systolic pressure was 75.0±9.6 vs 56.2±5.1 mmHg in control and diabetic groups, respectively. During ischemia and reperfusion, LV systolic pressure tended to be high but not significantly in diabetic compared to control rabbits (Fig. 2A). Heart rate was 273.8±11.6 vs 236.6±4.2 beats/min in control and diabetic groups, respectively, before ischemia. Heart rate during ischemia and reperfusion had a tendency to decrease, but not significantly in diabetic compared to control rabbits (Fig. 2B). Rate pressure product (RPP) was 24012±2460 vs 13286±1167

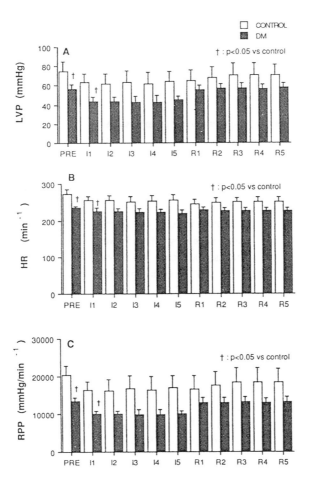

Figure 2. Hemodynamic changes during ischemia followed by reperfusion. Before the onset of ischemia, left ventricular systolic pressure was 75.0 ± 9.6 vs 56.2 ± 5.1 mmHg in control and diabetic groups, respectively. During ischemia and reperfusion. LV systolic pressure (LVP) tended to be high, but not significantly in diabetic compared to control rabbits (Fig. 2A). Heart rate (HR) was 273.8 ± 11.6 vs 236.6 ± 4.2 beats/min in control and diabetic groups, respectively, before ischemia. HR during ischemia and reperfusion tended to decrease, but not significantly in diabetic compared to control rabbits (Fig. 2B). Rate pressure product (RPP) was 20412 ± 2460 vs 13286 ± 1167 mmHg/min in control and diabetic groups, respectively. In early ischemic phase, RPP was small in diabetic compared to control rabbits (9932 ± 900 vs 16458 ± 2192 mmHg/min. $p<0.05$, respectively). During reperfusion, RPP was smaller in diabetic than in control rabbits but statistically not significant (Fig. 2C). Values are means ± SEM. †$p<0.05$ compared with control rabbits. *$p<0.05$ compared with pre-ischemic state.

mmHg/min in control and diabetic groups, respectively. In the early ischemic phase, RPP was small in diabetic compared to control rabbits (9932±90 vs 6458±2192 mmHg/min, p<0.05, respectively) (Fig. 2C). In diabetic groups, RPP was smaller than pre-ischemic value until early reperfusion but statistically not significant.

Metabolic Changes During Ischemia and Reperfusion

High energy phosphate metabolites: Representative results of ^{31}P-MRS obtained from the left ventricular myocardium during pre-ischemic, ischemia and reperfusion periods of control group are shown in Fig. 3.
Phosphocreatinine, Pi and ATP levels were not significantly different between control and diabetic hearts under pre-ischemic condition (Fig. 4). Control hearts had reduced levels of PCr in early ischemia, and diabetic had reduced in late ischemia (Fig. 5A). Recovery of PCr was higher in diabetic hearts when compared to control hearts, but this difference did not reach statistical significance. The changes of ATP levels did not occur during ischemia and reperfusion in both groups (Fig. 5B). Inorganic phosphate (Pi) in diabetic was higher than in control during ischemia and reperfusion. In early ischemia Pi level in diabetic was 146 ± 35.1% of pre-ischemic value (p<0.05) (Fig. 5C). The phosphorylation potential is an important measure of the energy status of the cell and can be used to determine the adequacy of energy reserves for vital cell functions. The PCr/Pi ratio has been suggested to be closely related to the ATP/ADP ratio (4,5). Figure 6 shows a significant decrease in PCr/Pi ratio in diabetic heart during ischemia and poor recovery in diabetic during reperfusion. The intracellular pH was significantly lower during ischemia and reperfusion in both groups (Fig. 7).

Risk area after coronary occlusion

Risk area of diabetic rabbits was similar to that of control rabbits (Table 2). Body weight and left ventricular weight were smaller in diabetic than in control rabbits though significantly.

Discussion

The rabbit is an appropriate animal for this study because diabetes does not accelerate atherogenesis in rabbits fed on a normal diet. Also, because the rabbit possesses characteristics desirable in laboratory model including reasonable size and long life, it is an interesting model for the longitudinal

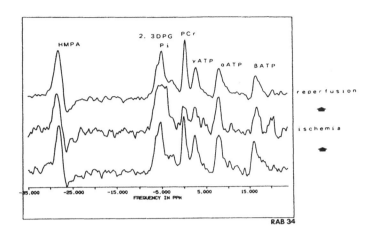

Figure 3. A typical series of P-31 NMR spectroscopy obtained from the left ventricular myocardium during pre-ischemic, ischemia and reperfusion periods of control group. Peak assignments: HMPA, Hexamethylphosphoric triamide; 2,3DPG, 2,3-diphosphoglycerate; Pi, inorganic phosphate; a, ß, r - AATP, resonances of each of the three phosphates of the ATP molecule.

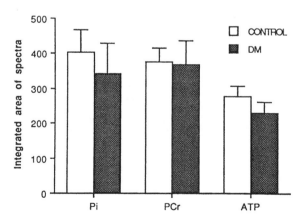

Figure 4. High energy phosphate contents in non-ischemic hearts. Phosphocreatinine, Pi and ATP levels were not significantly different between control and diabetic hearts under pre-ischemic condition. Values indicated integrated areas for that peak in absolute units. Values are means ± SEM.

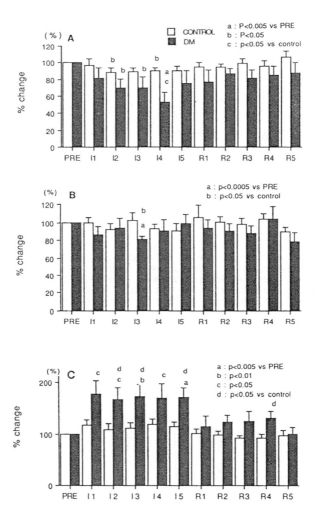

Figure 5. The changes of PCr during ischemia and reperfusion. Control hearts had reduced levels of PCr in early ischemia and diabetic had reduced levels in late ischemia (Figure 5A). Recovery of PCr was smaller in diabetic hearts when compared to control hearts, but this difference did not reach statistical significance. Figure 5B. The changes of ATP during ischemia and reperfusion. The changes of ATP levels did not vary during ischemia and reperfusion in both groups. Figure 5C. The changes of Pi during ischemia and reperfusion. Inorganic phosphate (Pi) in diabetic was higher than in control during ischemia and reperfusion. In early ischemia Pi level in diabetic was 178 ± 61.7% of pre-ischemic value ($p<0.05$). Values are means ± SEM.

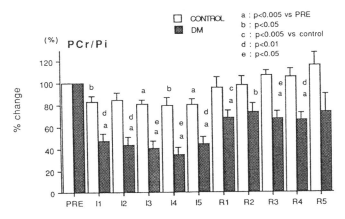

Figure 6. The changes of PCr/Pi during ischemia and reperfusion. The PCr/Pi ratio has been, suggested to be closely related to the ATP/ADP ratio. It shows a significant decrease in PCr/Pi ratio in diabetic heart during ischemia and poor recovery in diabetic during reperfusion. Values are means ± SEM.

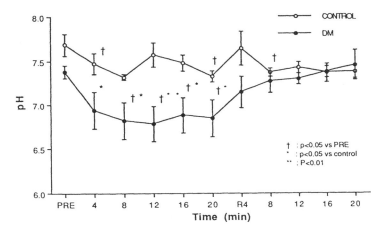

Figure 7. Intracellular pH was measured using chemical shift of intracellular Pi. Diabetic rabbits showed marked decrease in pH during ischemia. Values are means ± SEM.

Table 2. Coronary Occlusion in Intact Rabbits

Variable	Normal	Diabetic
Body weight (kg)	2.9 ± 0.2	2.8 ± 0.2
Left ventricular weight (g)	4.36 ± 0.26	3.84 ± 0.17
risk region (g)	1.76 ± 0.06	1.67 ± 0.25
% risk region (%)	44.3 ± 1.84	43.2 ± 4.93

Values are means ± SEM.

study of the effect of diabetes on atherosclerosis (6). Furthermore, rabbit heart size was appropriate for 20 mm surface coil with 30 mm bore magnet size. The recent advances in the application of ^{31}P-MRS to intact living cells and perfused organ systems in several laboratories has demonstrated its value in following details of metabolism of phosphate-containing molecules. ^{31}P-MRS has been used to observe high energy phosphate metabolism in heart in living rate (7), living rabbit (8), pig (9,10), dog (11) and perfused rabbit heart (12,13). The phosphorylation potential is an important measure of the energy status of the cell and can be used to determine the adequacy of energy reserves for vital cell functions. A reduction of PCr/Pi reflects an impairment in oxidative metabolism of the myocardium.

Diabetic myocardium has more frequent congestive heart failure than normal myocardium independent of any vascular disease in ischemia and reperfusion. It is suggested that this is due to a reduced Ca^{++} ATPase (14,15), an increase in free radical production (16) and intracellular acidosis (17, 18), changes of contractile proteins (19) and an increase in concentration of free fatty acids (20). The energy production and utilization may be a factor for it (21,22). In Vogel et al (23), HEP were decreased to the same extent in normal and diabetic rabbit. In terms of the use of HEP for maintaining cellular functions during ischemia this discrepancy may exist because measurements of nucleotide concentrations do not reflect either extent of ATP utilization or synthesis (24). Glycogenolysis during ischemia is the major H^+ and lactate may cause failure of functional recovery (25). The poor prognosis for myocardial infarction in diabetic patient without acidosis may not be related to a myocardial defect that increased sensitivity to ischemia but rather to other factors, such as pre-existing cardiomyopathy, impaired infarct healing, or increased severity of coronary artery disease. Although in the clinical setting many diabetic patients have mild ketosis, we cannot neglect this ketotic effect.

Limitation

First, the closer relation between high energy phosphates and sub-endocardial compared with sub-epicardial blood flow are, in part, a function of the NMR acquisition parameters. Metabolism in the sub-endocardium should be more sensitive to coronary stenosis.

Secondly, the actual volume and location of tissue contributing to the spectra could not be precisely defined using a surface coil. While use of an open-chest preparation eliminated the problem of contamination by non-cardiac tissues, potential contamination by signal from non-ischemic tissue remained a concern. This was avoided by placing a small surface coil in the center of a large ischemic region. Furthermore, the effect of contamination by signal from non-ischemic tissue would have been to underestimate the degree of metabolic abnormality during ischemia and thus diminish the observed metabolic changes.

Thirdly, the resonance in the PME region due to 2,3-DPG made the measurement of Pi intensity and chemical shift difficult under control conditions. Katz et al. (26) reported a small contribution from 2,3-DPG and phosphodiesters in the blood could be detected.

Summary

These findings suggest that abnormal HEP metabolism cannot all explain diabetic myocardial mechanical impairment induced by ischemia in the open chest rabbits. Reduced intracellular pH in the ischemic diabetic myocardium is more closely related to mechanical function than abnormalities of HEP metabolism.

References

1. Kannel WB, Hjortland M, Castelli WP: Role of diabetes in congestive heart failure: The Framingham Study. Am J Cardiol 34:29-34;1974.
2. Bhimji S, Godin VD, McNeill JH: Biochemical and functional changes in hearts from rabbits with diabetes. Diabetologia 28:452-7;1985.

3. Flaherty JT, Weisfeldt ML, Bulkley BH, Gardner TJ, Gott VL, Jacobus WE: Mechanism of ischemic myocardial cell damage assessed by phosphorus-31 nuclear magnetic resonance. Circulation 65:561-570;1982.
4. Ambrosio G, Jacobus WE, Bergman CA, Weisman HF, Becker LC: Preserved high energy phosphate metabolic reserve in grobally "stunned" hearts despite reduction of basal ATP content and contractility. J Mol Cell Cardiol 19:953-64;1987.
5. Chance B, Eleff S, Leigh JS, Sokolow D, Sapega A: Mitochondrial regulation of phosphocreatine/inorganic phosphate ratios in exercising human muscles: A gated P^{31}-NMR study. Proc Natl Acad USA 11:6714-6718;1981.
6. Zhao ZH, Watschinger B, Brown CD, Beyer MM, Friedman EA: Variations of susceptibility to alloxan induced diabetes in the rabbit. Horm Metabol Res 19:534-7;1987.
7. Bittle JA, Balschi JA, Ingwall JS: Contractile failure and high-energy phosphate turnover during hypoxia:P^{31}-NMR surface coil studies in living rat. Circ Res 60:871-8;1987.
8. Kavanaugh KM, Aisen AM, Fechner KP, Chenevert TL, Dunham WR, Buda AJ, Arbor A: Regional metabolism during coronary occlusion, reperfusion, and reocclusion using phosphorus-31 nuclear magnetic resonance spectroscopy in the intact rabbit. Am Heart J 117:53-9;1989.
9. Camacho SA, Lanzer P, Toy BJ, Gober J, Valenza M, Botvinick EH, Weiner MW: In vivo alternations of high-energy phosphates and intracellular pH during reversible ischemia in pigs: A ^{31}P magnetic resonance spectroscopy study. Am Heart J 116:701-8;1988.
10. Schaefer S, Camacho A, Gober J, Obregon RG, DeGroot MA, Botvinik EH, Massie B, Weiner MW: Response of myocardial metabolites to graded regional ischemia: P^{31} NMR spectroscopy of pocine myocardium in vivo. Circ Res 64:968-976;1989.
11. Guth BD, Martin JF, Heusch G, Ross J: Regional myocardial blood flow, function and metabolism using P^{31} nuclear magnetic resonance spectroscopy during ischemia and reperfusion in dogs: J Am Coll Cardiol 10:673-81;1987.
12. Freeman D, Mayr H, Schmidt P, Roberts JD, Bing RJ: Advantages of perfluorochemical perfusion in the isolated working rabbit heart preparation using P^{31}-NMR. Biochemica et Biophysica Acta 927:350-358;1987.

13. Gard JK, Kichura GM, Ackerman JJH, Eisenberg JD, Billadello JJ, Sobel BE, Gross RW: Quantitative P^{31} nuclear magnetic resonance analysis of metabolite concentrations in langendorff-perfused rabbit hearts. Biophys J 48:803-13;1985.
14. Fein FS, Kornstein LB, Strobeck JE, Capasso JM, Sonnenblick EH: Altered myocardial mechanics in diabetic rats. Circ Res 47:922-33;1980.
15. Fein FS, Green BM, Zola B, Sonnenblick EH: Reversibility of diabetic cardiomyopathy with insulin in rabbits. Am J Physiol 250:H108-13;1986.
16. Pieper GM: Superoxide dismutase plus catalase improves post-ischaemic recovery in the diabetic heart. Cardiovasc Res 22:916-26;1988.
17. Pieper GM: Functional and metabolic stunning of the isolated diabetic heart. Fed Proc 46:1259;1987.
18. Kupriyanov VV, Lakomkin VL, Steinschneider AY, Severina MY, Kapelko VI, Ruuge EK, Saks VA: Relationships between pre-ischemic recovery of rat heart. J Mol Cell Cardiol 20:1151-62;1988.
19. Schaffer SW, Mozaffari MS, Artman M, Willson GL: Basis for myocardial mechanical defects associated with non-insulin dependent diabetes. Am J Physiol 256:E25-30;1989.
20. Pieper GM, Salhany JM, Murray WJ, Wu ST, Eliot RS: Abnormal phosphocreatine metabolism in perfused diabetic hearts. Biochem J 210:477-81;1983.
21. Allison TB, Bruttig SP, Class MF, Eliot RS, Shipp JC: Reduced high-energy phosphate levels in rat hearts. 1. Effects of alloxan diabetes. Am J Physiology 230:1744-50;1976.
22. Malloy CR, Matthews PM, Smith MB, Radda GK: Influence of propranolol on acidosis and high energy phosphates in ischemic myocardium of the rabbit. Cardiovascular Research 20:710-20;1986.
23. Vogel WM, Apstein CS: Effects of alloxan-induced diabetes on ischemia-reperfusion injury in rabbit hearts. Circ Res 62:975-82;1988.
24. Lewandowski ED, Devous MD, Nunnally RL: High-energy phosphates and function in isolated, working rabbit hearts. Am J Physiol 253:H1215-23;1987.
25. Nayler WG: Protection of the myocardium against post-ischemic reperfusion damage. J Thorac Cardiovasc Surg 84:897-905,1982.
26. Katz LA, Swain JA, Portman MA, Balaban RS: Intracellular pH and inorganic phosphate content of heart in vivo: a P^{31}-NMR study. Am J Physiol 255:H189-96;1988.

Characterization of Beta-Adrenoceptors in Sinoatrial Node and Left Ventricular Myocardium of Diabetic Rat Hearts by Quantitative Autoradiography

K. Saito[1], A. Kuroda[2], H. Tanaka[2]

Health Service Center of National Institute of Fitness and Sports in Kanoya, JAPAN[1]. First Department of Internal Medicine of Faculty of Medicine, Kagoshima University, Kagoshima, JAPAN[2].

Introduction

Although it has been reported that the response of catecholamines to myocardial contractility and heart rate are reduced in diabetic animals (1-6), very little is known about the beta-adrenoceptors in the conduction system of diabetic animals (7). We characterized beta-adrenoceptors in sinoatrial node (SA) and left ventricle of diabetic rat hearts by quantitiative autoradiography.

Methods

Male Wistar rats weighing approximately 150g were randomly separated into control and diabetic groups. Diabetic groups received an intravenous injection of 0.1M citrate-buffered streptozotocin (STZ) at a dosage of 65 mg/Kg body weight. Control animals received a similar injection of vehicle alone. These animals were kept for 3 weeks under normal laboratory conditions with access to water and rat chow ad libitum and then sacrificed by decapitation at 9:00-11:00 AM after overnight fasting. Fasting blood glucose was measured by the glucose oxidase method and the value of blood sugar level of over 300 mg/dl was taken as a criteria of diabetes.

The SA node was dissected according to previous report (8). After opening the chest, we held up the right atrial appendage and cut out right atrium, including the junctional area to the superior vena cava. After that, the heart was immediately removed and a horizontal cut was made to separate the atria and proximal end of both ventricles from the rest of the heart. The

Nagano, M., Mochizuki, S., Dhalla, N.S. (eds.), CARDIOVASCULAR DISEASE IN DIABETES. Copyright © 1992. Kluwer Academic Publishers, Boston. All rights reserved.

dissected right atria, and the distal portion of the heart including the right and the left ventricle were frozen quickly by immersion in isopentane at -30°C, and stored not longer than 1 week at -70°C. Frozen, 16 um-thick sections were cut in a cryostat at -20°C. Sections containing the sinoatrial node were identified by staining with Karnovsky's solution to detect cholinesterase activity (9). Adjacent unstained sections containinig the SA node were thaw-mounted onto gelatin-coated glass slides and placed under vacuum at 4°C for no longer than 24 hrs prior to incubation. Sections were pre-incubated for 15 min at room temerature in 170 mM Tris-HCl buffer, pH 7.6, containing 10 uM phenylmethylsufonyl fluoride, 0.5 mM $MgCl_2$ and 0.01% ascorbate. To determine the total number of beta-adrenoceptors from the heart of 5 diabetic and 5 control rats, we labelled tissue sections in vitro by incubation for 150 min at room temperature in fresh buffer containing 400 pM ^{125}I iodocyanopindolol (spec. act. 2050 Ci/mmol, Amersham, Arlington Hgts, IL). This ligand concentration saturates beta-adrenoceptors in several peripheral tissues including the heart AV node (10,11,14). Non-specific binding was measured by incubating alternate sections under the same conditions with addition of 1 uM (-)-propranolol (ICI, Macclesfield, U.K.).

The percentages of beta-1-and beta-2-adrenoceptors were measured in alternate tissue sections from 5 individual rats incubated with 50 pM of ^{125}I iodocyanopindolol (CYP), with or without 100 nM CGP20712A for beta-1-over beta-2-adrenoceptors is approximately 10,000-fold and the use of 100 nM CGP20712A is sufficient for the estimation of the percentage of beta-1- and beta-2-adrenoceptors in membrane preparations (12) and by autoradiography (8,13-15). In each case, incubations were performed in parallel adjacent sections for total binding (incubated with 50 pM ^{125}I-CYP + 100 nM CGP20712A).

After incubation, the sections were rinsed in 170 mM Tris HCl buffer, pH 7.6, followed by two washes of 15 min each in the same buffer and a 30 sec rinse in cold distilled water. The sections were then dried under a cold stream of air, placed in x-ray cassettes together with ^{125}I-standards and opposed to Ultrofilm (LKB Industries, Rockville, MD) for 1 or 2 days. The films were then processed as described earlier (8,11,14,15). Optical densities on the areas corresponding to the SA node and left ventricle and ^{125}I-standards were quantified by computerized microdensitometry and binding data were calculated interpolation in the standard curve (8,11,14,15).

Specific binding of ^{125}I CYP to beta-1-adrenoceptors was defined as the difference between total and nonspecific + beta-2-adrenoceptor binding. Specific beta-2- adrenoceptor biinding was obtained by subtraction (8,13-15).

Results

Three weeks after STZ injection, diabetic rats showed significantly lower body weight and heart weight and higher blood glucose level (Table 1).

The SA node was localized between right atrium and superior vena cava and was stained heavily for acetylcholinesterase (Fig 1A). We measured the optical density that corresponded to beta-adrenoceptor binding in the heavily stained area surrounding SA node artery (Fig 1B).

Incubation of tissue section with 400 pM ^{125}I CYP demonstrated a high concentration of binding sites in the SA node in both of control and diabetic rats with relatively lower concentration in right atrium. However, the concentrations of ^{125}I CYP binding site in the SA node of diabetic rats (Fig B right) were lower than control rats (Fig 1B left).

The concentrations of 400 pM ^{125}I CYP binding sites in the left ventricle of diabetic rats were also lower than control rats (Table 2).

Incubation of adjacent tissue sections with 50 pM ^{125}I CYP with or without 100 nM CGP20712A, revealed that this beta-1-selective antagonist displaced about 65% of total number of binding sites in control (Fig 2(b) left) and 40% in diabetic rat (Fig 2(b) right). The mean value of proportion of beta-1/beta-2 in SA node and left ventricle were shown in Table 3. The SA node of control rats contained a higher proportion of beta-2-adrenoceptors than the left ventricle. This result confirms with previous report (8).

However, the SA node of diabetic rats contained lower proportion of beta-1-adrenoceptors than control rats. These findings indicate that reduction in beta-adrenoceptors of left ventricle and SA node of diabetic rats are mainly due to a decrease of beta-1-subtype.

Discussion

We demonstrated about 25% decrease in the ^{125}I CYP binding sites on the SA node and left ventricle isolated from the 3-wk-diabetic rats. Several researchers have demonstrated a significant decrease (20-50%) in beta-adrenoceptors of the diabetic rat hearts with no change in affinity (4,16-19). Our results of left ventricle confirm with their data. Savarese and Berkowitz

Table 1. General characteristics of experimental animals.

	Body Weight (g)	Heart Weight (g)	HW/BW (%)	Blood Sugar (mg/dl)
Control	315 ± 4	1.24 ± 0.04	0.39 ± 0.01	127 ± 5
Diabetes	186 ± 14*	0.76 ± 0.06*	0.41 ± 0.02	353 ± 9*

Values are mean ± S.E.M. for each of 5 rats.
* significantly (p<0.01) different from control.

Table 2. Beta-adrenoceptors in sinoatrial node and left ventricle of diabetic and control rats.

	400 pM ^{125}I CYP binding (fmol/mg protein)	
	SA Node	Left Ventricle
Control	96.0 ± 7.0	58.4 ± 3.4
DM	71.6 ± 2.6*	43.2 ± 2.2*

Values are mean ± S.E.M. for each of 5 rats.
* significantly (p<0.05) different from control.

(16) first reported a 28% decrease in ventricular beta-adrenoceptor number to accompany a 24% decrease in heart rate for the diabetic animals and suggested that a decrease in beta-adrenoceptors plays an important role in bradycardia of diabetic animals. In this study, we have demonstrated a significant decrease of beta-adrenoceptor number, especially beta-1-subtypes, in the SA node of diabetic rats. Our results support their hypothesis. The mechanism that causes beta-adrenoceptors decrease in diabetic rat heart, however, has been controversial. Several studies reported that the decrease in beta-adrenoceptors in diabetic heart could be explained by the secondary effects of the diabetic condition, such as increase in plasma catecholamine level, decrease in the plasma T_3 level and impaired body weight gain (16,18). However, several researchers recently reported that hypothyroidism and non-specific abnormalities of protein synthesis were not the primary causative

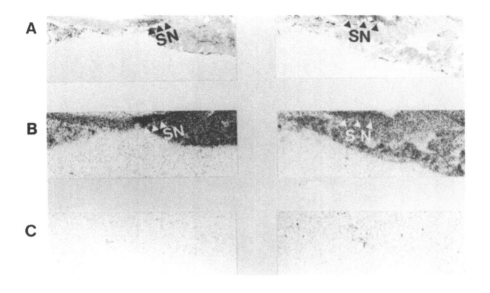

Figure 1. Autoradiographic localization of beta-adrenoceptor binding site in the sinoatrial node of a control (left) and a diabetic rat (right).
A: sections containing sinoatrial node were stained with Karnovsky's solution to detect the presence of acetylcholinesterase.
B: adjacent sections to A were incubated with 400 pM ^{125}I iodocyanopindolol.
C: adjacent sections to B were incubated with 400 pM ^{125}I iodocyanopindolol in the presence of 1 /uM (-)-propranolol. Calibration bar = 1 mm.

factor of decreasing beta-adrenoceptors in diabetic hearts (4,17,19,20). The decrease of beta-adrenoceptors in diabetic hearts may be explained by a 'down-regulation' and increased membrane lipid content (4). Alterations of cardiac automaticity, ultrastructure and enzyme activities have been also reported in the conduction system as well as working myocardium in diabetic animals (21,22). Our result showing a decrease in beta-adrenoceptors in SA node of diabetic heart may confirm with their results.

Summary

In this study, we demonstrated that the number of beta-adrenoceptors, mainly beta-1-subtype, were decreased in the SA node as well as left ventricle of diabetic rat hearts. These findings may lead to a better understanding in reduced response of catecholamines to myocardial contractility and heart rate in diabetic animals.

Table 3. Quantitative characterization of beta-adrenoceptor in the SA node and left ventricle of control and diabetic rats.

	SA node				Left Ventricle			
	beta-1	beta-2	total	beta-1/beta-2 (%)	beta-1	beta-2	total	beta-1/beta-2 (%)
Control	23.5 ± 1.4	22.8 ± 2.4	46.3 ± 3.1	51 ± 3/49 ±3	19.1 ± 2.2	10.6 ± 1.0	29.7 ± 2.4	64 ± 4/36 ± 4
DM	11.6 ± 0.9	24.1 ± 1.9	35.8 ± 2.6	33 ± 2/67 ± 2	9.8 ± 1.1	10.5 ± 0.5	20.2 ± 0.7	48 ± 4/52 ± 4
P	<0.01	NS	<0.05	<0.05	<0.05	NS	<0.05	<0.05

50 pM ^{125}I iodocyanopindolol binding (fmole/mg protein)

Values are mean ± S.E.M. for each of 5 rats.

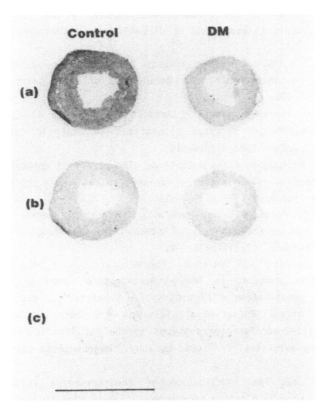

Figure 2. Autoradiographic localization of beta-adrenoceptor binding site in a rat heart.
A: were incubated as described in METHODS in the presence of 50 pM ^{125}I iodocyanopindolol.
B: adjacent sections to (a) were incubated with 50 pM ^{125}I iodocyanopindolol in the presence of 100 nM CGP 20712A.
C: adjacent sections to (B) were incubated 50 pM ^{125}I iodocyanopindolol in the presence of 1 uM (-)-propranolol. Calibration bar indicate 1 cm.

Acknowledgement

The authors thank Miss Hiromi Takada for her editorial assistance.

References

1. Foy JM and Lucas PD. Effect of experimental diabetes, food deprivation and genetic obesity on the sensitivity of pithed rats to autonomic agents. Br J Pharmacol 1976:57:229-234.

2. Fein FS, Kornstein LB, Strobeck JE, Capasso JM and Sonnenblick EH. Altered myocardial mechanics in diabetic rats. Circ Res 1980;47:922-933.
3. Penpargkul S, Schaible T, Yipintsoi T and Scheuer J. The effect of diabetes on performance and metabolism of rat hearts. Circ Res 1980;47:911-921.
4. Heyliger C, Pierce G, Singal P, Beamish R and Dhalla N. Cardiac alpha- and beta-adrenergic receptor alterations in diabetic cardiomyopathy. Basic Res Cardiol 1982;77:610-618.
5. Vadlamudi R, Rodgers R and McNeill J. The effect of chronic alloxan and streptozotocin-induced diabetes on isolated rat heart performance. Can J Physiol Pharmacol 1982;60:902-911.
6. Sunagawa R, Murakami K and Mimura G. Effects of adrenergic drugs on isolated and perfused hearts of streptozotocin-induced diabetic rats. Japan J Pharmacol 1987;44:233-240.
7. Saito K, Kuroda A and Tanaka H. Characterization of beta-1 and beta-2-adrenoceptor subtypes in the atrioventricular node of diabetic rat hearts by quantitative autoradiography. Submitted for publication.
8. Saito K, Torda T, Potter WZ and Saavedra JM. Characterization of beta-1- and beta-2-adrenoceptor subtypes in the rat sinoatrial and stellate ganglia by quantitative autoradiography. Neuroscience Lett 1989;96:35-41.
9. Karnovsky MJ. The localization of cholinesterase activity in rat cardiac muscle by electron microscopy. J Cell Biol 1964;23:217-223.
10. Lipe S and Summers RJ. Autoradiographic analysis of the distribution of beta-adrenoceptors in the dog splenic vasculature. Br J Pharmac 1986;87:603-609.
11. Saito K, Kurihara M, Cruciani R, Potter WZ and Saavedra JM. Characterization beta$_1$- and beta$_2$-adrenoceptor subtypes in the rat atrioventricular node by quantitative autoradiography. Cir Res 1988;62:173-177.
12. Dooley DJ, Bittiger H and Reymann NC CGP 20712 A: a useful tool for quantitating beta$_1$- and beta$_2$-adrenoceptors. Eur J Pharmacol 1986;130:137-139.
13. Molennar P, Canale E and Summers RJ. Autoradiographic localization of beta-1 and beta-2 adrenoceptors in guinea pig atrium and regions of the conducting system. J Pharmacol Exp Ther 1987;241:1048-1064.

14. Saito K, Potter WZ and Saavedra JM. Quantitative autoradiography of beta-adrenoceptors in the cardiac vagus ganglia of the rat. Eur J Pharmacol 1988;153:289-293.
15. Pinto JEB, Nazarali AJ, Torda T and Saavedra JM. Autoradiographic characterization of beta-adrenoceptors in rat heart valve leaflets. Am J Physiol 1989;256:H821-827.
16. Savarese JJ and Berkowitz BA. Beta-adrenergic receptor decrease in diabetic rat hearts. Life Sci 1979;25:2075-2078.
17. Williams RS, Schaible TF, Scheuer J and Kennedy R. Effects of experimental diabetes of adrenergic and cholinergic receptors of rat myocardium. Diabetes 1983;32:881-886.
18. Sundaresan PR, Sharma VK, Gingold SI and Banerjee SP. Decreased beta-adrenergic receptors in rat streptozotocin-induced diabetes: Role of thyroid hormone. Endocrinology 1984;114:1358-1363.
19. Atkins FL, Dowell RT and Love S. Beta-adrenergic receptors, adenylate cyclase activity and cardiac dysfunction in the diabetic rat. J Cardiovasc Pharmacol 1985;7:66-70.
20. Nishio Y, Kashiwagi A, Kida Y, Kodama M, Abe N, Saeki Y and Shigeta Y. Deficiency of cardiac beta-adrenergic receptor in streptozotocin-induced diabetic rats. Diabetes 1988;1181-1187.
21. Senges J, Brachmann J, Pelzer D, Hasslacher C, Weiher E and Kubler W. Altered cardiac automaticity and conduction in experimental diabetes mellitus. J Mol Cell Cardiol 1980;12:1341-1351.
22. Kuroda A, Saito K and Tanaka H. Histochemical studies of conduction system of diabetic rat hearts. Arch Histol Cytol. In press.

Effects of Zinc Deficiency on Heart Catecholamine Concentrations in Normal and Diabetic Rats

H. Fushimi, S. Ishihara, M. Kameyama, T. Minami[1] and Y. Okazaki[1]

Department of Medicine and Laboratory of Sumitomo Hospital,
[1]Department of Pharmacology, Kinki University, Osaka, JAPAN

Introduction

The mechanism of the diabetic autonomic neuropathy, a life threatening complication especially in heart, is not known. We have reported that plasma epinephrine and norepinephrine response to stress is decreased in a time-dependent manner in streptozotocin Wistar male diabetic rats (1), while tissue catecholamine concentrations are increased until 6 weeks of diabetes and then declined (Fig. 1). These results have suggested failure of catecholamine secretion as one of the causes of diabetic autonomic neuropathy. Urinary zinc excretion is markedly increased in diabetic patients and rats. It is also true in urine of diabetic rats on zinc deficiency diets (3). Therefore, in this paper, we studied the effects of zinc deficiency on catecholamine concentrations of plasma, kidney and heart of diabetic rats.

Material and Methods

Wistar male rats, 7 weeks old, were made diabetic by injecting streptozotocin 80 mg/kg body weight into the tail vein and fed standard laboratory chow (5.2 g/100g) or zinc deficiency diet (1.6 mg zinc/100g) for 7 weeks. Plasma glucose was measured by a glucose oxidase method. Catecholamines and dopamine were measured by a fully automatic high performance liquid column chromatography (4). Values were shown as Mean S.E.

Results

Control rats showed no significant decrease in plasma response of epinephrine by zinc deficiency diet (Table 1). Diabetic rats showed decreased plasma epinephrine response compared with control rats as previously reported (5) and zinc deficiency decreased plasma response even more in diabetic rats.

Nagano, M., Mochizuki, S., Dhalla, N.S. (eds.), CARDIOVASCULAR DISEASE IN DIABETES. Copyright © 1992. Kluwer Academic Publishers, Boston. All rights reserved.

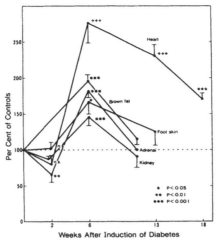

Fig. 1. Increase in catecholamine concentration of various tissues in diabetic rats after induction of diabetes.

Table 1. Effects of Zn Deficiency on Plasma Catecholamine Concentration of Control and Diabetic Rats After Stress.

			Epinephrine (ng/ml)	Norepinephrine
Control	(5)	− Zn	0.837 ± 0.101 ⎤ a	0.244 ± 0.015
		+ Zn	0.755 ± 0.218 ⎦	0.224 ± 0.006
Diabetic	(5)	− Zn	0.224 ± 0.147 ⎤ b	0.200 ± 0.022
		+ Zn	0.477 ± 0.075 ⎦	0.229 ± 0.041

a − P < 0.02   b − P < 0.05

Norepinephrine (main catecholamine of tissue except adrenal) concentrations of kidney as depicted in Table 2 were not significantly reduced in diabetic rats yet, but they were reduced significantly in diabetic rats on zinc deficiency diet compared with those on control diet and also in diabetic rats compared with control rats on zinc deficient diet.

Heart norepinephrine concentrations were still increasing (2), though not significantly, in Table 3 and zinc deficiency also resulted in similar effects.

Table 2. Effects of Zn Deficiency on Kidney Norepinephrine Concentration of Control and Diabetic Rats.

			Norepinephrine (n moles/g tissue)	
Control	(5)	- Zn	0.89 ± 0.07	⎤
		+ Zn	0.86 ± 0.05	⎦ a
Diabetic	(5)	- Zn	0.45 ± 0.02	⎤
		+ Zn	0.68 ± 0.07	⎦ b

a - $P < 0.001$ b - $P < 0.02$

Table 3. Effects if Zn Deficiency on Heart Norepinephrine Concentration of Control and Diabetic Rats.

			Norepinephrine (n moles/g tissue)	Dopamine (ng/g tissue)	
Control	(5)	- Zn	2.06 ± 0.04	8.91 ± 0.33	⎤
		+ Zn	2.00 ± 0.20	8.05 ± 0.55	⎦ a
Diabetic	(5)	- Zn	2.38 ± 0.13	11.01 ± 0.53	⎤
		+ Zn	2.44 ± 0.11	8.25 ± 0.68	⎦ b

a - $P < 0.001$ b - $P < 0.05$

However, dopamine (precurser of norepinephrine) concentration was increased significantly in diabetic rat hearts on zinc deficiency diet compared with those on control diet.

Discussion

Effects of zinc deficient diet was examined because zinc excretion was increased in diabetic rats compared with control rats and even more so on zinc deficient diet, and, therefore, unmarked deficiency might be accompanied in diabetic condition and might adversely affect the autonomic neuropathy, especially in heart.

The tissue catecholamine concentrations were increased markedly by 6 weeks of the diabetic stage and returned to basal levels at around 13 weeks (2). On the other hand, the levels of plasma catecholamine response to stress showed the stepwise reduction (1). These data suggested that diabetic rats have a smaller catecholamine response and that their ability to secrete catecholamines is impaired. Then, increased catecholamine synthesis may represent a compensation for difficulty in secretion and, for the time being, decompensation may occur, followed by a decrease in tissue concentration of catecholamines and loss of plasma catecholamine response. This could be one of the mechanisms of diabetic autonomic neuropathy. So far no objective data against this working theory have not been reported. According to this hypothesis, the stage of the diabetic rats used in this paper is a beginning of decompensation of catecholamine synthesis. The data that kidney norepinephrine concentrations of diabetic rats on zinc deficiency diet were already decreased significantly compared with those on control diet and with control rats on zinc deficiency diet seems to indicate that zinc deficiency may reduce catecholamine synthesis more markedly.

Dopamine, a precurser of catecholamine, in the diabetic hearts has not been reported yet in relation to diabetes, but the increase in concentration confirms some disturbance in synthesis of catecholamine.

Summary

Impaired secretion of catecholamine may be one of the causes of diabetic autonomic neuropathy. Zinc may accelerate it.

References

1. Fushimi H, Inoue T, Kishino B, Nishikawa M, Tochino Y, Funakawa S, Yamatodani A and Wada H. Abnormalities in plasma catecholamine response and tissue catecholamine accumulation in streptozotocin diabetic rats. A possible role for diabetic autonomic neuropathy. Life Sci. 1984;35: 1074-1081.
2. Fushimi H, Inoue, T Matsuyama Y, Kishino B, Kameyama M, Funakawa S, Tochino Y, Yamatodani A, Wada H, Minami T and Okazaki Y. Impaired catecholamine secretion as a cause of diabetic autonomic neuropathy. Diabetes Res Clin Pract 1988;4:303-307.
3. Fushimi H, Inoue T, Yamada Y, Horie H, Otsuka A, Tsujimura T, Kameyama M, Inoue K, Minami T and Okazaki Y. Zinc deficiency and its significance in

diabetes mellitus: Zinc deficiency exaggerates diabetic osteomalasia and nephropathy. in preparation.
4. Yamatodani A and Wada H. Automated analysis for plasma epinephrine and norepinephrine by liquid chromatography, including a sample cleanup procedure. Clin Chem 1981;27:1983-1987.
5. Fushimi H, Inoue T, Namikawa H, Kishino B, Nishikawa M, Tochino Y, Funakawa S, Yamatodani A and Wada H. Decreased response of plasma catecholamines in the diabetic rats. Endocrinol Jpn 1982;29:593-596.

Atrial Natriuretic Peptide in Plasma and Atrial Auricles of the Non-Obese Diabetic (NOD) Mouse

S. Yano, Y. Kobayashi, K. Tanigawa, S. Suzuki, T. Shimada,
S. Morioka, Y. Kato and K. Moriyama

*Fourth Department of Internal Medicine, Department of Pharmacology,
First Department of Internal Medicine, Institute of Experimental Animals,
Shimane Medical University, Izumo, 693, JAPAN.*

Introduction

Decompensated diabetes mellitus (DM) is associated with abnormalities in fluid and electrolyte balance (1,2,3). Alterations in the renin-angiotensin-aldosterone system and vasopressin have been observed both in human with DM (4,5) and in rats treated with the diabetogenic agent, streptozotocin (STZ) (6,7,8).

Since atrial natriuretic peptide (ANP) is a hormone released by atrial myocytes in response to acute (9) and chronic (10) extracellular volume expansion, ANP levels both in plasma and the atrial auricle should be changed in severe stages of ill DM. Plasma ANP levels in humans with DM and diabetic animals have been studied previously (11,12,13), however, results regarding changes in plasma ANP levels are inconclusive.

In the present study, non-obese diabetic (NOD) mice, which are a model for human type 1 DM (14), were used. Plasma and right atrial auricular ANP levels were measured by radioimmunoassay (RIA) as well as by immunohistochemistry, transmission and scanning electron microscopy were applied to observe morphological changes in the right atrial auricles.

Method

The female NOD mice were obtained from our own breeding colony in the Institute of Experimental Animals, Shimane Medical University. These animals were housed at 24°C under 12-hour light (8 a.m. to 8 p.m.) - 12-hour dark cycles and given free access to water and chow pellets (MF, Oriental Yeast

*Nagano, M., Mochizuki, S., Dhalla, N.S. (eds.), CARDIOVASCULAR
DISEASE IN DIABETES. Copyright © 1992. Kluwer Academic Publishers,
Boston. All rights reserved.*

Co., LTD.) which contains 60% carbohydrate, 13% fat and 27% protein.

Changes on Water Metabolism with DM state

Twenty female mice were used for the study on water metabolism with aging. The amounts of water intake, food intake and urinary volume were measured in each mice kept in an aluminum metabolic cage for 24 hours from 11 weeks of age.

Urinary glucose levels were measured by the glucose oxidase method using a kit (Glu-Lq, Dia-iatron). The NOD mice were divided into three groups according to urinary glucose concentrations at around 25 weeks of age. The first group was the control group (NOD-N) which mice were normoglycemic at around 25 weeks of age. The second group (NOD-A) mice were those whose urinary glucose level began to increase more than 14 mM and maintained the higher levels within 1 month. The third group (NOD-C) mice had high urinary glucose levels for more than 1 month. The body weight (BW) began to decrease with the development of DM. Some mice, with DM for more than 1 month and BW decreased markedly, could not adapt to the metabolic cage.

Changes of ANP with DM state

From 15 weeks of age, the urinary glucose levels of the other female NOD were tested every three to four days by using Diastix (Miles-Sankyo Co., LTD.). BW were also measured.

At 25 weeks of age the animals were anesthetized with an intraperitoneal injection of sodium pentobarbital (0.1 mg per gram BW). The blood was drawn into a syringe from the left cervical artery and transferred into cooled test-tubes. The test-tubes for plasma ANP RIA contained both 15 mg EDTA and aprotinin (1,000 kallikrein-inhibitor units). Plasma glucose levels were measured by the glucose oxidase method. Plasma sodium was determined by using a flame photometer (Hitachi type 750). Plasma osmolality (Posmol) was estimated by the following formula: Posmol (mmol/kg) = 2(sodium)meq/L+(glucose)mM (15).

The NOD mice were divided into three groups according to plasma glucose concentrations and BW loss. The first group, normoglycemic mice was the control group (NOD-N). The urinary glucose in this group had remained negative (< 5.6 mM) prior to sacrifice, and plasma glucose concentrations at sacrifice were less than 11.2 mM. This group corresponded with NOD-N group in the study on water metabolism. The second group (NOD-M) included mice whose urinary glucose had shown positive (> 14 mM) within the last month prior to sacrifice and whose plasma glucose levels at sacrifice was over 11.2 mM. The percent BW loss was calculated with the formula (Maximum BW - BW at sacrifice/Maximum BW x 100). It was less than 20% in NOD-M mice. The NOD-M mice were considered to correspond with NOD-A mice in the study on water metabolism. The third group (NOD-H) mice had high plasma glucose concentrations of > 33.6 mM, and their percent BW loss as over 20%. The NOD-C mice in the study on water metabolism were considered to locate between NOD-M and NOD-H groups in the study on ANP.

The right auricles were divided into 4 pieces. The first piece was used for immunohistochemistry by the Peroxidase-anti-peroxidase (PAP) method (16) using anti-human antiserum (Peptide Institute Inc.) diluted to 1:400. After processing with the PAP method, the specimens were stained with hematoxylin.

The second piece of each auricle was used for the transmission electron microscopic (TEM) study. The third sections were prepared for scanning electron microscope (SEM). They were processed by the Aldehyde-Osmium-DMSO-Osmium (A-O-D-O) method (17). The fourth pieces were frozen and stored at -80°C for RIA. The ANP concentration was measured by following the RIA procedures described by Nakao et al (18). The atrial auricular ANP levels in the NOD-N and NOD-H mice were used for immunohistochemistry. The anti-human ANP antiserum was used at 1:25,000 final dilution. Synthetic rat ANP (Peptide Institute Inc.) was used as a standard. Protein content of auricular sample was measured by Lowry's method (19). For plasma RIA, anti human/rat ANP antiserum kindly donated by Dr. Nakao, Kyoto University, was used at 1:200,000 final dilution, because plasma ANP could not be detected using the antiserum from the Peptide Institute.

The data are expressed as means ± S.E. The statistical analysis of the data was performed by one-way analysis of variance, and the significance was determined by the Scheffe's method for the two comparisons. The Student's unpaired t test was used for analysis of atrial auricular ANP levels between NOD-N and NOD-H. The statistical significance was defined as $p < 0.05$.

Results
Changes on water metabolism with DM state

Development of DM in some NOD female mice with aging was shown in Figure 1. About 40% of female mice showed higher urinary glucose levels after 15 weeks of age. At beginning, water intake, urinary volume and food intake were

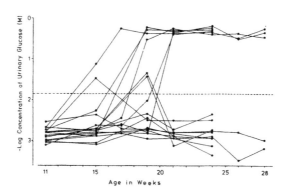

Figure 1. Changes of urinary glucose concentration of 16 female NOD mice during aging. Six mice showed higher urinary glucose levels (> 14 mM) between 15 and 21 weeks of age and higher urinary glucose levels (300-600 mM) was maintained for a long time. Three mice showed higher urinary glucose levels once, however, the levels recovered to lower levels again. Seven mice did not show higher urinary glucose levels throughout the experiment.

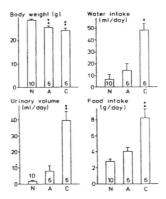

Figure 2. Comparisons in body weight, water intake, urinary volume and food intake among different groups of the female NOD mice. N, A, C: normoglycemic, acute hyperglycemic (changed and the state was maintained within 1 month) and chronic hyperglycemic (the state was maintained over 1 month) NOD mice. Values are the mean and the vertical bars indicate S.E. Numbers in or above the columns indicate the number of animals. * $p < 0.05$, ** $p < 0.01$, NOD-N vs. NOD-A or NOD-C. Water intake, urinary volume and food intake of NOD-C group was significantly larger than those of NOD-A group ($p < 0.01$).

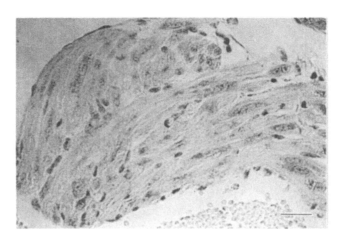

Figure 3. Immunohistochemical staining of right atrial auricle in the NOD-H mouse. Most myocyte particularly near the pericardium exhibit an intense reaction. Immunoreactive material is accumulated around the nuclease. Bar = 200 um.

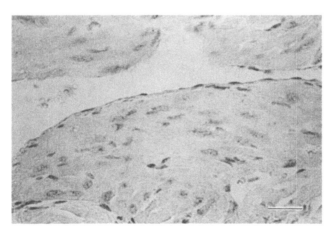

Figure 4. Immunohistochemical staining of right atrial auricle in the NOD-N mouse. The staining around the nucleus is less than the NOD-H group. Bar = 200 um.

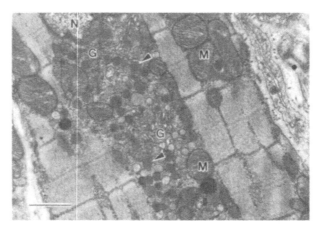

Figure 5. An electron micrograph of the NOD-H mouse atrial cardiocyte, illustrating marked number of atrial granules (arrowheads). Extensive stacks of Golgi cisternae (G) are observed. N: nucleus. M: mitochondria. Bar = 1 um.

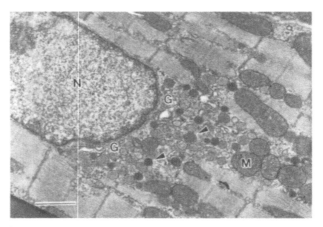

Figure 6. Ultrastructure of NOD-N mouse atrial myocyte. Number of atrial granules (arrowheads) appears to be less than that in the NOD-H mouse. Abbreviations are the same as those in Figure 5. Bar = 1 um.

Table 1. General characteristics of three groups of the NOD mice.

	NOD-N	NOD-M	NOD-H
Number of animals	10	5	5
BW (g)	25.9 ± 0.1	26.0 ± 0.2	16.8 ± 0.2 #,**
P-glucose (mM)	9.7 ± 0.1	20.9 ± 0.4 #	46.4 ± 0.8 #,*

NOD-N, M, H: normo, moderate, hyperglycemic NOD mice. BW: body weight. P-glucose: plasma glucose. Values are means ± S.E. # $p < 0.01$, NOD-N vs. NOD-M or NOD-H. * $p < 0.05$, ** $p < 0.01$, NOD-M vs. NOD-H.

Table 2. Plasma osmolarity and related variables in the NOD mice.

	NOD-N	NOD-M	NOD-H
Number of animals	10	5	5
Hct (%)	36.3 ± 0.1	37.0 ± 0.8	45.3 ± 0.5 *
Plasma sodium (meq/L)	140.7 ± 0.2	140.1 ± 0.3	141.1 ± 0.2
Posmol (mmol/kg)	289.9 ± 0.4	309.4 ± 0.5	319.4 ± 0.7 **,#

NOD-N, M, H: normo, moderate, hyperglycemic NOD mice. Hct: hematocrit. Posmol: plasma osmolarity. Values are means ± S.E. * $p < 0.05$, ** $p < 0.01$, NOD-N vs. NOD-H. # $p < 0.01$, NOD-M vs. NOD-H.

Table 3. The number of granules in a atrial auricular myocyte section.

	NOD-N	NOD-H
Number of animals	4	4
Number of cells	80	80
Number of granules	36.5 ± 0.2	82.9 ± 0.4 *

NOD-N, H: normo, hyperglycemic NOD mice. Values are means ± S.E. * $p < 0.01$, NOD-N vs. NOD-H.

Table 4. ANP levels in plasma and right atrial auricle.

	NOD-N	NOD-M	NOD-H
Number of animals	10	4	4
Plasma ANP (pg/ml)	143.5 ± 1.0	92.0 ± 1.5*	54.7 ± 2.5 **
Auricular ANP (mg/g)	13.4 ± 0.2		27.6 ± 0.4 *

NOD-N, M, H: normo, moderate, hyperglycemic NOD mice. Values are means ± S.E.
** $p < 0.01$, NOD-N vs. NOD-H. * $p < 0.05$, NOD-N vs. NOD-M and 3 NOD-N vs. NOD-H.

not significantly different in acute hyperglycemic mice (NOD-A) group compared with normoglycemic mice (NOD-N) group (Fig. 2). BW was slightly but significantly lighter in NOD-A mice in this series of experiments. Then, BW decreased significantly and water intake, urinary volume and food intake increased markedly in chronic hyperglycemic state (NOD-C). Urinary glucose levels showed a plateau in chronic hyperglycemic state between 300 to 600 mM, which was more than 100-fold higher than normoglycemic mice. In some mice, transient high urinary glucose state was observed and they were excluded from NOD-A group.

Changes of ANP with DM state

Body weights and plasma glucose concentrations of the 3 groups in ANP study were shown in Table 1.

The NOD-H mice lose almost 30% of their BWs and their plasma glucose concentrations were 5-fold higher than the NOD-N mice. In the NOD-M mice, BWs were not significantly different from those in the NOD-N mice, but plasma glucose concentrations were significantly higher compared to the NOD-N mice.

Table 2 shows the hematocrit, plasma sodium and calculated plasma osmolality of the 3 groups. Hematocrit in the NOD-H group was significantly higher than in the NOD-N group. Plasma sodium levels did not change among the three groups. Calculated plasma osmolality was significantly higher in the NOD-H groups than in both the NOD-M and the NOD-N groups. In contrast, the values for calculated plasma osmolality in the NOD-M mice exhibited no significant difference from those in the NOD-N mice.

The PAP method with anti-human ANP antiserum resulted in the perinuclear

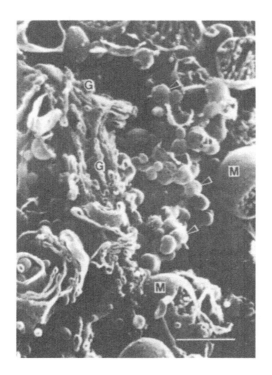

Figure 7. Scanning electron micrograph of NOD-H mouse. Numerous atrial granules (arrowheads) were observed in the perinuclear zone of the myocyte. G: golgi complex. N: nucleus. M: mitochondria. Bar = 1 um.

area of the bilateral auricular cells being stained brown. The right auricle was stained either the same or a little bit more intensely compared with the left auricle. In the NOD-H group, the tissue appeared to be stained more intensely than in the NOD-N group (Fig. 3). This might have resulted from expansion in the size of the immunoreactive perinuclear zones. In the NOD-N group. The specimens had narrow regions which were deeply stained (Fig. 4). The intensity of the staining in the NOD-M mice varied from light to dark one.

In the TEM study, auricular specific granule in the right atrial auricles had a limiting membrane and sometimes had a lucent area between the limiting membrane and the core (Figs. 5,6). The granules were distributed at the perinuclear region of the atrial auricular cells. The total number of granules per a section of a myocyte in the NOD-H mice significantly increased compared with that in the NOD-N mice (Table 3). The Golgi complex was developed at the perinuclear region of the auricular cells of the NOD-H mice as well as the NOD-N mice (Figs. 5,6).

The auricular specific granules were observed three-dimensionally by SEM. The NOD-H mice had many granules in the perinuclear area, which is consistent with the results of the immunohistochemistry and TEM (Fig. 7).

Table 4 shows plasma and right auricular ANP levels in the three different glycemic states. Plasma ANP levels were significantly lower in the NOD-H mice and in the NOD-M mice than in the NOD-N group. The right auricular ANP levels per tissue protein in the NOD-H mice increased to more than 2 fold of those in the NOD-N mice.

Discussion

The structure of the mouse pre-ANP has been clarified from the cDNA analysis, and was classified as rat type (20,21). The plasma ANP level has been measured by RIA and the concentrations ranged 100-200 pg/ml in normal humans, and 200-400 pg/ml in rats (19,22). Plasma ANP levels in normoglycemic NOD mice was 143.5 ± 10.1 pg/ml in the present study, which is consistent with the ANP levels in humans and rats.

There have been some reports regarding the plasma ANP levels in DM (11,12,13). Ortola et al (12) reported the plasma ANP levels doubled in diabetic state rats which had been treated 2 weeks prior with STZ. They speculated that moderate hyperglycemia, with its attendant chronic volume expansion, stimulates atrial ANP release, and the elevated plasma ANP levels might contribute to the hyperfiltration observed in diabetes (10,23). In contrast, Hebden et al (13) demonstrated that plasma-ANP levels were unchanged in rats at 1, 3, 6 and 12 weeks after STZ injection. These results disagree with the present results. While Ortola et al (12) and Hebden et al (13) tested plasma ANP levels in normo- and moderate glycemic diabetic rats, the present study used severely ill diabetic mice with hyperglycemia and hyperosmolality.

The calculated osmolality was significantly higher in the NOD-H group than the NOD-N group. It has been observed that an increase in extracellular osmolality is capable of increasing circulating ANP levels (24,25). Gibbs showed that high concentrations of NaCl and KCl stimulated ANP levels more than the glucose levels did (24). The plasma sodium levels in the three groups did not show statistical significance. The decrease of plasma ANP levels in the NOD-H mice does not appear to be related to the plasma hyperosmolality.

Marked increase in water intake and urinary volume in chronic DM state mice observed in the present study was considered to be due to severe osmotic diuresis. Judging from the present results, the maximum urinary glucose concentration of mice may be ranged from 300 to 600 mM. Chronic DM state may result the enhancement of food intake and the reduction of BW. It is possible to speculate that decreased ANP secretion in the NOD-H mice was produced by a homeostatic mechanism which protects from water depletion observed in the present study. In the dehydrated state, plasma ANP levels were markedly decreased in rats (26,27). Marked fluid restriction may have been caused by significant decreases in atrial pressure, although atrial pressure was not measured in this study.

A recent study by Zisfein et al (28) showed that levels of stored ANP in atria measured by RIA did not change even with marked volume depletion. In our study, both tissue ANP levels by RIA and the intense immunohistochemical staining of auricles were increased in the NOD-H mice. An increase of atrial granules in the NOD-H mice was observed in TEM and SEM study. Two-fold increase of the number of atrial granules seemed to be consitent with the increase of ANP concentration measured by RIA. Development of the Golgi complex in myocyte of the NOD-H mice suggested that synthesis of ANP was not inhibited completely. Reduction of plasma ANP levels in the NOD-H mice may result in an increase of tissue ANP levels.

In conclusion, the present study demonstrated that severely ill NOD mice have decreased circulating ANP levels and elevated tissue ANP levels.

Summary

Atrial natriuretic peptide (ANP) levels in plasma and right atrial auricles were examined in the decompensated diabetic state by using non-obese diabetic (NOD) mouse as a model of type 1 diabetes mellitus (DM). Severely ill mice, which had blood glucose levels of > 33.6 mM and showing marked body weight loss (NOD-H), had a higher increase of calculated plasma osmolality (319.4 ± 6.7 mmol/kg) than the age-matched normoglycemic NOD (NOD-N) mice (289.9 ± 3.5 mmol/kg) ($p < 0.01$). The plasma ANP levels decreased determined by radioimmunoassay (RIA) to an average of 54.7 pg/ml in the NOD-H mice compared to 143.5 pg/ml in the NOD-N mice (p < 0.01). The right auricles in the NOD-H mice showed an intense immunohistochemical staining by anti-human ANP antiserum. The ANP levels by RIA in the right auricles were 27.6 mg/g protein in the NOD-H mice and 13.4 mg/g protein in the NOD-N mice. An increase of auricular specific granules in the NOD-H mice was found by transmission and scanning electron microscopy. These findings suggested that the secretion of plasma ANP was inhibited and that the storage of atrial auricular ANP increased to adjust or counter-balance the marked dehydration in the deteriorated diabetic state.

Acknowledgments

This work was supported in part by a research grant to Y. Kobayashi from the Ministry of Education, Science and Culture, Japan.

References

1. Rose BD. Clinical physiology of acid-base and electrolyte disorders. McGraw-Hill Book Co., New York: 1977;27.
2. Christrieb AR, Long R, and Underwood RH. Renin-angiotensin-aldosterone system, electrolyte homeostasis and blood pressure in alloxan diabetes. Nature 1985;314:264-266.
3. Hebden RA, Gardiner SM, Bennett T, and MacDonald IA. The influence of streptozotocin-induced diabetes mellitus on fluid and electrolyte handling in rats. Clin. Sci. 1986;70:111-117.
4. Zerbe RL, Vicicor F, and Robertson GL. Plasma vasopressin in uncontrolled diabetes mellitus. Diabetes 1979;28:503-508.
5. Morimoto S, Uchida K, Kikoshi H, Hosojima H, Yamamoto I, and Azukizawa S. Responsiveness of plasma aldosterone to antiotensin II in patients with diabetes mellitus. Endocrinol. Jpn. 1983;30:671-678.
6. Van Itallie CM, and Fernstrom JD. Osmolal effects on vasopressin secretion in the streptozotocin-diabetic rat. Am. J. Physiol. 1982;42:E411-E417.
7. Funakawa S, Okahara T, Imanishi M, Komori T, Yamamoto K, and Tochino Y. Renin-angiotensin system and prostacyclin biosynthesis in streptozotocin diabetic rats. Eur. J. Pharmacol. 1983;94:27-33.
8. Kigoshi T, Imaizumi M, Azukizawa S, Yamamoto I, Uchida K, Konishi F, and Morimoto S. Effects of angiotensin II, adrenocorticotropin, and

potassium on aldosterone production in adrenal zona glomerulosa cells from streptozotocin-induced diabetic rats. Endocrinology 1986; 118:183-188.
9. Lang RE, Tholken H, Canten D, Luft FC, Ruskoaho H, and Unger TH. Atrial natriuretic factor: A ciruclating hormone stimulated by volume loading. Nature 1985;314:264-266.
10. Tanaka I, Misono K, and Inagami T. Atrial natriuretic factor in rat hypothalamus, atria and plasma: Determination by specific radioimmunoassay. Biochem. Biophys. Res. Commun. 1984;124:663-668.
11. Kahn JK, Grekin RJ, Shenker Y, and Vinik AI. Plasma levels of immunoreactive atrial natriuretic hormone in patients with diabetes mellitus. Regul. Peptides 1986;15:323-332.
12. Ortola FV, Ballerman BJ, Anderson S, Mendez RE, and Brenner BM. Elevated plasma atrial natriuretic peptide levels in diabetic rats. J. Clin. Invest. 1987;80:670-674.
13. Hebden RA, and McNeil JH. Concentration(s) of natriuretic hormone in the plasma of rats with streptozotocin-induced diabetes mellitus. Life Sci. 1988;42:1789-1795.
14. Makino S, Kunimoto K, Muraoka Y, Mizushima Y, Katagiri K, and Tochino Y. Breeding of a nonobese diabetic strain of mice. Exp. Anim. 1980;29:1.
15. Ederman IS, Liebman J, O'Meara MP, and Birkenfeld LW. Interrelations between serum sodium concentration, serum osmolarity and total exchangeable sodium, total exchangeable potassium and total body water. J. Clin. Invest. 1958;37:1236-1256.
16. Sternberger LA, Hardy PH, Cuculis JJ, and Meyer HG. The unlabeled antibody enzyme method of immunochemistry. Preparation and properties of soluble antigen-antibody complex (horseradish peroxidase-antihorseradish peroxidase) and its use in identification of spirochetes. J. Histochem. Cytochem. 1970;18(5):315-333.
17. Tanaka K, and Mitsushima A. A preparation method for observing intracellular structures by scanning electron microscopy. J. Microsc. 1984;133:213.
18. Nakao K, Sugawara A, Morii N, Sakamoto M, Suda M, Soneda J, Ban T, Kihara M, Yamori Y, Shimokura M, Kiso Y, and Imura H. Radioimmunoassay for α-human and rat atrial natriuretic polypeptide. Biochem. Biophys. Res. Commun. 1984;124:815-821.

19. Lowry OH, Rowebroush NJ, Farr AL, and Randall RJ. Protein measurement with Folin phenol reagent. J. Biol. Chem. 1951;193:265.
20. Seidman C. The structure of rat preproatrial natriuretic factor as defined by a complementary DNA clone. Science 1984;225:324.
21. Oikawa S, Imai M, Inuzawa C, Tawaragi Y, Nakazato H, and Matsuo H. Structure of dog and rabbit precursors of atrial natriuretic polypeptides deduced from nucleotide sequence of cloned cDNA. Biochem. Biophys. Res. Commun. 1985;132:892-899.
22. Miyata A, Kangawa K, and Matsuo H. Molecular forms of atrial natriuretic peptides in rat tissues and plasma. J. Hypertension 1986;4(suppl 2):9-11.
23. Ballermann BJ, Bloch KD, Seidman JG, and Brenner BM. Atrial natriuretic peptide transcription, secretation, and glomerular receptor activity during mineralocorticoid escape in the rat. J. Clin. Invest. 1986;78:840-843.
24. Gibbs DM. Noncalcium-dependent modulation of in vitro atrial natriuretic factor release by extracellular osmolarity. Endocrinology 1987;120:194-197.
25. Naruse K, Naruse M, Obana K, Brown AB, Shibasaki T, Demura H, Shizume K, and Inagami T. Right and left atrium share a similar mode of secreting atrial natriuretic factor in vitro in rats. J. Hypertension 1986;4 (suppl 6):497-499.
26. Takayanagi R, Tanaka I, Maki M, and Inagami T. Effects of changes in water-sodium balance on levels of atrial natriuretic factor messenger RNA and peptide in rats. Life Sci. 1985;36:1843-1848.
27. Kohno M, Glegg K, Sambhi M, Eggena P, and Barrett J. Immunoreactive atrial natriuretic polypeptide in plasma of volume-depleted rats. Clin. Res. 1985;36:1843-1848.
28. Zisfein JB, Matsueda GR, Fallon JT, Bloch KD, Seidman CE, Seidman JG, Homcy CJ, and Graham RM. Atrial natriuretic factor: Assessment of its structure in atria and regulation of its biosynthesis with volume depletion. J. Mol. Cell. Cardiol. 1986;18:917-929.

D. PHARMACOLOGICAL AND THERAPEUTIC ASPECTS OF DIABETIC HEART

Effects of Beta-Adrenoceptor Blocking Agents on Myocardium Isolated From Experimentally Diabetic Rats

F. Nagamine, R. Sunagawa, K. Murakami, M. Sakanashi* and G. Mimura

*The Second Department of Internal Medicine and *The Department of Pharmacology, School of Medicine, Faculty of Medicine, University of the Ryukyus, 207 Uehara, Nishihara-cho, Okinawa 903-01, JAPAN*

Introduction

It is well known that patients with diabetes mellitus are frequently associated with atherosclerotic diseases such as hypertension and/or ischemic heart diseases (1-4). Recently, there are reports that some cases with diabetic cardiomyopathy have no obvious genesis but are accompanied with chronic congestive heart failure (5,6). In experimentally diabetic animals, it has been noted that chronotropic and inotropic actions of beta-adrenoceptor stimulating agents (beta agonists) diminished in isolated myocardium (7-9), and concomitant decrease in the number of beta-adrenoceptor might be responsible for these reduced myocardial functions (7-9). On the other hand, beta-adrenoceptor blocking agents (beta blockers) have generally been used for the therapy of hypertension and/or ischemic heart diseases accompanied with diabetes mellitus (10,11). When beta blockers are administered to patients with diabetic mellitus, their influences on lipids metabolism, hypoglycemia and/or secretion of insulin have been taken into account (12,13), but this is not the case with respect to myocardial function. If the decrease in the number of beta adrenoceptor is related to reduced myocardial function, then great attention must be paid to the use of beta blockers in diabetic patients. In the present study, therefore, to evaluate experimentally the influence of beta-blockers on diabetic myocardium, effects of propranolol with $beta_1$ and $beta_2$ adrenoceptor blocking activity as a standard beta blocker, and atenolol with $beta_1$ adrenoceptor blocking activity as a cardioselective beta blocker on isoproterenol-induced responses of both atrial and papillary muscles isolated from experimentally diabetic rats were examined.

Nagano, M., Mochizuki, S., Dhalla, N.S. (eds.), CARDIOVASCULAR DISEASE IN DIABETES. Copyright © 1992. Kluwer Academic Publishers, Boston. All rights reserved.

Methods
Induction of diabetes

Male Sprague-Dawley rats (Clea Japan, Tokyo, Japan), weighing 200-260 g, were randomly separated into two groups: the control group (n=18) and the diabetic group (n=17). In approximately half the rats of each group (n=9 in the control group and n=8 in the diabetic group), effects of propranolol were examined. In remaining rats (n=9 in both control and diabetic groups), effects of atenolol were examined. After an overnight fast, the diabetic group was treated with a single intravenous injection of streptozotocin (60 mg/kg, Sigma, St. Louis, MO, USA) which was dissolved in physiological saline solution immediately before use, and the control group was injected with buffered vehicle. The diabetic state was assessed when nonfasting blood glucose value was more than 350 mg/dl at 3 days after streptozotocin i.v. Animals were fed an ordinary rat chow (Clea Japan, CE-2) and water ad libitum for 6 weeks.

Preparation of right atrial and papillary muscles and measurement of cardiac parameters

At 6 weeks after vehicle or streptozotocin i.v., animals were anesthetized with an intraperitoneal injection of sodium pentobarbital (30 mg/kg). The abdomen was opened, and 3-5 ml of blood were rapidly collected from the inferior vena cava. Immediately after a thoracotomy, the heart was removed in a beaker containing oxygenated Krebs-Henseleit solution of the following composition (mmol/l): NaCl, 120.0; KCl, 4.8; $CaCl_2$, 1.25; $MgSO_4$, 1.2; KH_2PO_4, 1.2; $NaHCO_3$, 25.0; and glucose 11.0. The right ventricular papillary muscle was carefully dissected from the ventricle, and one end of papillary muscle was attached to a stimulating electrode assembly and the other end was connected to a force-displacement transducer (Nihon Kohden, TB-611T, Tokyo, Japan). The atrium was carefully dissected from the right ventricle and remaining fat and aorta was trimmed off. One end of the atrium was attached to a tissue-holder and the other end was connected to a force-displacement transducer (Nihon Kohden, TB-611T). Thus, isolated myocardial preparations were suspended in a 20 ml organ bath filled with Krebs-Henseleit solution (pH 7.4) which was maintained at 37°C and continuously aerated with a gas mixture of 95% O_2 and 5% CO_2. Krebs-Henseleit solution in the organ bath was replaced every 15 min and these preparations were allowed to equilibrate for 1 hour. Resting tension in right atrial and papillary muscles was adjusted at 300 mg and maintained throughout the experiment. Beating rate (R) in the right atrium and isometric force development (F) and its first derivative (±dF/dt) in the papillary muscle under pacing (voltage; 10-15% above threshold, duration; 1-5 msec) at a constant rate of 3.3 Hz (200 beats/min) using an electronic stimulator (Nihon Kohden, SEN-3201) were recorded. R was counted continuously by a cardiotachometer (Nihon Kohden, AT-600G) triggered by the developed force of the right atrium. The first derivatives of force development (±dF/dt) of the papillary muscle were derived from differentiating the force development signal using an electronic differentiator (Nihon Kohden, ED-601G). All parameters were recorded on a heat-pen writing polygraph (Nihon Kohden, WT-685G) and stored on a tape using a data-recorder (Sony Magmescale, A-47; Sony, Tokyo, Japan).

The drugs used in the present study were as follows: dl-isoproterenol hydrochloride (Nikken Kagaku, Tokyo, Japan), dl-propranolol hydrochloride (ICI Pharma, Osaka, Japan) and atenolol (ICI Pharma, Osaka, Japan).

Experimental protocol and calculation of ED_{50} value and pA_2 value

After all parameters were equilibrated, an experiment was started. Isoproterenol was dissolved in physiological saline solution and cumulatively added to the organ bath in a volume less than 0.2 ml. Chronotropic and inotropic effects of isoproterenol on the right atrial and papillary muscles were observed and expressed as percent changes in R, F and ±dF/dt when the maximum increases in each parameter were defined as 100%. Thus, cumulative concentration response curves of R, F, or ±dF/dt were obtained. As an index of affinity, values of mean effective dose (ED_{50}) for R, F or ±dF/dt were geometrically derived from these concentration response curves. Muscle preparations were then washed out several times and equilibrated for 1 hour. Thereafter, beta blockers at a certain concentration were added and concentration response curves of each preparation for isoproterenol were again obtained 30 min after addition of these beta blockers. Furthermore, preparations were once again washed out and concentration response curves for isoproterenol were taken after addition of beta-blockers of 10-fold higher concentration than the first one. pA_2 values were calculated from these concentration response curves after confirming the same slope (=1) of the line for beta-agonist and beta-blockers. At the end of experiment, the right atrial and papillary muscles were removed from the organ bath and their wet weights were measured.

Table 1. General features of control and diabetic rats.

	C group (n=18)	DM group (n=17)
Plasma glucose (mg/dl)	146.6 ± 2.9	552.7 ± 17.7**
Plasma glycosylated hemoglobin (%)	5.0 ± 0.1	14.2 ± 0.3**
Body weight (g)	468.7 ± 7.9	287.7 ± 10.4**
Heart weight (g)	1.1 ± 0.0	0.9 ± 0.0**
Right atrium weight (mg)	86.2 ± 2.4	71.4 ± 2.6**
Papillary muscle weight (mg)	41.4 ± 2.4	35.5 ± 1.9

C: control. DM: diabetes mellitus. Each value represents mean ± SEM. n = number of rats. ** $P < 0.01$ versus the corresponding control value. From Nagamine et al (24).

Blood analysis

Plasma glucose levels were measured by a glucose oxidase method (14) and plasma glycosylated hemoglobin levels were measured by an affinity column method (15,16).

Statistical analysis

The data were expressed as mean ± SEM and the statistical analysis of the data was done with non-paired Student's t-test. A P value less than 5% was defined as significant difference.

Results

Values of plasma glucose, plasma glycosylated hemoglobin, body weight and wet heart weight

Values of plasma glucose, glycosylated hemoglobin, body weight and wet weights of heart, right atrial muscle and papillary muscle of the control and diabetic groups at 6 weeks after vehicle or streptozotocin i.v. are summarized in Table 1. Plasma glucose and glycosylated hemoglobin levels were significantly higher in the diabetic group than in the control group ($P < 0.01$). Body weight and wet weights of the heart and the right atrium were significantly lower in the diabetic group than in the control group ($P < 0.01$). Though wet weight of the right papillary muscle was lower in the diabetic group in the control group, there was no statistical significance.

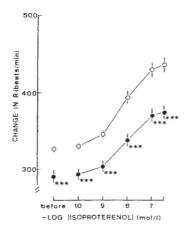

Figure 1. Effects of isoproterenol on beating rate (R) of isolated right atria from control (open circles, n=18) and diabetic (closed circles, n=17) rats. Each point represents mean ± SEM. *** P < 0.01 versus the corresponding control value. The points at "before" show the basal beating rate. From Nagamine et al (24).

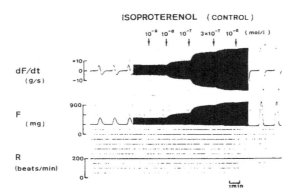

Figure 2. Typical recording of effects of isoproterenol on isolated papillary muscle from the control rat. ±dF/dt: first derivative of force development. F: myocardial force development. R: beating rate by pacing. The papillary muscle was paced at a constant rate of 200 beats/min.

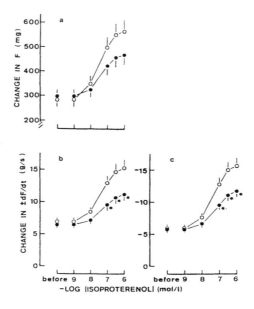

Figure 3. Effects of isoproterenol on myocardial force development (F, panel a) and first derivatives of F (+dF/dt, panel b and -dF/dt, panel c) of isolated papillary muscle from control (open circles, n=13) and diabetic (closed circles, n=15) rats. Each point represents mean ± SEM. * $P < 0.05$ versus the corresponding control value. The values at "before" show the basal force development, the basal +dF/dt and the basal -dF/dt, respectively. From Nagamine et al (24).

Basal values of R, F, +dF/dt and -dF/dt in a steady state

Basal values of R, F, +dF/dt and -dF/dt in a steady state are 326.8 ± 4.1 beats/min, 278.8 ± 32.2 mg, 6.9 ± 0.6 g/sec and -5.9 ± 0.6 g/sec in the control group and 290.6 ± 8.2 beats/min, 297.2 ± 27.8 mg, 6.4 ± 0.5 g/sec and -5.8 ± 0.5 g/sec in the diabetic group, respectively. Basal value of R was significantly lower in the diabetic group than in the control group ($P < 0.001$). Basal F and basal ±dF/dt were not different between groups.

Chronotropic effects in right atrium and inotropic effects in right ventricular papillary muscle of isoproterenol

Concentration response curves of R by cumulative administrations of isoproterenol in right atria are shown in Figure 1. Increases in R by

Table 2. ED_{50} values (mol/l) of right atrial and papillary muscles to isoproterenol.

	R	F	+dF/dt	-dF/dt
C group	5.31×10^{-9} (4.40 - 6.41) (n=18)	2.92×10^{-8} (2.12 - 4.03) (n=13)	4.24×10^{-8} (3.69 - 4.86) (n=13)	4.37×10^{-8} (3.60 - 5.25) (n=13)
DM group	5.73×10^{-9} (4.73 - 6.89) (n=17)	3.97×10^{-8} (3.24 - 4.86) (n=15)	4.92×10^{-8} (4.04 - 6.00) (n=15)	6.17×10^{-8}* (4.84 - 7.85) (n=15)

C: control. DM: diabetes mellitus. Each value represents geometric mean ED_{50} and their 95% confidence intervals (in parentheses). n = number of preparations. * $P < 0.05$ versus the corresponding control value. R: beating rate of right atrium. F: myocardial force development of papillary muscle. +dF/dt: positive first derivative of force development. -dF/dt: negative first derivative of force development. From Nagamine et al (24).

isoproterenol were concentration dependent in both control and diabetic groups. The maximum response of R to isoproterenol was significantly lower in the diabetic group than in the control group (the control group; 436 ± 10 beats/min, the diabetic group; 375 ± 9 beats/min, $P < 0.001$). Typical responses of the papillary muscle to isoproterenol were illustrated in Figure 2. Increases in F and ±dF/dt by isoproterenol were concentration dependent, and increases of ±dF/dt by isoproterenol (10^{-7} - 10^{-6} mol/l) in the diabetic group were significantly smaller than those in the control group (Fig. 3, $P < 0.05$). The maximum responses of +dF/dt (the control group; 15.1 ± 1.4 g/sec, the diabetic group; 11.2 ± 1.0 g/sec, $P < 0.05$) and -dF/dt (the control group; -15.7 ± 1.3 g/sec, the diabetic group; -11.8 ± 0.9 g/sec, $P < 0.05$) to isoproterenol (10^{-6} mol/l) were significantly smaller in the diabetic group than in the control group. The maximum response of F to isoproterenol (10^{-6} mol/l) was also smaller in the diabetic group than in the control group, but there was no significant difference between two groups. ED_{50} values of -dF/dt for isoproterenol were significantly greater in the diabetic group than in the control group. However, ED_{50} values of R, F and +dF/dt tended to be greater in the diabetic group but were not statistically different between two groups (Table 2).

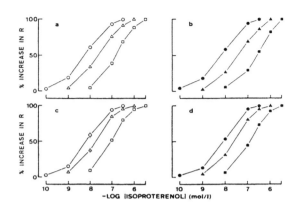

Figure 4. Effects of propranolol (panels a and b, circles: control, triangles: 10^{-8} mol/l, squares: 10^{-7} mol/l) and atenolol (panels c and d: circles: control, triangles: 10^{-7} mol/l, squares: 10^{-6} mol/l) on isoproterenol-induced percent increases in beating rate (R) of right atria of control (open symbols, propranolol and atenolol: n=9) and diabetic (closed symbols, propranolol: n=8, atenolol: n=9) rats. Each point represents mean ± SEM. SEM values are included in each symbol since they are smaller than the size of symbol. From Nagamine et al (24).

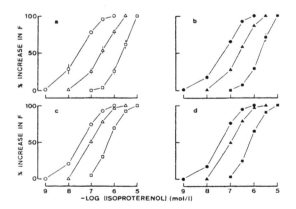

Figure 5. Effects of propranolol (panels a and b, circles: control, triangles: 10^{-8} mol/l, squares: 10^{-7} mol/l) and atenolol (panels c and d, circles: control, triangles: 10^{-7} mol/l, squares: 10^{-6} mol/l), on isoproterenol-induced percent increases in myocardial force development (F) of right ventricular papillary muscle from control (open symbols, propranolol: n=5, atenolol: n=7) and diabetic (closed symbols, propranolol: n=5, atenolol: n=9) rats. Each point represents mean ± SEM. SEM values are included in each symbol since they are smaller than the size of symbol. From Nagamine et al (24).

Table 3. pA_2 values of beta blockers.

	R	F	+dF/dt	-dF/dt
Propranolol-treated				
C group	8.72 ± 0.23 (0.9) (n=9)	8.36 ± 0.26 (1.0) (n=5)	8.79 ± 0.17 (1.0) (n=5)	8.73 ± 0.08 (1.0) (n=5)
DM group	8.71 ± 0.08 (0.9) (n=8)	9.00 ± 0.19 (0.9) (n=5)	8.45 ± 0.09 (0.9) (n=5)	8.40 ± 0.17 (1.0) (n=5)
Atenolol-treated				
C group	7.11 ± 0.11 (0.9) (n=9)	7.27 ± 0.10 (1.0) (n=7)	7.24 ± 0.08 (0.9) (n=7)	7.25 ± 0.09 (0.9) (n=7)
DM group	7.19 ± 0.08 (0.9) (n=9)	7.12 ± 0.06 (1.0) (n=9)	7.12 ± 0.05 (0.9) (n=9)	7.19 ± 0.08 (1.0) (n=9)

C: control group. DM: diabetes mellitus. Each value represents geometric mean pA_2 value ± SEM. Value of slope of the line for beta-agonist and beta-blocker is given in parentheses. n = number of preparations. R: beating rate of right atrium. F: myocardial force development of papillary muscle. +dF/dt: positive first derivative of force development. -dF/dt: negative first derivative of force development. From Nagamine et al (24).

Effects of beta-blockers on isoproterenol-induced responses in isolated right atrial and papillary muscles

Concentration response curves of R for isoproterenol after administrations of propranolol (10^{-8} mol/l and 10^{-7} mol/l) and atenolol (10^{-7} mol/l and 10^{-6} mol/l) are shown in Figure 4. The concentration response curves of R were shifted to the right by propranolol (10^{-8} mol/l and 10^{-7} mol/l) and atenolol (10^{-7} mol/l and 10^{-6} mol/l) in both control and diabetic groups, and the pA_2 values of propranolol and atenolol were not different between two groups (Table 3). Propranolol and atenolol similarly shifted the concentration response curves of F (Fig. 5) and ±dF/dt for isoproterenol to the right, and pA_2 values in each parameter were not different between two groups (Table 3).

Discussion

It has been well documented that streptozotocin selectively destroys the beta cells of the pancreas (17), resulting in reduction of insulin levels, and reveals a pathogenic state of diabetes mellitus such as hyperglycemia, hypoinsulinemia, hyperglycosylated hemoglobinemia, low body weight and low heart wet weight (8,9,18-20). Thus, streptozotocin has generally been used as a drug to induce experimentally a diabetic state. Similarly, in our experimentally diabetic model, streptozotocin induced a diabetic state: body weight and wet weights of the heart and the right atrium in diabetic rats were lower than those of control rats, and glycosylated hemoglobin level, which reflects the mean plasma glucose level during past 4 to 8 weeks (21), and plasma glucose levels were higher in the diabetic group than in the control group.

The present results in experimentally diabetic rats at 6 weeks after streptozotocin injection showed that the basal value of R in the right atrium was less frequent than that in control rats, but the basal F and the basal ±dF/dt in the right ventricular papillary muscle were not different between two groups. This less frequent R in the atrium coincided with other results that the basal value of R in the right atrium decreased in isolated myocardium of experimentally diabetic animals (7,9,18,22). On the other hand, in contrast to the present result, Fein et al (19) reported that the basal value of -dF/dt decreased more markedly than that of +dF/dt in the left ventricular papillary muscle of the diabetic rat. Discrepancy of the results of Fein et al (19) and our study might be related to differences in the experimental methods. For example, sex of rats, period from streptozotocin injection to a start of experiment, temperature, glucose and calcium concentrations in the medium, resting tension and/or stimulating frequency. They were female Wistar rats, 5 - 30 weeks, 30°C, 5.5 mmol/l, 0.6 - 2.4 mmol/l, 1.0 g and 0.1 - 0.8 Hz in Fein et al (19) study, and male Sprague-Dawley rats, 6 weeks, 37°C, 11.0 mmol/l, 1.25 mmol/l, 0.3 g and 3.3 Hz in our study, respectively.

In the present study, increases in R by isoproterenol were concentration dependent in both control and diabetic groups, but the maximum response of R was smaller in the diabetic group than in the control group. ED_{50} values of R were not significantly different between two groups in this study. These were in accordance with the results reported by Ramanadham and Tenner (9) and Ojewole (18) that the maximal responses of R to isoproterenol or norepinephrine were smaller in diabetic animals than in control ones, but the chronotropic sensitivity of right atrium for isoproterenol mediated by beta-receptor was not different between control and diabetic animals. Thus, the present results concerning R in the atrium of diabetic rats were almost similar to those observed in the previous works. However, the reason for the decreased R in diabetic rats was not clarified in this study.

In the right ventricular papillary muscles, increases in F by isoproterenol (10^{-8} mol/l - 10^{-6} mol/l) tended to be smaller in the diabetic group than in the control group and increases in +dF/dt and -dF/dt by isoproterenol (10^{-7} mol/l - 10^{-6} mol/l) were significantly less in the diabetic group than in the control group. ED_{50} values for isoproterenol were not different between two groups in F and +dF/dt except for -dF/dt: ED_{50} value of -dF/dt was significantly higher in the diabetic group than in the control group. These results show that affinity of beta receptors on the papillary muscle to isoproterenol may not be altered between control and diabetic states, but the relaxant velocity (-dF/dt) decreases in the diabetic state. In isolated and perfused rat hearts in our previous study (20), it was observed that responsiveness of F to isoproterenol and norepinephrine was lower in the diabetic group than in the control group, and -dF/dt was more easily influenced by the diabetic condition, being similar to the present results. This is consistant with the reports of Heyliger et al (8) and Ramanadham and Tenner (9). For example, Heyliger et al (8) have reported no alteration of affinity to beta receptors and depression of responsiveness to beta agonist in isolated ventricular papillary muscle from the diabetic heart when compared with the results in the control heart. The possibility that the lower body weight in the diabetic group may influence the depressed F and ±dF/dt is not completely denied in this study, although it has been shown that malnutrition is not the primary factor responsible for changes in cardiac performance observed after the streptozotocin treatment in pair-fed animals (19,23).

Thus, the present results suggest that the depressed responsiveness of diabetic hearts such as less increases in F and ±dF/dt by isoproterenol may be due to the decrease in the number of beta-adrenoceptors, while the function of receptors, at least affinity, would be intact even under the present diabetic state judging from no change in ED_{50} and pA_2 values of R, F and ±dF/dt for isoproterenol or beta blockers, except for ED_{50} value of -dF/dt for isoproterenol. Since pA_2 values in R, F and ±dF/dt were not different between two groups, it is considered that propranolol and atenolol exert the same beta-adrenoceptor blocking potency in both diabetic and non-diabetic rat hearts.

Summary

Effects of propranolol and atenolol on isoproterenol-induced responses of isolated atrial and papillary muscles from experimentally diabetic rats were examined. Male Sprague-Dawley rats were divided into the diabetic group (DM) which received streptozotocin 60 mg/kg i.v. and the control group (C) which received vehicle i.v. At 6 weeks after, the right atrial or right ventricular papillary muscle was isolated, and beating rate (R) in the atrium or isometric force development (F) and its first derivatives (±dF/dt) in the papillary muscle under pacing were recorded. Basal R was less frequent in DM than in C, but ED_{50} values for isoproterenol-induced chronotropy were not different between two groups. Basal F and basal ±dF/dt were not different between two groups, but isoproterenol-induced increases in F and ±dF/dt were less in DM than in C. ED_{50} values in F and +dF/dt were not different between both groups. Propranolol and atenolol shifted concentration response curves of R, F and ±dF/dt for isoproterenol to the right in both groups. pA_2 values of propranolol and atenolol in each parameter were not different between two groups. Results indicate that propranolol and atenolol exert the same beta-adrenoceptor blocking potency in both diabetic and non-diabetic hearts of rats.

References
1. Modan M, Halkin H, Almog S, Lusky A, Eshkol A, Shefi M, Shitrit A and Fuchs Z. Hyperinsulinemia. A link between hypertension obesity and glucose intolerance. J Clin Invest 1985;75:809-817.
2. Kessler II. Mortality experience of diabetic patients. A twenty-six year follow-up study. Am J Med 1971;51:715-724.
3. Garcia MJ, McNamara PM, Gordon T and Kannell WB. Morbidity and mortality in diabetics in the Framingham population. Sixteen year follow-up study. Diabetes 1974;23:105-111.
4. Kannel WB and McGee DL. Diabetes and cardiovascular disease. The Framingham study. JAMA 1979;241:2035-2038.

5. Rubler S, Dlugash J, Yuceoglu YZ, Kumral T, Branwood AW and Grish A. New type of cardiomyopathy associated with diabetic glomerulosclerosis. Am J Cardiol 1972;30:595-602.
6. Hamby RI, Zoneraich S and Sherman L. Diabetic cardiomyopathy. JAMA 1974;229:1749-1754.
7. Savarese JJ and Berkowitz BA. ß-adrenergic receptor decrease in diabetic rat hearts. Life Sci 1979;25:2075-2078.
8. Heyliger CE, Pierce GN, Singal PK, Beamish RE and Dhalla NS. Cardiac alpha- and beta-adrenergic receptor alterations in diabetic cardiomyopathy. Basic Res Cardiol 1982;77:610-618.
9. Ramanadham S and Tenner TE Jr. Alterations in cardiac performance in experimentally-induced diabetes. Pharmacology 1983;27:130-139.
10. Nieman LK and Davis PJ. Hypertension in diabetes mellitus. NY State J Med 1983;83:688-691.
11. ß-Blocker Heart Attack Trial Research Group. A randomized trial of propranolol in patients with acute myocardial infarction. JAMA 1982;247:1707-1714.
12. Byers SO and Friedman M. Insulin hypoglycemia enhanced by beta adrenergic blockade. Proc Soc Exp Biol Med 1966;122:114-115.
13. Weinberger MH. Antihypertensive therapy and lipids. Evidence, mechanisms and implications. Arch Intern Med 1985;145:1102-1105.
14. Raabo E and Terkildsen TC. On the enzymatic determination of blood glucose. Scand J Clin Lab Invest 1960;12:402-407.
15. Bunn HF, Shapiro R, McManus M, Garrick L, McDonald MJ, Gallop PM and Gabbay KH. Structural heterogeneity of human hemoglobin A due to nonenzymatic glycosylation. J Biol Chem 1979;254:3892-3898.
16. Klenk DC, Hermanson GT, Krohn RI, Fujimoto EK, Mallia AK, Smith PK, England JD, Wiedmeyer HM, Little RR and Goldstein DE. Determination of glycosylated hemoglobin by affinity chromatography: Comparison with colorimetric and ion-exchange methods, and effects of common interferences. Clin Chem 1982;28:2088-2094.
17. Rerup CC. Drugs producing diabetes through damage of the insulin secreting cells. Pharmacol Rev 1970;22:485-518.
18. Ojewole JAO. The influence of streptozotocin-induced diabetes on myocardial contractile performance in vitro. Meth Find Exp Clin Pharmacol 1985;7:119-124.

19. Fein FS, Kornstein LB, Strobeck JE, Capasso JM and Sonnenblick EH. Altered myocardial mechanics in diabetic rats. Circ Res 1980;47:922-933.
20. Sunagawa R, Murakami K, Mimura G and Sakanashi M. Effects of adrenergic drugs on isolated and perfused hearts of streptozotocin-induced diabetic rats. Jpn J Pharmacol 1987;44:233-240.
21. Koenig RJ, Peterson CM, Jones RL, Saudek C, Lehrman M and Cerami A. Correlation of glucose regulation and hemoglobin A_{1c} in diabetes mellitus. N Engl J Med 1976;295:417-420.
22. Foy JM and Lucas PD. Comparison between spontaneously beating atria from control and streptozotocin-diabetic rats. J Pharm Pharmacol 1978;30:558-562.
23. Penpargkul S, Schaible T, Yipintsoi T and Scheuer J. The effect of diabetes on performance and metabolism of rat hearts. Circ Res 1980;47:911-921.
24. Nagamine F, Murakami K, Mimura G and Sakanashi M. Effects of beta-adrenoceptor blocking agents on isolated atrial and papillary muscles from experimentally diabetic rats. Jpn J Pharmacol 1989;49:67-76.

Effects of Autonomic Agents on Isolated and Perfused Hearts of Streptozotocin-Induced Diabetic Rats

R. Sunagawa, F. Nagamine, K. Murakami, G. Mimura and M. Sakanashi*

The Second Department of Internal Medicine and *The Department of Pharmacology, School of Medicine, Faculty of Medicine, University of the Ryukyus, 207 Uehara, Okinawa 903-01, JAPAN

Introduction

Although it has been reported that myocardial contractility is reduced in diabetic animals (1-6), very little is known about cardiac responses to administered adrenergic and cholinergic agents. The present study, therefore, was designed to investigate the myocardial contractile response of perfused hearts isolated from experimental diabetic rats and insulin-treated diabetic rats to adrenergic and cholinergic agents.

Materials and Methods

Induction of experimental diabetes

Effects of adrenergic agents were investigated in male Sprague-Dawley rats weighing 200-260 g. Rats were randomly separated into three groups; control (C, n=13) group, diabetes mellitus (DM, n=17) group, and diabetes mellitus treated with insulin (DMI, n=15) group. In approximately half of the rats in each group (n=6 in C, n=8 in DM, and n=7 in DMI), effects of isoproterenol (ISO) and calcium chloride ($CaCl_2$) were examined. In the remaining rats (n=7 in C, N=9 in DM, and n=8 in DMI), effects of norepinephrine (NE) and aminophylline (AMI) were examined. Effects of acetylcholine (ACh) were investigated in other male Sprague-Dawley rats weighing 180-210 g; these rats were also separated into three groups; C group (n=7), DM group (n=6), and DMI group (n=9). After an overnight fast, DM and DMI groups were made diabetic with a single intravenous injection of STZ (60 mg/kg) which was dissolved immediately before use. C group was injected with buffered vehicle. The diabetic state was assessed by measurement of

Nagano, M., Mochizuki, S., Dhalla, N.S. (eds.), CARDIOVASCULAR DISEASE IN DIABETES. Copyright © 1992. Kluwer Academic Publishers, Boston. All rights reserved.

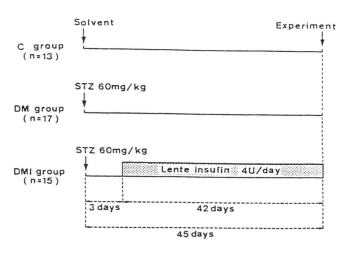

Scheme. Induction of experimental diabetes

STZ = streptozotocin. C = age-matched control; DM = STZ-induced diabetics; DMI = insulin-treated diabetics. Number of rats is given in parentheses. From Sunagawa et al. (21,22).

nonfasting plasma glucose levels 3 days after STZ injection. Subsequently, the rats in DMI group were treated with 4 U of Lente insulin (Insulin Novo Lente[R] MC, Novo Industry A/S) subcutaneously every day for 42 days (Scheme). Animals were maintained on ordinary rat chow (Clea Japan, CE-2) and water ad libitum for 45 days. Experiments were performed at 45 days after injection of STZ.

Perfusion of the heart

After an overnight fast, animals were anesthetized with sodium pentobarbital 30 mg/kg i.p. The abdomen was opened, and blood was collected rapidly from inferior vena cava. Immediately after thoracotomy, the heart was removed and chilled in Krebs-Henseleit solution of the following composition (mM): NaCl 120.0, KCl 4.8, $CaCl_2$ 1.25, $MgSO_4$ 1.2, KH_2PO_4 1.2, $NaHCO_3$ 25.0, and glucose 11.0. The heart was transferred to non-recirculating Langendorff apparatus and perfused with the Krebs-Henseleit solution (pH 7.4), which was maintained at 37°C and continuously aerated with a gas mixture of 95% O_2 + 5% CO_2, at a constant flow rate to maintain a perfusion pressure of 50 mmHg by means of a microtube pump (Eyela, MP-3). In the hearts in which effects of adrenergic agents were examined, the flow rates (ml/min) of each group were 9.8 ± 0.8 in C (n=13), 6.9 ± 0.8 in DM (n=17), and 8.5 ± 0.4 in DMI group (n=15), respectively. On the other hand, in the hearts in which effects of cholinergic agents were examined, the flow rates (ml/min) of each group were 11.5 ± 0.8 in C (n=7), 6.9 ± 0.4 in DM (n=6), and 10.5 ± 0.7 in DMI group (n=9), respectively. Perfusion pressure was monitored through a tube connected to the aortic cannula by means of an electronic manometer (Nihon Kohden, TP-101T). The heart was preloaded with a resting tension of 1.0 g. Myocardial developed tension (T) was isometrically measured through a hook attached to the apex of the heart by means of a force-displacement transducer (Nihon Kohden, TB-611T). The first derivative of myocardial developed tension (dT/dt) was derived from differentiating the developed tension signal using an electronic differentiator (Nihon Kohden, ED-601G). Heart rate was counted continuously with a cardiotachometer (Nihon Kohden, AT-600G) triggered by the developed tension. When the effects of adrenergic agents were examined, the heart was paced at a constant rate of 300 beats/min with rectangular pulses of 0.5 msec in duration and twice threshold voltage derived from an electronic stimulator (Nihon Kohden, MSE-3R) through a pair of platinum electrodes attached on the surface of the right atrium. The purpose of pacing was to remove influence of the heart rate. Pacing at 300 beats/min for about 120 min did not produce any remarkable changes in T or dT/dt in each group. On the other hand, when the effects of ACh were examined, the heart was not paced but spontaneously beating. All the parameters were recorded on a heat-pen writing polygraph (Nihon Kohden, WT-645G).

Experimental protocol

After all the parameters were equilibrated for about 20 min under these conditions, experiments were started. Drugs were dissolved in physiological saline solution, and injected into a rubber tube connected to the perfusion apparatus near the aortic cannula in a volume of 0.1 ml. Injection of the solvent in a volume of 0.1 ml did not produce any remarkable changes in all the parameters in this study. A cumulative dose-response curve was obtained by increasing concentrations of each drug in the perfusion medium. At the end of the experiment, each heart was carefully removed from the perfusion apparatus, and wet heart weight was measured. The drugs used in the present study were as follows: 1-isoproterenol hydrochloride (ISO, Nikken Kagaku), dl-norepinephrine hydrochloride (NE, Sankyo), calcium chloride (CaCl$_2$, Wako), aminophylline (AMI, Eisai), and acetylcholine chloride (ACh, Daiichi).

Blood analysis

Plasma insulin was measured by a radioimmunoassay method employing antibody-coated beads to separate bound and unbound radiolabeled insulin (7), using rat insulin as a standard. Plasma glucose levels were measured by the glucose oxidase method (8). Glycosylated hemoglobin levels were measured by the affinity column method (9,10).

Statistical significance

The data were expressed as mean ± S.E.M. of percent change from each predrug value, and the statistical analysis of the data was done with Student's t-test and chi-square test. P value less than 5% was defined as significant difference.

Results

Plasma glucose, plasma insulin, glycosylated hemoglobin, body weight, and wet heart weight

The general features (plasma glucose, plasma insulin, glycosylated hemoglobin, body weight, and wet heart weight) of C, DM, and DMI groups at the time of experiment are summarized in Table 1. Plasma glucose levels in DM group were significantly higher than in C group. While the plasma glucose levels in DMI group were significantly lower than in DM group, those in DMI group were significantly higher than in C group. Plasma insulin levels in DM group were significantly lower than in C group. Though plasma insulin levels in DMI group were higher than in DM group, there was no statistical significance. Glycosylated hemoglobin levels showed the similar pattern of changes in C, DM and DMI groups to plasma glucose levels. Body weight and wet heart weight in DM group were significantly lower than in C group, and body weight in DMI group was significantly higher than in DM group (Table 1).

Basal values of myocardial developed tension, +dT/dt and -dT/dt

Steady state values of each cardiac parameter of each group are summarized in Table 2.

Table 1. General features of control, diabetic and insulin-treated diabetic rats.

1) Rats in which effects of adrenergic agents were examined.

	Plasma glucose (mg/dl)	Plasma insulin (ng/ml)	Body weight (g)	Heart weight (g)
C group (n=13)	142.4 ± 8.7	1.6 ± 0.3	423.8 ± 5.7	1.1 ± 0.0
	**	**	**	**
DM group (n=17)	499.3 ± 15.6	0.6 ± 0.1	218.1 ± 8.9	0.8 ± 0.0
	xx **	*	xx **	xx
DMI group (n=15)	370.6 ± 27.6	0.9 ± 0.1	360.1 ± 8.4	1.1 ± 0.1

C = age-matched control; DM = streptozotocin-induced diabetics; DMI = insulin-treated diabetics. Each value represents mean ± S.E.M. Number of rats is given in parentheses. Significantly different from control value at $^*p < 0.05$ and $^{**}p < 0.01$. Significantly different from diabetic value at $^{xx}p < 0.01$. Because experiments were performed after an overnight fast, the rats of DMI group were withdrawn from insulin 18 hours prior to experiments to avoid the hypoglycemic shock. From Sunagawa et al. (21).

2) Rats in which effects of ACh were examined.

	Plasma glucose (mg/dl)	Glycosylated hemoglobin (%)	Body weight (g)	Heart weight (g)
C group (n=7)	116.0 ± 4.9	3.9 ± 0.1	397.9 ± 9.0	1.0 ± 0.1
	**	**	**	*
DM group (n=6)	480.1 ± 31.0	16.0 ± 0.4	250.9 ± 19.1	0.8 ± 0.2
	xx *	xx **	xx	xx
DMI group (n=9)	204.6 ± 34.8	5.8 ± 0.4	381.7 ± 8.3	1.1 ± 0.0

Explanation is the same as for the above table. From Sunagawa et al. (22).

Table 2. Steady state values of each cardiac parameter of control, diabetic and insulin-treated diabetic rats.

1) Rats in which effects of adrenergic agents were examined.

		Myocardial developed tension (g)	+dT/dt (g/sec)	-dT/dt (g/sec)
C	group (n=13)	4.16 ± 0.24	87.98 ± 10.42	60.84 ± 9.00
DM	group (n=17)	4.13 ± 0.19	72.78 ± 7.26	47.14 ± 4.20
DMI	group (n=15)	4.41 ± 0.24	98.86 ± 12.11	63.81 ± 7.13 ˣ

C = age-matched control; DM = streptozotocin-induced diabetics; DMI = insulin-treated diabetics. Each value represents mean ± S.E.M. Number of rats is given in parentheses. Significantly different from diabetic value at $^x p < 0.05$. From Sunagawa et al. (21).

2) Rats in which effects of ACh were examined.

		Myocardial developed tension (g)	+dT/dt (g/sec)	-dT/dt (g/sec)
C	group (n=7)	5.08 ± 0.14	125.8 ± 7.0	94.4 ± 2.9
DM	group (n=6)	4.79 ± 0.20	100.1 ± 4.1 *	60.2 ± 5.1 **
DMI	group (n=9)	5.47 ± 0.34	126.4 ± 9.2 ˣ	95.2 ± 8.9 ˣˣ

Explanation is the same as for the above table. Significantly different from control value at $^* p < 0.05$ and $^{**} p < 0.01$. Significantly different from diabetic value at $^x p < 0.05$ and $^{xx} p < 0.01$. From Sunagawa et al. (22).

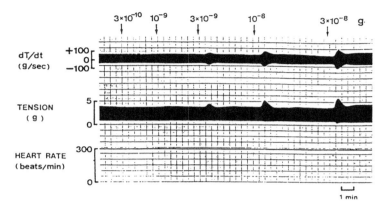

Figure 1. Typical recording of the effects of bolus injections of isoproterenol on an isolated and perfused heart from a control rat. dT/dt: first derivative of myocardial developed tension. The heart was paced at a constant rate of 300 beats/min. From Sunagawa et al. (21).

Effects of drugs on myocardial developed tension

Cumulative administrations of adrenergic agents produced dose-dependent increases in maximal developed tension (T) of isolated and perfused hearts of each group. Figure 1 shows a typical recording of the effects of bolus injection of ISO on a control rat heart. ISO 3×10^{-10} g did not change T (Fig. 1 and 2).

Percent increases in T by ISO 10^{-9} - 3×10^{-8} g in DM group were significantly lower than in C group. On the other hand, percent increases in T by ISO 3×10^{-9} - 3×10^{-8} g in DMI group were significantly greater than in DM group, and these increases in DMI group were almost the same as in C group (Fig. 2).

Percent increases in T by NE 10^{-8} - 3×10^{-8} g were not significantly different among three groups. However, percent increases in T by NE 10^{-7} - 10^{-6} g in DM group were significantly lower than in C group. Though percent increases in DMI group were greater than in DM group, those were not statistically significant (Fig. 3).

Percent increases in T by $CaCl_2$ 1.1×10^{-4} - 2.2×10^{-3} g were not significantly different among three groups except the value by $CaCl_2$ 5.6×10^{-4} g (Fig. 4). Furthermore, percent increases in T by AMI 0.31×10^{-3} - 5.00×10^{-3} g were also not significantly different among three groups (Fig. 5).

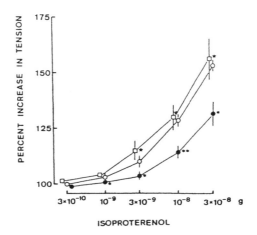

Figure 2. Effects of isoproterenol on percent increase in myocardial developed tension of isolated and perfused hearts from control (0-0, n=6), diabetic (●-●, n=8), and insulin-treated diabetic (□-□, n=7) rats. Each value represents mean ± S.E.M. Significantly different from control value at $^*p < 0.05$ and $^{**}p < 0.01$. Significantly different from diabetic value at $^*p < 0.05$. From Sunagawa et al. (21).

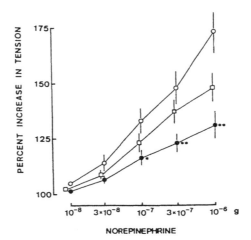

Figure 3. Effects of norepinephrine on percent increase in myocardial developed tension of isolated and perfused hearts from control (0-0, n=7), diabetic (●-●, n=9), and insulin-treated diabetic (□-□, n=8) rats. Each value represents mean ± S.E.M. Significantly different from control value at $^*p < 0.05$ and $^{**}p < 0.01$. From Sunagawa et al (21).

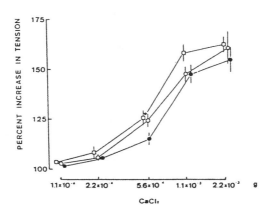

Figure 4. Effects of CaCl$_2$ on percent increase in myocardial developed tension of isolated and perfused hearts from control (0-0, n=6), diabetic (●-●, n=8), and insulin-treated diabetic (□-□, n=7) rats. Each value represents mean ± S.E.M. Significantly different from the diabetic value at * $p < 0.05$. From Sunagawa et al. (21).

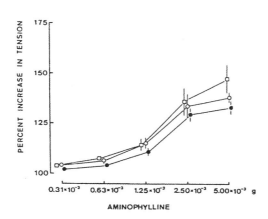

Figure 5. Effects of aminophylline on percent increase in myocardial developed tension of isolated and perfused hearts from control (0-0, n=7), diabetic (●-●, n=9), and insulin-treated diabetic (□-□, n=8) rats. Each value represents mean ± S.E.M. From Sunagawa et al. (21).

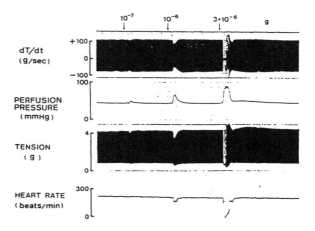

Figure 6. Typical recording of the effects of bolus injections of acetylcholine on a perfused heart isolated from a control rat. dT/dt: first derivative of myocardial developed tension. From Sunagawa et al. (22).

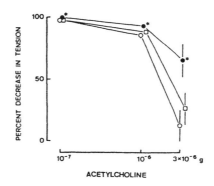

Figure 7. Effects of acetylcholine on percent decrease in myocardial developed tension of perfused hearts isolated from control (O-O, n=7), diabetic (●-●, n=6), and insulin-treated diabetic (□-□, n=9) rats. Each value represents mean ± S.E.M. Significantly different from control value at *p < 0.05. From Sunagawa et al. (22).

Figure 6 shows a typical recording of the effects of bolus injections of ACh on a control rat heart (Fig. 6). Percent decreases in T by ACh 10^{-7} - 3×10^{-6} g in DM group were significantly smaller than in C group, and those in DMI group tended to be greater than in DM group (Fig. 7).

Effects of drugs on +dT/dt

To evaluate effects of drugs on myocardial contraction velocity (+dT/dt) and rate of relaxation (-dT/dt), percent changes in the first derivative of T (+dT/dt) by each drug were measured. Percent increases in +dT/dt by ISO $3 \times 10^{-9} - 3 \times 10^{-8}$ g, NE $10^{-8} - 10^{-6}$ g and $CaCl_2$ $2.2 \times 10^{-4} - 2.2 \times 10^{-3}$ g tended to be lower in DM group than ion C and DMI groups, and the difference of change by ISO 10^{-8} g was significant statistically. Percent increases in +dT/dt by AMI $1.25 \times 10^{-3} - 5.00 \times 10^{-3}$ g were significantly lower in DM group than in C group, and those in DMI group tended to be greater than in DM group. Percent decreases in +dT/dt ACh $10^{-7} - 3 \times 10^{-6}$ g were not significantly different among three groups except the value by ACh 3×10^{-6} g in DM group. Percent changes in -dT/dt by each drug in DM group were lower than in C group, and differences of percent increases and percent decreases were statistically significant at NE $10^{-7} - 10^{-6}$ g and ACh $10^{-7} - 3 \times 10^{-6}$ g, respectively. Percent changes in -dT/dt by each drug in DMI group were greater than in DM group, and percent increases and percent decreases were significantly different at NE $3 \times 10^{-7} - 10^{-6}$ g and ACh $10^{-7} - 10^{-6}$ g, respectively.

Effects of ACh on heart rate

Chronotropic responsiveness of the heart to ACh was examined in each group. Resting heart rates in DM group were less than in C group, and those in DMI group were more than in DM group (Table 3). Administration of ACh 3×10^{-6} g produced a transient cardiac arrest in some hearts of each group, and incidence of the transient cardiac arrest in DM group was significantly less than in both C and DMI groups (Table 3).

Discussion

In the present study, steady state basal values of myocardial developed tension, +dT/dt and -dT/dt were not significantly different among three groups. In isolated ventricular papillary muscle and isolated perfused working heart preparations of diabetic rats, the decrease in myocardial contractility has been observed (1-6). Discrepancy of the present results from those in previous studies may be due to differences in experimental conditions such as isolated and perfused heart preparations or loading conditions, suggesting less myocardial damages in the present experimental conditions.

Table 3. Effects of acetylcholine on heart rate of control, diabetic, and insulin-treated diabetic rats.

		Resting heart rate (beats/min)	Transient cardiac arrest by ACh 3×10^{-6} g (number of case)	Incidence of transient arrest (%)
C	group (n=7)	248.9 ± 7.6	6	85.7
DM	group (n=6)	207.5 ± 20.9	1	16.7 *
DMI	group (n=9)	236.2 ± 9.0	6	66.7

C = age-matched control; DM = streptozotocin-induced diabetics; DMI = insulin-treated diabetics. Number of rats is given in parentheses. Significantly different from control value at * $p < 0.05$ (chi-square test). From Sunagawa et al. (22).

As shown previously (11), STZ selectively destroys the beta cells of pancreas and causes an absolute or relative reduction in insulin levels. In the present experiment, plasma insulin levels were significantly lower in DM group than in C group, and significantly recovered in DMI group, indicating that the low insulin levels in DM group most probably result from STZ-induced insulin deficiency.

In this experimental model, influences of direct STZ-induced cardiac toxicity and altered thyroid hormone levels on cardiac function must be considered (12). However, as shown in the present results, percent increases in tension by $CaCl_2$ and AMI were not significantly different among C, DM, and DMI groups. Fein et al. (13) studied animals given insulin or various thyroid hormones and provided evidence that neither depressed thyroid hormone levels nor STZ-induced cardiac toxicity is responsible for the myocardial mechanical dysfunction in animals. Therefore, the above possibilities may be ruled out.

The possible reasons of high plasma glucose levels of DMI group in spite of treatment with insulin in this study will be as follows: because the rats of DMI group were withdrawn from insulin 18 hours prior to experiments to avoid the hypoglycemic shock (1). Therefore, the plasma glucose levels of DMI group were transiently elevated at the time of experiment. In fact, glycosylated hemoglobin levels which reflect the mean glucose levels during the past 4 to 8 weeks (14) were significantly lower in DMI group than in DM group. From this, it can be expected that, in our experimental models the plasma glucose levels in DM group were maintained under hyperglycemic conditions and those in DMI group, under similar conditions to those in C group.

In the present study, body weight in DM group was significantly lower than in C and DMI groups. However, it is unlikely that this decrease in body weight influences the depressed myocardial contractile response, since it has been demonstrated using pair-fed animals that malnutrition was not the primary factor responsible for changes observed in cardiac performance after STZ treatment (1,2). The present results of no changes in percent increase in tension by $CaCl_2$ and AMI also support this view.

Though percent increases in tension by ISO and NE were significantly lower in DM group than in C group, those by $CaCl_2$ and AMI were not significantly different among three groups, suggesting that adrenergic receptor-mediated contractile response is specifically depressed in the diabetic hearts at 45 days after injection of STZ, when myocardial contractile response is assessed by the percent increase in tension. This suspicion is supported by reports of Heyliger et al. (3) and Atkins et al. (15). Atkins et al. (15) studied the relationship of cardiac function to the beta-adrenergic receptor and/or adenylate cyclase activity in open-chest anesthetized diabetic rats, and observed that the activity of adenylate cyclase by ISO stimulation was significantly depressed in DM group despite of no change in adenylate cyclase activity by NaF and forskolin. They proposed that beta-adrenergic receptor number in cardiac membranes from diabetic rats is significantly reduced, and this view is supported by the previous findings reported by Savarese et al. (16) and Williams et al. (17). This also may account for the present results that percent increases in tension by AMI were not significantly different among three groups. Furthermore, in the present experiments, percent increases in tension by $CaCl_2$ were also not different among three groups, suggesting that calcium channel-mediated contractile response is not depressed in the diabetic hearts at 45 days after STZ injection.

Percent decreases in maximal developed tension and those in heart rate induced by ACh in DM group were significantly smaller than in C group, suggesting that cholinergic receptor-mediated cardiac responsiveness would be significantly depressed in the diabetic hearts.

Foy and Lucas (18) reported that 1 to 2 week alloxan- and STZ-induced diabetes produced a reduced sensitivity to the depressor effect of ACh in pithed rats. On the other hand, Vadlamudi et al. (19) studied effect of carbachol on perfused working hearts and observed that diabetic rat hearts at 100 days after induction of diabetes exhibited a reduced responsiveness to the negative inotropic effect of carbachol when compared with control rat hearts. The present results obtained from the diabetic rat hearts at 45 days agree with the findings of Foy and Lucas (17) and the report by Vadlamudi et al. (18). Thus, it is likely that the diabetic conditions will induce the reduction in responsiveness of postsynaptic cholinergic receptors to exogenously administered cholinergic drugs, resulting in depression of ACh-induced negative inotropic action in DM group.

Very little is known about the chronotropic effects of exogenously administered cholinergic agonists on the heart in experimentally induced diabetes. In the present results, percent decrease in heart rate by ACh was significantly smaller in DM group than in C group. Furthermore, incidence of the transient cardiac arrest by ACh in DM group was significantly less than in C group, meaning that the responsiveness of the heart to the negative chronotropic action of cholinergic agonist is depressed in the diabetic rats.

The percent changes in +dT/dt and -dT/dt by each drug including $CaCl_2$ and AMI showed a tendency to be smaller in DM group than in C group. In general, it has been established experimentally that myocardial maximal developed tension is not related to its maximal shortening velocity (20). Therefore, if there was no agreement with the results between tension and ±dT/dt, it may not always be unreasonable. Alternatively, it is speculated that ±dT/dt is more easily influenced than tension under the certain pathophysiological conditions.

In conclusion, the present results indicate that adrenergic and cholinergic receptor-mediated cardiac responsiveness are significantly depressed in the diabetic hearts and that these depressed responsiveness in DM group can be reversed by insulin therapy.

Summary

To evaluate responses of the diabetic heart to autonomic agents, effects of isoproterenol (ISO), norepinephrine (NE) and acetylcholine (ACh) on perfused hearts isolated from streptozotocin (STZ)-induced diabetic rats and insulin-treated diabetic rats were examined. Male Sprague-Dawley rats were divided into control (C)-group, diabetes mellitus (DM)-group, and diabetes mellitus treated with insulin (DMI)-group. C group was injected with buffered vehicle. DM and DMI groups were injected intravenously with 60 mg/kg STZ at the first day. Three days after STZ injection, DMI group was subsequently treated with 4 U of Lente insulin subcutaneously every day. At 45 days after injection of STZ, experiments were performed using a Langendorff perfused heart preparation. In the evaluation of effect of adrenergic agents, the heart was paced at 300 beats/min and myocardial developed tension (T) was measured isometrically. In the evaluation of effect of ACh, spontaneous heart rate and T were measured. Plasma glucose values (mg/dl) were 116.0 ± 4.9 to 142.4 ± 8.7 in C, 480.1 ± 31.0 to 499.3 ± 15.6 in DM, and 204.6 ± 34.8 to 370.6 ± 27.6 in DMI group, respectively. The order of percent increases in T induced by ISO ($3 \times 10^{-9} - 3 \times 10^{-8}$ g) was C = DMI >> DM, and that by NE($10^{-7} - 10^{-6}$ g) was C > DMI > DM. The order of percent decreases in T and heart rate by ACh heart rate by ACh ($10^{-7} - 3 \times 10^{-6}$ g) was C > DMI > DM. On the other hand, percent increase in T induced by $CaCl_2$ ($1.1 \times 10^{-4} - 2.2 \times 10^{-3}$ g) or aminophylline (AMI, $0.31 \times 10^{-3} - 5.00 \times 10^{-3}$ g) was not significantly different among three groups. These results suggest that both adrenergic and cholinergic receptor-mediated cardiac responsiveness are significantly depressed in the diabetic heart.

References

1. Fein F, Kornstein L, Strobeck J, Capasso J and Sonnenblick E. Altered myocardial mechanics in diabetic rats. Circ Res 1980;47:922-933.
2. Penpargkul S, Schaible T, Yipintsoi T and Scheuer J. The effect of diabetes on performance and metabolism of rat hearts. Circ Res 1980;47:911-921.
3. Heyliger C, Pierce G, Singal P, Beamish R and Dhalla N. Cardiac alpha- and beta-adrenergic receptor alterations in diabetic cardiomyopathy. Basic Res Cardiol 1982;77:610-618.

4. Vadlamudi R, Rodgers R and McNeill J. The effect of chronic alloxan and streptozotocin-induced diabetes on isolated rat heart performance. Can J Physiol Pharmacol 1982;60:902-911.
5. Fein F and Sonnenblick E. Diabetic cardiomyopathy. Progr Cardiovas Dis 1985;27:255-270.
6. Tahiliani A and McNeill J. Diabetes-induced abnormalities in the myocardium. Life Sci 1986;38:959-974.
7. Catt K and Tregear G. Solid-phase radioimmunoassasy in antibody-coated tubes. Science 1967;158:1570-1572.
8. Raabo E and Terkildsen T. On the enzymatic determination of blood glucose. Scand J Clin Lab Invest 1960;12:402-407.
9. Bunn H, Shapiro R, McManus M, Garrick L, McDonald M, Gallop P and Gabby K. Structural heterogeneity of human hemoglobin A due to non-enzymatic glycosylation. J Biol Chem 1979;254:3892-3898.
10. Klenk D, Hermanson G, Krohn R, Fujimoto E, Mallia A, Smith P, England J, Wiedmeyer H, Little R and Goldstein D. Determination of glycosylated hemoglobin by affinity chromatography: Comparison with colorimetric and ion-exchange methods, and effects of common interferences. Clin Chem 1982;28:2088-2094.
11. Rerup C. Drugs producing diabetes through damage of the insulin secreting cells. Pharmacol Rev 1970;22:485-518.
12. Malhotra A, Penpargkul S, Fein F, Sonnenblick E and Scheuer J. The effect of streptozotocin-induced diabetes in rats on cardiac contractile proteins. Circ Res 1981;49:1243-1250.
13. Fein F, Strobeck J, Malhotra A, Scheuer J and Sonnenblick E. Reversibility of diabetic cardiomyopathy with insulin in rats. Circ Res 1981;49:1251-1261.
14. Bunn H. Evaluation of glycosylated hemoglobin in diabetic patients. Diabetes 1981;30:613-617.
15. Atkins F, Dowell R and Love S. ß-adrenergic receptors, adenylate cyclase activity, and cardiac dysfunction in the diabetic rats. J Cardiovasc Pharmacol 1985;7:66-70.
16. Savarese J and Berkowitz B. ß-adrenergic receptor decrease in diabetic rat hearts. Life Sci 1979;25:2075-2078.
17. Williams R, Schaible T, Scheuer J and Kennedy R. Effects of experimental diabetes on adrenergic and cholinergic receptors of rat myocardium. Diabetes 1983;32:881-886.

18. Foy J and Lucas P. Effect of experimental diabetes, food deprivation and genetic obesity on the sensitivity of pithed rats to autonomic agents. Br J Pharmacol 1976;57:229-234.
19. Vadlamudi R and McNeill J. Effect of alloxan- and streptozotocin-induced diabetes on isolated rat heart responsiveness to carbachol. J Pharmacol Exp Ther 1983;225:410-415.
20. Katz A. Physiology of the Heart. pp. 73-88, Raven Press, New York, 1984.
21. Sunagawa R, Murakami K, Mimura G and Sakanashi M. Effects of adrenergic drugs on isolated and perfused hearts of streptozotocin-induced diabetic rats. Jap J Pharmacol 1987;44:233-240.
22. Sunagawa R, Nagamine F, Murakami K, Mimura G and Sakanashi M. Effects of dobutamine and acetylcholine on perfused hearts isolated from streptozotocin-induced diabetic rats. Arzneim-Forsch/Drug Res 1989;39(I):470-474.

Insulin-Like Actions of Vanadyl Sulfate Trihydrate in Streptozotocin-Diabetic Rats

Margaret C. Cam and John H. McNeill

Division of Pharmacology and Toxicology, Faculty of Pharmaceutical Sciences
The University of British Columbia, Vancouver, B.C. Canada V6T 1W5

Introduction

Vanadium is a ubiquitous group V transitional element (atomic weight 50.94). An essential trace nutrient in chicks, dietary deficiencies were observed to result in decreased body and feather growth although in rats, impaired reproductive ability, the sole consequence of vanadium lack is seen only after four generations (1). In humans, the total vanadium pool is estimated to range between 100-200 ug although symptoms of deficiency have not yet been established (2). Vanadium exists in several valence forms (-1 to +5) and in red blood cells and adipocytes is converted intracellularly from vanadate (VO_3^-, +5) to vanadyl (VO^{2+}, +4) (3).

Several laboratories have now reported the insulin-like activity of vanadium both in vitro and in vivo. Among its recognized effects in isolated tissues are increased glucose uptake and stimulation of glycogen synthesis in rat diaphragm, liver and fat cells (4), enhanced glucose transport and oxidation in rat adipocytes and skeletal muscle (5,6,7) activation of glycolysis in rat liver (8), inhibition of lipolysis (9) and activation of lipogenesis in rat adipocytes (10), inhibition of hepatic cholesterol and phospholipid synthesis (11,12), insulin receptor activation (13) and down-regulation (14,15). In addition, its insulin-mimetic actions have been correlated with a rise in tyrosine phosphorylation of the insulin receptor 95 kd subunit (16,17), although some controversy still exists regarding the significance of this finding, including a possible direct intracellular involvement (18,19,20,21). Furthermore, significant differences between certain metabolic effects of insulin and vanadium have also been demonstrated *in vitro* (7,22,23).

Nagano, M., Mochizuki, S., Dhalla, N.S. (eds.), CARDIOVASCULAR DISEASE IN DIABETES. Copyright © 1992. Kluwer Academic Publishers, Boston. All rights reserved.

The first recorded use of vanadium in diabetes transpired in 1899 when Lyonnet et al (24) observed a decrease in urine glucose in 2 out of 3 diabetic patients who were administered sodium vanadate. In 1985, a study on the *in vivo* insulin mimetic actions of vanadium in animals was first performed in our lab by Heyliger et al (25), who managed to depress elevated glucose levels in streptozotocin (STZ)-diabetic rats by adding sodium orthovanadate (Na_3VO_4, 0.6 and 0.8 mg/ml) into the drinking water for 4 weeks. In addition, it prevented the development of cardiac functional abnormalities in the diabetic rats. However it was subsequently observed that at a concentration of 0.8 mg/ml, vanadate was toxic to the animals, resulting in severe diarrhea and death due to dehydration in some animals. Similarly, Meyerovitch et al (26) reported that at 0.8 mg/ml sodium metavanadate ($NaVO_3$), which had effectively reduced hyperglycemia in STZ-diabetic rats, adversely altered liver and kidney function, and intake ultimately resulted in death. In a more recent study by Brichard et al (27), glucose-lowering effects were accompanied by severe dehydration in rats treated with 0.5 mg/ml Na_3VO_4.

Recently, Paulson et al (28) reported the absence of vanadate toxicity at concentrations of 0.8 mg/ml when buffered at pH 7.0, where it was proposed some vanadate would exist as vanadyl. Furthermore, the vanadyl ion has been reported to have an LD_{50} 6 to 10 times greater than vanadate (29). Hence, our laboratory has been interested in determining the effectiveness of vanadyl in the chronic oral treatment of STZ-diabetic rats. Various properties which are inherently deviant in diabetes were assessed including body weight, food and fluid intake, several metabolic and hormonal plasma parameters, heart function, glycerol output from isolated adipose tissue, glucose and insulin response to the oral glucose tolerance test, islet cell number and insulin content, and pancreatic insulin secretion.

Methods

Treatment and Maintenance. For these studies, male Wistar rats weighing between 170-200 g were used. One group was made diabetic by a single injection of streptozotocin (60 mg/kg i.v.) while a control group received only the vehicle (0.1 mol/L citrate buffer, pH 4.5). After 3 days blood glucose was measured using a glucometer, and rats with glucose levels > 13.75 mmol/L were considered diabetic and further subdivided into two groups. One was given plain water (STZ) while the other (STZ-T) was supplied with tap water containing vanadyl sulfate trihydrate (VST). Control rats were similarly grouped into treated (CON-T) and non-treated (CON) groups. One set of control and diabetic animals was maintained for 10 weeks prior to tissue analysis. The treated animals CON-T (n=8) and STZ-T (n=11) received VST 1.0 mg/ml throughout the entire study period. A separate set of controls and diabetics was kept for 16 weeks. Treated animals in this group were subjected to 3 weeks of vanadyl treatment followed by a 13-week withdrawal period prior to sacrifice. The STZ-T rats were administered VST in varying concentrations, (mg/ml): 0.25 (n=8), 0.50 (n=9), 0.75 (n=9) and 1.00 (n=9).

Working Heart Perfusion (detailed in ref. 30). Immediately following sacrifice, the heart was isolated and placed in an oxygen-rich buffer. Heart function was examined using a working heart apparatus (31). Left ventricular developed pressure (LVDP), rate of ventricular force development (+dP/dt) and relaxation (-dP/dt) were assessed at left atrial filling pressures 5.0 - 22.5 cm H_2O.

Isolated Cardiac Tissue Preparation (detailed in ref. 32). Inotropic sensitivity of myocardial tissue was measured after completion of the working heart study. A piece of right ventricular tissue was mounted onto two platinum electrodes, while the other was fixed to a force transducer. The strips were electrically stimulated, basal developed force (BDF) and inotropic responses were recorded at various doses of Ca^{++} added to the bath.

Incubation of Epididymal Adipose Tissue and Preparation of Extracts (detailed in ref. 30). Lipolytic activity was based on glycerol release as described previously (33). Following sacrifice of the animals, epididymal fat pads were removed and incubated in the presence or absence of insulin (45 min). The pads were homogenized and extraction performed through centrifugation.

Glycerol Output from Adipose Tissue (detailed in ref. 30). Following removal of incubated adipose tissue, samples of the incubation medium were treated and centrifuged prior to storage. Glycerol output was measured on deproteinized samples using commercial kits (34).

Incorporation of ^{32}P into Proteins of Adipose Tissue Supernatant Fractions (detailed in ref. 30). Samples of the protein-containing supernatant fraction extracted from adipose were reacted with [^{32}P]ATP for 10 min. Protein pellets recovered through centrifugation were digested and subjected to electrophoresis using the discontinuous pH gel system (35,36). Autoradiographs were prepared and the extent of ^{32}P incorporation into phosphoproteins and protein content of gels was subsequently measured by densitometry.

OGTT (detailed in ref. 37). Rats were fasted overnight at the conclusion of the 16-week study, and administered a dose of 1 g/kg gluocse by oral gavage. Blood samples were then collected at various times for plasma glucose and insulin determinations.

Pancreas Perfusion. Insulin secretion from isolated perfused pancreas was stimulated with perfusate containing 300 mg/dl glucose with gastric inhibitory peptide (GIP) as a gradient (0-1 ng/ml) described by Pederson et al (38).

Islet Immunohistochemistry (detailed in ref. 37). Immunocytochemical staining was performed on samples from head, body and tail of the pancreas collected after perfusion study.

Islet Cell Quantification (detailed in ref. 37). The total islet cell area and area percent occupied by immunoreactive insulin cells were calculated for 75 islets per pancreas using a computerized morphometrics system.

Plasma Analysis. Blood was collected into heparinized tubes at time of sacrifice and centrifuged for 5 minutes (3,000 xg, 4°C). The plasma fraction was removed and stored at -80°C until assays were performed using standard commercial kits: glucose, triglyceride, cholesterol, and phospholipid (Boehringer Mannheim) and insulin, T_3 and T_4 (Amersham).

Vanadium Determination. Kidney and plasma levels were determined by methods previously described (13).

Statistical Analyses. All results are expressed as average ± S.E.M. Geometric mean effective concentration (EC_{50}) values were used to express changes in sensitivity (39). The data were analyzed using ANOVA followed by Duncan's and/or Newman-Keuls tests. Significant differences between values for glycerol output was assessed using the Student's unpaired t-test. $P < 0.05$ was considered significant.

Results

Ten-week study (ref. 30)

Body weight did not increase in STZ-T rats relative to the STZ group whereas CON-T rats exhibited lowered body weights in comparison to CON albeit remaining higher than both diabetic groups. As expected, the STZ group consumed abnormally high volumes of fluid, while in both sets of treated animals, fluid intake did not differ significantly to CON. Average vanadyl dose (mg/kg body weight/day) which was significantly higher for STZ-T during the first week subsequently became equivalent to CON-T values for the remaining treatment period (30).

The characteristic symptoms of diabetes, hyperglycemia and hypoinsulinemia were observed in the STZ rats. On the other hand, plasma glucose values in the STZ-T animals were normalized in spite of low insulin, while in CON-T was unchanged from control values (ref. 30, Table 1). Interestingly, a significant drop in circulating insulin was also noted in the CON-T group. Overall, plasma insulin was not different among groups CON-T, DIA and DIA-T (30).

A significantly lowered heart weight was observed in STZ-T, CON-T and STZ groups as compared to CON; however, the ratio of heart to body weight was only significantly higher in STZ, indicative of cardiac hypertrophy in this group. Furthermore, heart function as measured by +dP/dt, -dP/dt, and LVDP although equal in all groups in the lower atrial filling pressures, was significantly decreased in the STZ group at a higher filling pressures of 17.5 to 22.5 cm H_2O, while STZ-T and CON-T groups did not show any significant difference to CON (30).

Other plasma parameters which are significantly altered in the STZ group were found to be normalized in diabetic rats by treatment with vanadyl and unchanged in CON-T (ref. 30, Table 1). Plasma T_4, which was significantly depressed in the STZ group was returned to control levels in the STZ-T group. As well, lipid levels were correspondingly improved with vanadyl treatment: plasma triglycerides, cholesterol, and phospholipid levels in this group did not significantly deviate from control (30).

Rate of lipolysis was measured by glycerol output from isolated adipose tissue. STZ values were, as anticipated, increased to twice the normal levels but were considerably reduced after treatment with vanadyl. Control animals did not demonstrate a further drop in lipolytic activity as a result of treatment. Tissue-responsiveness to insulin was found to be significant (32-38%) and similar in all groups.

Protein phosphorylation was analyzed in isolated adipose tissue in order to ascertain to some degree the mechanism of action of vanadyl on fat metabolism at the intracellular level. Strong evidence exists for the role of phosphorylation of key regulatory proteins in the hormonal action of insulin, effects which have at least been shown to be mediated through protein kinases

Table 1. Various plasma parameters recorded at end of 10-week maintenance period (Data calculated from ref. 30)

Group	n	Glu (mM)	T_4 (nM)	TG (mM)	Chol (mM)	Ins (uU/ml)
CON	10	7.2 ± 0.9	59 ± 3	1.5 ± 0.28	1.52 ± 0.11	87.1 ± 12.9
CON-T	7	7.2 ± 0.7	57 ± 3	1.01 ± 0.34	1.34 ± 0.13	43.1 ± 13.4[b]
STZ	11	25.1 ± 0.7[a]	34 ± 2[a]	2.38 ± 0.27[a]	1.89 ± 0.10[a]	17.9 ± 3.6[b]
STZ-T	11	8.7 ± 0.7	51 ± 4	1.49 ± 0.28	1.36 ± 0.11	23.9 ± 4.7[b]

* Values are presented as means ± S.E.
a Significantly different from all other groups (p < 0.05)
b Significantly different from control (p < 0.05)

and/or protein phosphatases (40). The phosphoprotein profile presented seven major ^{32}P-labeled protein subunits which were consistent, having the approximate M_r values (x10^{-3}) of 120, 105, 90, 73, 65, 54 and 46. In addition, a substantial number of minor ^{32}P-labeled protein subunits was observed. ^{32}P incorporation into subunits of M_r 65,000 and 46,000 were elevated in the STZ group (146 +/- and 153 +/- 4% of the control, respectively), alterations which were no longer apparent after treatment (30).
Sixteen-week study (results from ref. 32 & 37)

The percentage of animals which developed euglycemia at the end of the 13-week withdrawal period was 25% (2/8) in 0.25 mg/ml, 43% (3/7) in 0.50 mg/ml, 83% (5/6) in 0.75 mg/ml, and 60% (3/5) in 1.00 mg/ml (Table 2). An increase in the effectiveness of vanadyl treatment was accompanied by a rise in mortality rate with progressive concentrations of vanadyl in the drinking water. In the range of concentrations tested, the 0.75 mg/ml group had the highest rate of response while in the 1.00 mg/ml concentration, effectiveness dropped and mortality rate rose. Death ensued as a result of diarrhea, followed by dehydration and hypoglycemia (due to deficient food intake) or from refusal to drink (encountered at a concentration of 1.00 mg/ml). Body weights of rats in the STZ-T group were significantly higher than the untreated STZ rats, but remained lower than the control group (32).

Plasma parameters such as elevations in plasma glucose and lipids (triglycerides, cholesterol and phospholipids) and depressions in thyroid

Table 2. Concentration-dependent effects of vanadyl treatment in STZ-diabetic rats[*]. (Data calculated from ref. 32)

Vanadyl Concentration (mg/ml)	Survival Rate (%)	Percent Euglycemic[a]		
		During Treatment[b]	1 day w.d.[c]	13 week w.d.[d]
0.25 (n=8)	100	38	25	25
0.50 (n=9)	78	100	71	43
0.75 (n=9)	67	100	100	83
1.00 (n=9)	56	100	60	60

* Values are means ± S.E.
a Percentage of euglycemic animsla with respect to number of surviving animals (blood glucose concentrations < 8 mM)
b Blood glucose concentrations measured between 2-3 weeks following initiation of treatment
c After three weeks of treatment, vanadyl was withdrawn (w.d.) and glucose levels taken the following day
d At time of sacrifice (13 weeks post 3-week treatment period)

hormones (T_3 and T_4) were corrected. More significantly and in contrast to previous observations (30), resting insulin levels in the responding animals of the STZ-T group were found to be normal (32).

In the cardiac and adipose tissue experiments, seven STZ-T rats which were euglycemic at the end of 16 weeks were pooled and assessed as one group. Cardiac function as measured by left ventricular filling pressure (LVDP), and rates of contraction (+dP/dt) and relaxation (-dP/dt) was compared between groups at atrial filling pressures between 5.0 and 22.0 cm H_2O. At atrial pressures above 15.0 cm H_2O, cardiac performance was diminished for the STZ group, while the STZ-T group showed increasingly improved myocardial performance which was not different from control at 20 and 22.5 cm H_2O. Heart weight was similar with all three groups, however, body weight was significantly lower in the diabetic groups, thus heart to body weight ratios were higher for STZ and STZ-T groups (32).

Rates of glycerol release from epidydymal fat pads were significantly elevated in the STZ group in the absence of drugs (basal), or in the presence

Table 3. Basal and peak glucose levels and integrated insulin responses to oral glucose challenge[a]. (Data calculated from ref. 37)[*]

Group	Basal glucose[b] (mmol/L)	Peak glucose (mmol/L)	Integrated insulin response[c]
CON (n=11)	6.49 ± 0.50	15.76 ± 0.05	8.2 ± 2.1
STZ (n=14)	18.26 ± 2.78	> 25.0	1.7 ± 0.5
STZ-T (n=11)	6.88 ± 0.55	17.59 ± 0.94	2.8 ± 0.4

[*] Values are means ± S.E.
[a] Rats were administered 1 g/kg gavage of glucose solution
[b] Plasma glucose measured at time 0 after 12 hr fast
[c] Values are expressed as $U \cdot ml^{-1} \cdot 180$ min

of insulin and/or epinephrine. As recorded in the 10-wk chronic study (30), basal glycerol release and rate of lipolysis in response to either agent in the STZ-T group was decreased to normal levels (32).

Basal developed force (BDF) was significantly higher in the STZ group, and the Ca^{++} concentration-response curve was shifted to the left, indicating supersensitivity of the tissue to inotropic effects of Ca^{++}, as reflected in a lower geometric EC_{50} value. On the other hand, values obtained from the STZ-T group indicated that tissue sensitivity was restored to normalcy (32).

All STZ-T animals from groups given 0.75 and 1.00 mg/ml vanadyl concentrations were euglycemic at the end of the 16-week study and were subjected to an OGTT. Peak plasma glucose obtained after a 1 g/kg oral bolus of glucose was slightly higher in STZ-T than control, however integrated glucose response was not different between the two groups. Although glucose tolerance was normalized by vanadyl treatment, insulin response though slightly greater than in the STZ group, was not nearly as substantial as the CON group (ref. 37, Table 3). In addition, insulin levels were dramatically lowered after overnight fasting in the STZ-T animals and were found to be similar to STZ values without a detrimental effect of basal glucose (37).

Insulin release from the pancreas in response to stimulation by GIP/glucose was assessed (ref. 37, Table 4). Although insulin response was considerably higher in the STZ-T group (10 x STZ), it was nevertheless only

Table 4. Islet area, insulin content and insulin response from isolated pancreas to 16.65 mMol (300 mg/dl) glucose*. (Data calculated from ref. 37)

Group	Islet area (um^2)	Insulin %	Integrated insulin response[a]
CON	8630 ± 704[b]	83 ± 1[b]	364 ± 54
STZ	685 ± 86[c]	25 ± 2[c]	4.6 ± 0.21
STZ-T	5856 ± 540[d]	74 ± 1.5[d]	45 ± 11

* Values are means ± S.E.
a Data expressed as mU·ml^{-1}·40 min
b $P < 0.05$ vs. 16-week STZ rats
c $P < 0.05$ vs. controls
d $P < 0.05$ vs. both control and STZ

12% of the CON response. Pancreatic islet cell area and insulin-content quantification revealed that although treatment with vanadyl had remarkably protected the pancreas from destruction by STZ, insulin release from the pancreas to glucose challenge in the STZ-T rats did not match that of the CON group (37).

Vanadium levels were measured on the tissue and blood of STZ-T rats (n=11) collected at the time of sacrifice. Vanadium was found in low amounts in the kidney (0.85 ± 0.23 uM) and was undetectable in blood (37).

Discussion

Various studies in the past have demonstrated numerous insulin-like actions of vanadium *in vitro*. Because of the hydrophilic properties of vanadium salts and its ready absorption in the GI tract, it was questioned earlier whether vanadium could in fact be useful in the chronic oral treatment of STZ-diabetic animals. This has been confirmed in several experiments which utilized the vanadate (+5) form of vanadium (25-28,41). However, administering this form of the element has been repetitively shown to result in the death of some animals due to severe diarrhea or the refusal of some animals to drink (unpublished observations). Clearly, toxicity was a serious concern with regard to its applicability to humans. Since vanadyl had been reported to be far less toxic than vanadate, it was decided to examine the effectiveness of vanadyl as a safer alternative in the chronic treatment of

STZ-diabetic rats.

Depression of myocardial function is well-recognized as a secondary complication of STZ-induced diabetes (42). As well, abnormally high lipolytic activity of adipose tissues alone and in the presence of insulin is characteristically seen (43). Both myocardial contractile performance and adipose tissue functions were normalized in the STZ-T group from both the 10- and 16-week study rats (30,32). In addition, plasma parameters such as T_4, triglycerides, and cholesterol were restored to control levels. In both groups, the low to undetectable levels of vanadium found in blood and tissues of STZ-T rats suggest that the insulin-like properties of orally administered vanadyl are apparent not only following acute treatment but are prolonged and apparent for a significant time long after treatment has ceased.

Several observations have led to some possible explanations for the continued effects of vanadyl during treatment and more remarkably, during the post-withdrawal period. One noteworthy difference between the 10-wk and 16-wk STZ-T groups was that while the former exhibited hypoinsulinemia, the latter had normal resting insulin values (as opposed to fasting insulin which was found to be similar to STZ levels). Additional *in vitro* experiments revealed normal tissue function in spite of low endogenous levels of insulin (30). Furthermore, although the amount of insulin released *in vivo* from the pancreas following an oral glucose (1 g/kg) challenge in the 16-wk STZ-T group did not rise to normally required levels, integrated glucose response was found to be normal (37). The same phenomenon has been reported using the i.v. route to administer glucose, thus ruling out possible influences in oral glucose absorption (27,44). From analyses of these data, one can postulate that vanadyl may have two principal mechanisms of action: 1) acutely and chronically, it may work as a supplement to insulin and/or it increases the sensitivity of various tissues to low levels of insulin, without developing excessive responses in these tissues, resulting in hypoglycemia with increasing levels of the hormone and 2) during the withdrawal period, by normalizing resting plasma levels of insulin, it chronically improves all other diabetic abnormalities, thus protecting cardiac and other tissues from the progressive degeneration which develops in the STZ-diabetic rats.

Many *in vitro* studies support the possibility that either replacement of insulin or the enhancement of tissue sensitivity to insulin might have developed as a result of vanadyl treatment. In addition to the normalized tissue functions and plasma parameters observed in the presence of hypoinsulinemia (30), the idea of enhanced tissue sensitivity is further substantiated by the normal rise in plasma glucose accompanied by consistently low plasma insulin following an oral glucose challenge in STZ-T rats, and the disability of the pancreas in this group to release insulin in response to glucose (37). This concept is also congruent with a study by Meyerovitch et al (26) which demonstrated a doubling of hexose uptake in the liver and muscle tissues *in vivo* in control and diabetic rats treated with vanadate. However, it was also pointed out that these actions are in part vanadate-specific and unlike insulin which fails to influence sugar transport in the liver (26). An increase in insulin receptor autophosphorylation by vanadium although presented *in vitro* (16,17), has been contradicted *in vivo* (20). Recently, it has also been shown that the antilipolytic activity of vanadate *in vitro* does not coincide with an insulin-like increase in cellular tyrosine phosphorylation in both intensity and specificity (19). Thus, it remains unclear whether vanadyl *in vivo* mimics or merely enhances insulin activity perhaps by an intracellular mechanism(s). In one study (30), it was found at least to correct the changes in protein phosphorylation seen in STZ.

Normalizations in the lipid and hormonal profile, namely, hyperlipidemia and hypothyroidism, could account for the absence of cardiomyopathy in the treated diabetic animals (45,46). This gives rise to a possibility that the improvements maintained in the normoinsulinemic 16-wk STZ-T rats may in fact be secondary to a separate and unique property of vanadium. From the immunohistochemical data, it was observed that progressive degeneration of pancreatic ß-cells from the cytotoxic effect of STZ had in fact been prevented to some extent by vanadyl treatment (37). Hence, the apparent preservation of islet cell viability and the improved insulin content in these cells may be a critical addendum to the antidiabetogenic actions of vanadyl in the STZ-diabetic rat. There are two observations however which cast some doubt to the actual significance of this phenomenon. Firstly, despite the near normal insulin content, pancreatic ß-cells in the STZ-T rats remained insensitive to stimulation by glucose (37). Moreover, the 10-wk chronically treated (STZ-T) rats displayed normal plasma and tissue characteristics in spite of being hypoinsulinemic (30). Furthermore, partially (90%) pancreatectomized rats were also shown recently to develop euglycemia from vanadate treatment (47). Hence, it is perhaps only in the extended period following discontinuation of treatment that the cytoprotective property of this unique element becomes important in maintaining the existing, improved metabolic and physiologic status of the treated STZ-diabetic rat.

Endogenous insulin was dramatically reduced in the CON-T group to half of control levels (30), confirming our earlier work with vanadate (25). Nevertheless, euglycemia was found to be maintained consistently in these animals. Hence it was postulated that vanadyl inhibits insulin release from the islet cells of the pancreas. As mentioned earlier, it is possible that vanadyl has, by substituting for insulin and/or amplifying the effects of endogenous insulin *in vivo* as described *in vitro*, successfully produced a euglycemic state in the hypoinsulinemic animal (30). In either case, the development of a homeostatic condition with less demand for circulating insulin may have subsequently contributed to a negative feedback of insulin secretion from the pancreatic ß-cells (30). Moreover, an apparent normalization of resting insulin levels in the STZ-T rats after long-term withdrawal from treatment lends support to the notion that when additional "insulin" in the form of vanadyl is no longer provided, this indirect inhibition, or possibly a more direct suppression of insulin release is removed (32).

An "Achilles Heel" inherent in the methodology of these studies, however, was that treatment was initiated 3 days after the STZ-injection, a time at which spontaneous reversal of the diabetic state may still occur. Ongoing studies have since demonstrated the comparable effectiveness of vanadyl (0.75 mg/ml) at treatment initiation times of up to three weeks post-induction of diabetes. Several questions still need to be addressed, however, regarding the actual properties of vanadyl *in vivo*, its cellular and/or intracellular involvement which produces insulin-like actions and whether these properties can in fact be maintained indefinitely.

Summary

The compilation of studies presented here has confirmed the effectiveness of oral vanadyl treatment in alleviating diabetes-induced changes in several plasma parameters and tissue deficiencies independent of insulin levels. The apparent persistence in effect after a long period of withdrawal from treatment has also been demonstrated. Chronic maintenance of euglycemia and preventions of ensuing hyperglycemia following an oral glucose challenge, both of which are produced without the apparent normalization of insulin levels, points to the supplementary action of vanadyl as an insulin-substitute or as agent which enhances tissue sensitivity to insulin, potentially through intracellular mechanisms. Most significantly, vanadyl treatment was shown to preserve myocardial and adipose tissue function in the STZ-diabetic rat and protect the pancreas from the cytotoxic properties of STZ. Overall, it has been demonstrated that vanadyl sulfate trihydrate, orally administered to the STZ-diabetic rat can effectively correct the various abnormalities associated with the diabetic state. Future applications of these findings to the disease condition in humans remain to be seen.

Acknowledgements

This research was funded in part by grants from the Canadian Diabetes Foundation, Alfred and Agnes Woods Research Fund, Medical Research Council of Canada, and British Columbia Health Care Research Foundation.

References

1. Hopkins LL and Mohr HE. The biological essentiality of vanadium. In: Newer trace elements in nutrition. (edited by Mertz W and Cornatzer WE) New York: Dekker, 1971, pp. 195-213.
2. Byrne AR and Kosta L. Vanadium in foods and in human body fluids and tissues. Sci Total Environ 1978;10:17-30.
3. Degani H, Gochin M, Karlish SJD and Schecter Y. Electron paramagnetic resonance studies and insulin-like effects of vanadium in rat adipocytes. Biochemistry 1981;20:5795-5799.
4. Tolman EL, Barris E, Burns M, Pansini A and Partridge R. Effects of vanadium on glucose metabolism in vitro. Life Sci 1979;25:1159-1164.
5. Dubyak GR and Kleinzeller A. The insulin-mimetic effects of vanadate in isolated rat adipocytes. Dissociation from effects of vanadate as a (Na^+-K^+)-ATPase inhibitor. J Biol Chem 1980;255:5306-5312.
6. Schecter Y and Karlish SJD. Insulin-like stimulation of glucose oxidation in rat adipocytes by vanadyl (IV) ions. Nature (Lond) 1980;284:556-558.
7. Clark AS, Fagan JM and Mitch WE. Selectivity of the insulin-like actions of vanadate on glucose and protein metabolism in skeletal muscle. Biochem J 1985;232:273-276.

8. Gomez-Foix AM, Rodriguez-Gil JE, Fillat C and Guinovart JJ. Vanadate raises fructose 2,6'-bisphosphate concentrations and activates glycolysis in rat hepatocytes. Biochem J 1988;255:507-512.
9. Duckworth WC, Solomon SS, Liepnieks J, Hamel FG, Hand S and Peavy DE. Insulin-like effects of vanadate in isolated rat adipocytes. Endocrinology 1988;122:2285-2289.
10. Schecter Y and Ron A. Effect of depletion of phosphate and bicarbonate ions on insulin action in rat adipocytes. J Biol Chem 1986;261:14945-14950.
11. Curran GL. Effects of certain transition group elements on hepatic synthesis of cholesterol in the rat. J Biol Chem 1954;210:765-770.
12. Snyder F and Cornatzer WE. Vanadium inhibition of phospholipid synthesis and sulphydryl activity in rat liver. Nature (Lond) 1968;182:462.
13. Tracey AS and Gresser MJ. Interaction of vanadate with phenol and tyrosine: implications for the effects of vanadate on systems regulated by tyrosine phosphorylation. Proc Natl Acad Sci USA 1986;83:609-613.
14. Marshall S and Monzon R. Down-regulation of cell-surface insulin receptors in primary cultured rat adipocytes by sodium vanadate. Endocrinology 1987;121:1116-1122.
15. Torossian K, Freedman D and Fantus IG. Vanadate down-regulates cell surface insulin and growth hormone receptors and inhibits insulin receptor degradation in cultured human lymphocytes. J Biol Chem 1988;263:9353-9359.
16. Tamura S, Brown TA, Dubler RE and Larner J. Insulin-like effect of vanadate on adipocyte glycogen synthase and on phosphorylation of 95,000 dalton subunit of insulin receptor. Biochem Biophys Res Commun 1983;113:80-86.
17. Tamura S, Brown TA, Whipple JH, Fujita-Yamaguchi Y, Dubier RE, Cheng K and Larner J. A novel mechanism for the insulin-like effect of vanadate on glycogen synthase in rat adipocytes. J Biol Chem 1984;259:6650-6658.
18. Green A. The insulin-like effect of sodium vanadate on adipocyte glucose transport is mediated at a post-insulin-receptor level. Biochem J 1986;238:663-669.

19. Bernier M, Laird DM and Lane MD. Effect of vanadate on the cellular accumulation of pp15, an apparent product of insulin receptor tyrosine kinase action. J Biol Chem 1988;263:13626-13634.
20. Mooney RA, Bordwell KL, Luhowskyj S and Casnellie JE. The insulin-like effect of vanadate on lipolysis in rat adipocytes is not accompanied by an insulin-like effect on tyrosine phosphorylation. Endocrinology 1989;124:422-429.
21. Strout HV, Vicario PP, Saperstein R and Slater EE. The insulin-mimetic effect of vanadate is not correlated with insulin receptor tyrosine kinase activity nor phosphorylation in mouse diaphragm in vivo. Endocrinology 1989;124:1918-1924.
22. Bosch F, Arino J, Gomez-Foix AM and Guinovart JJ. Glycogenolytic, noninsulin-like effects of vanadate on rat hepatocyte glycogen synthase and phosphorylase. J Biol Chem 1987;262:218-222.
23. Jackson TK, Salhanick AI, Sparks JD, Sparks CE, Bolognino M. and Amatruda JM. Insulin-mimetic effects of vanadate in primary cultures of rat hepatocytes. Diabetes 1988;37:1234-1240.
24. Lyonnet B, Martz F and Martin E. L'emploi therapeutique des derives du vanadium. La Presse Medicale 1899;7:191-192.
25. Heyliger CE, Tahiliani AG and McNeill JH. Effect of vanadate on elevated blood glucose and depressed cardiac performance of diabetic rats. Science 1985;227:1474-1477.
26. Meyerovitch J, Farfel Z, Sack J and Schecter Y. Oral administration of vanadate normalizes blood glucose levels in streptozotocin-treated rats. Characterization and mode of action. J Biol Chem 1987;262:6658-6662.
27. Brichard SM, Okitolonda W and Henquin JC. Long term improvement of glucose homeostasis by vanadate treatment in diabetic rats. Endocrinology 1988;123:2048-2053.
28. Paulson DJ, Kopp SJ, Tow JP and Peace DG. Effects of vanadate on in vivo myocardial reactivity to norepinephrine in diabetic rats. J Pharmacol Exp Ther 1987;240:529-534.
29. Hudson TGF. Vandium, Toxicology and Biological Significance. New York: Elsevier, 1964.
30. Ramanadham S, Mongold JJ, Brownsey RW, Cros GH and McNeill JH. Oral vanadyl sulfate in treatment of diabetes mellitus in rats. Am J Physiol 1989;257:904H-911H.

31. Vadlamudi RVSV, Rodgers RL and McNeill JH. The effect of chronic alloxan- and streptozotocin-induced diabetes on isolated rat heart performance. Can J Physiol Pharmacol 1982;60:902-911.
32. Ramanadham S, Brownsey RW, Cros GH, Mongold JJ and McNeill JH. Sustained prevention of myocardial and metabolic abnormalities in diabetic rats following withdrawal from oral vanadyl treatment. Metabolism 1989;38:1022-1028.
33. Brownsey RW and Denton RM. Evidence that insulin activates fat cell acetyl-CoA carboxylase by increased phosphorylation at a specific site. Biochem J 1982;202:77-86.
34. Garland PB and Randle PJ. A rapid enzymatic assay for glycerol. Nature (Lond) 1962;196:987-988.
35. Laemmli UK. Cleavage of structural proteins during the assembly of the head of bacteriophage T4. Nature (Lond) 1970;227:680-685.
36. Brownsey RW, Edgell NJ, Hopkirk TJ and Denton RM. Studies on insulin-phosphorylation of acetyl-CoA carboxylase, ATP-citrate lyase and other proteins in rat epidydymal tissue. Biochem J 1984;218:733-743.
37. Pederson RA, Ramanadham S, Buchan AMJ and McNeill JH. Long-term effects of vanadyl treatment on streptozotocin-treated diabetes in rats. Diabetes 1989;38:1390-1395.
38. Pederson RA, Buchan MAJ, Zahedi-Asl S, Chan CB and Brown JC. Effect of jejunoileal bypass in the rat on the enteroinsular axis. Regul Pept 1982;5:53-63.
39. Fleming WW, Westfall DD, De La Lande IS and Jellet LB. Log-normal distribution of equieffective doses of norepinephrine and acetylcholine in several tissues. J Pharmacol Exp Ther 1972;181:339-345.
40. Brownsey RW, Edgell NJ, Hopkirk TJ and Denton RM. Studies on insulin-stimulated phosphorylation of acetyl-CoA carboxylase, ATP-citrate lyase and other proteins in rat epididymal adipose tissue. Biochem J 1984;218:733-743.
41. Bendayan M and Gingras D. Effect of vanadate administration on blood glucose and insulin levels as well as on the exocrine pancreatic function in streptozotocin-diabetic rats. Diabetologia 1989;32:561-567.
42. Vadlamudi RVSV, Rodger RL and McNeill JH. The effect of chronic alloxan- and streptozotocin-diabetes on isolated rat heart performance. Can J Physiol Pharmacol 1982;60:902-911.

43. Saudek CD and Eder HA. Lipid metabolism in diabetes mellitus. Am J Med 1979;66:843-852.
44. Blondel O, Bailbe D and Portha B. In vivo insulin resistance in streptozotocin-diabetic rats - evidence for reversal following oral vanadate treatment. Diabetologia 1989;32:185-190.
45. Feuvray FS, Idell-Wagner JA and Neely JR. Effects of ischemia on rat myocardial function and metabolism in diabetes. Circ Res 1979;44:322-329.
46. Pittman CS, Suda AK, Chambers JB and Ray GY. Impaired 3,5,3'-triiodothyronine (T_3) production in diabetic patients. Metabolism 1979;28:333-338.
47. Rossetti L and Laughlin MR. Correction of chronic hyperglycemia with vanadate, but not with phlorizin, normalizes in vivo glycogen repletion and in vitro glycogen synthase activity in diabetic skeletal muscle. J Clin Invest 1989;84:892-899.

Different Cardiac Effects of Hypoglycaemic Sulphonylurea Compounds

Z. Aranyi, G. Ballagi-Pordány, M.Z. Koltai, G. Pogátsa

National Institute of Cardiology, Budapest P. Box: 88 HUNGARY 1450

Introduction

The result of the UGDP study (1) suggested that the increased cardiovascular mortality among diabetics could be related to tolbutamide treatment. The mortality of diabetics in coronary care units is known to be significantly higher than that of metabolically healthy patients (2). The hypoglycaemic sulphonylureas alter the electrical and mechanical functions of the heart directly under "in vitro" (3,4) and "in vivo" conditions (5,6,7). Lasseter et al. (8) and Crass et al. (9) suggested that the increase in Purkinje fibers automaticity, myocardial contractile force, and the elevation of arterial blood pressure induced by hypoglycaemic sulphonylureas might be responsible for the development of increased cardiovascular mortality in diabetics. It was also demonstrated that a second generation sulphonylurea compound, glibenclamide, decreases the automaticity and the conduction time in the Purkinje fibers (3) and did not elevate the arterial blood pressure (5) in contrast to the first generation sulphonylureas (Figure 1). Furthermore, it was demonstrated that in diabetic patients tolbutamide and carbutamide enhanced while glibenclamide did not influence the incidence of digitalis intoxication, or that of multifocal ventricular ectopic beats during digitalis therapy (10). Koltai et al. (11) documented further that the incidence of lethal and nonlethal myocardial infarction is increased in tolutamide, chlorpropamide and carbutamide treated diabetics. Balant (12) demonstrated first that the hypoglycaemic sulphonylureas can be divided into first and second generation preparations according to their chemical structures and their efficacies. The aim of our present work was to investigate whether or not the cardiovascular effects differ among the diabetic human and animal subjects treated with first or second generation sulphonylurea compounds.

Nagano, M., Mochizuki, S., Dhalla, N.S. (eds.), CARDIOVASCULAR DISEASE IN DIABETES. Copyright © 1992. Kluwer Academic Publishers, Boston. All rights reserved.

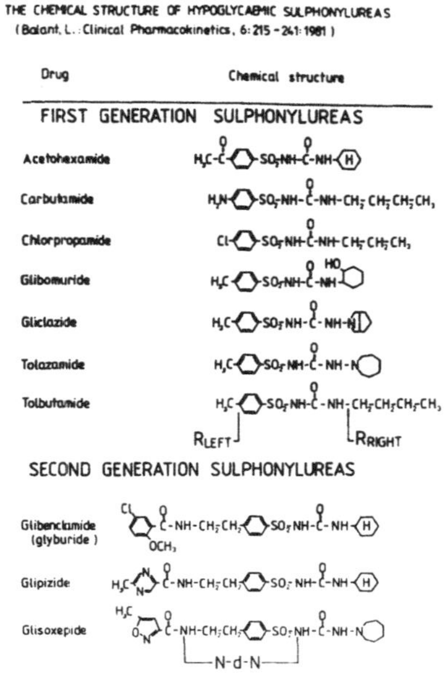

Figure 1. The chemical structure of hypoglycaemic sulphonylureas.

Methods

In the diabetic outpatient clinic of the National Institute of Cardiology alterations of survival time and metabolic variables as well as the incidence of cardiovascular risk factors were investigated among the differently treated diabetics. The date of these diabetics are:

	All	Men	Women
Number of patients	967	444	523
Mean age of patients, (year)	55 ± 1	54 ± 1	55 ± 1
Therapy: diet alone	164	99	65
insulin	320	127	193
oral antidiabetic drugs	463	218	245
first generation sulphonylureas:			
carbutamide	80	36	44
chlorpropamide	33	10	23
gliclazide	2	1	1
tolbutamide	105	56	49
second generation sulphonylureas:			
glibenclamide	243	115	128

The effect of different sulphonylureas on strophanthidine cardiotoxicity were investigated in 255 male, New Zealand, white rabbits anaesthetized with intravenously administered sodium pentobarbital (133 umol/kg). Body weight was between 1.6 - 3.5 kg. The animals received the sulphonylureas in a dose of 0.01 - 1000 umol/kg and the solvents of these drugs intravenously in a 1 ml/kg volume. The hypoglycaemic effect was counteracted by an intravenous administration of 0 - 2.5 mmol/kg glucose adjusted to the amount of sulphonylureas. Two hours after the pretreatment of sulphonylureas 23 umol/kg/min strophanthidine was infused intravenously under continuous ECG monitoring until the onset of the first ventricular ectopic beat and thereafter until that of ventricular fibrillation. The cumulative dose of strophanthidine was calculated (13).

The effect of different sulphonylureas on the arrhythmogenety of myocardial infarction was investigated in 306 male Wistar rats, weighing 150 - 250 grams according to the method of Lepran and his coworkers (14). A week after the insertion of a loop of yarn under the anterior descending branch of left coronary artery the animals were treated intraperitoneally with different sulphonylureas in a dose of 0.01 - 1000 umol/kg and solvents of these drugs in a volume of 1 ml/kg. The hypoglycaemic effect was prevented by simultaneous intraperitoneal administration of 0 - 2.5 mmol/kg glucose appropriated to the amount of sulphonylureas. Thirty minutes after sulphonylurea pretreatment, the coronary artery was occluded under ECG control by the loop of yarn and the number of left ventricular ectopic beats as well as the duration of transitional ventricular fibrillation were registered on a tree-channel ECG during the first 30 minutes. Thereafter the size of myocardial infarction was measured following formaldehyde fixation by gravimetric method (15).

The haemodynamic effects of different sulphonylureas were tested partly in 30 healthy mongrel dogs of both sexes, weighing 8.9 - 22.4 kg and partly in 30 male New Zealand white rabbits, weighing 1.8 - 3.4 kg. Both kinds of animals were anaesthetized intravenously with sodium pentobarbital (133 umol/kg), intubated endotracheally and ventilated artificially. The chest was opened, and an electromagnetic blood flowmeter (Gould SP 2200) was placed on the aortic root to measure cardiac output. Mean arterial blood pressure was measured intrafemorally by a Statham P23D transducer. An isometric transducer was sewn into the anterior wall of the left ventricle for measuring myocardial contractile force. Cardiac work was calculated by multiplying the heart rate and mean arterial blood pressure. The animals were treated with different sulphonylureas in a dose of 0.4 - 1184 umol/kg and with the solvents of these drugs intravenously in a volume of 3 ml/kg. The hypoglycaemic effect was prevented by simultaneous administration by 0 - 2.5 mmol/kg glucose appropriated to the amount of sulphonylureas (16,17).

Investigating the effect of different sulphonylureas on the vagus nerve tone, 36 healthy mongrel dogs of both sexes weighing 7 - 15 kg were anesthetized intravenously by pentobarbital (133 umol/kg). The vagus nerve was exposed and cut. The distal end was stimulated electrically with 2 V and increasing square wave frequencies (1,2,4,8,16 Hz). Arterial blood pressure was measured intrafemorally by a Statham P23D transducer. The heart rate was registered on a three-channel ECG. Different sulphonylureas were administered in a dose of 0.01 - 1000 umol/kg intravenously as well as solvents of these drugs in a volume of 1 ml/kg.

The different sulphonylureas were solved as sodium salts in a mixture of 10% ethanol and 10% polyethylenglycol in water; the pH of the solution was 8.0.

Results

In the diabetic patients acute myocardial infarction occurred in 43 cases of diabetics treated with first generation sulphonylureas and their survival was found to be 5 ± 1 years. Among the diabetic patients treated with glibenclamide, a second generation sulphonylurea compound, acute myocardial lesion could be detected in 25 individuals surviving for 9 ± 1 years. Forty-four of insulinized diabetics and 25 of those on diet and regime alone had acute myocardial infarction with similar survivals of 9 ± 1 and 9 ± 2 years respectively. Thus, only the survival of diabetic patients suffering from myocardial infarction and treated with first generation sulphonylureas proved to be markedly shorter. Acute myocardial lesion could be observed at a similar age and after a similar duration of diabetes in diabetics treated with the first and second generation of sulphonylurea compounds. In insulinized patients, the first acute myocardial infarction occurred at a younger age and following a longer duration of diabetes. On the contrary, in diabetics kept only on diet and regime, the acute myocardial infarction could be observed at older age but after a shorter duration of diabetes (Figure 2).

Smoking habits were significantly greater, while duration of treatment, body mass index and arterial blood pressure were markedly lower in diabetics

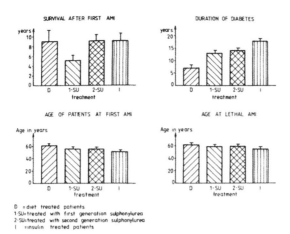

Figure 2. Survival, duration of diabetes, age of patients at first and at lethal acute myocardial infarction.

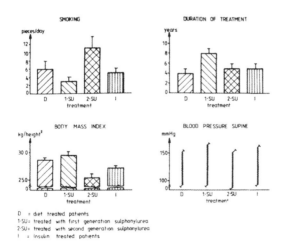

Figure 3. Distribution of risk factors in diabetic patients.

treated with glibenclamide compared to those treated with first generation sulphonylureas (Figure 3).

At the beginning of the observation, data of diabetics suffered later from acute myocardial infarction, do not differ notably among the patients treated with different antidiabetic drugs. However, also in this case, the incidence of arrhythmias was higher (23 - 30 per cent) in the group of patients treated with the first generation of sulphonylurea compounds than in the other groups (0 - 14 per cent).

In the cardiac state following the development of acute myocardial infarction, differences were found only in the appearance of an apicobasal discrepancy in the lungs ($P < 0.05$) between the groups of patients treated with the first generation of sulphonylurea compounds (2 per cent) or with glibenclamide (24 per cent). The incidence of supraventricular (30 and 4 per cent, respectively) and ventricular (23 and 0 per cent, respectively) ectopic beats were greater ($P < 0.05$) in the group of patients treated with first generation sulphonylurea compounds. The frequency of anginal attacks was considerably ($P < 0.05$) greater in the group of diabetics treated with glibenclamide (56 per cent) than in groups of those treated with the first generation of sulphonylurea compounds (35 per cent). Accordingly, the difference in cardiac state following the development of acute myocardial infarction could not explain the shorter survival in the patients treated with first generation sulphonylurea compounds. The parameters of the carbohydrate metabolism were found to be considerably higher only in the insulinized group (Figure 4). The level of serum triglyceride was found to be higher in diabetics treated with glibenclamide, while that of HDL-cholesterol in diabetic patients on first generation sulphonylurea therapy (Figure 5).

Discussion

Almost all of the diabetic patients controlled regularly in the outpatient clinic of the National Institute of Cardiology showed some manifestations of heart and vascular disorders as complications of diabetes mellitus. Their existence could serve an explanation for the more than 50 per cent of death in the diabetics during the 22 years of observation.

In contrast to the observation of Laube and Krausch (18) we did not find a decreased HDL-cholesterol level in the diabetics treated with sulphonylureas, however, the cited work did not give any reference to the generation of the applied sulphonylurea compounds.

Hypoglycaemic sulphonylurea compounds have been demonstrated firstly by Christlieb (19) and Wales (20) to induce hypertension. Further, it was demonstrated that carbutamide, gliclazide and glibenclamide do not influence similarly the blood pressure in experimental animals, and these data are referring to a group specific property of sulphonylurea compounds responsible

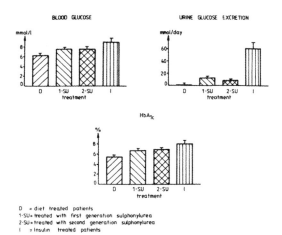

Figure 4. Variables of carbohydrate metabolism in diabetic patients.

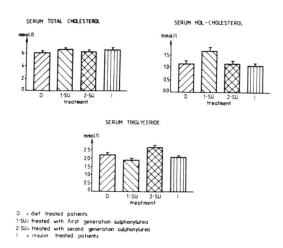

Figure 5. Variables of lipid metabolism in diabetic patients.

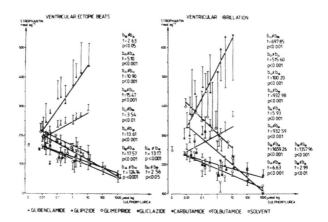

Figure 6. Effects of hypoglycaemic sulphonylureas on strophanthidine toxicity in rabbits.
On the left part of figure 6 the dose-response curves of amounts of strophanthidine evoking the first ventricular ectopic beat and on the right part of this figure those evoking ventricular fibrillation were presented under the influence of pretreatments with different sulphonylureas. The figure demonstrates that first generation sulphonylureas increase, while second generation sulphonylureas diminish strophanthidine toxicity.

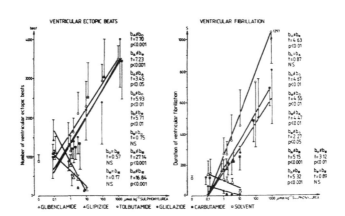

Figure 7. Effects of hypoglycaemic sulphonylureas on arrhythmogenicity induced by myocardial infarction in rats.
The left part of Figure 7 demonstrates the dose-response curves of the number of ventricular ectopic beats and the right part of this figure the cumulative time of transitional ventricular fibrillation during the first 30 minutes after infarction under the influence of pretreatment with different sulphonylureas. The first generation sulphonylureas enhance, while the second generation sulphonylureas decrease the number of ectopic beats and the cumulative time of ventricular fibrillation.

341

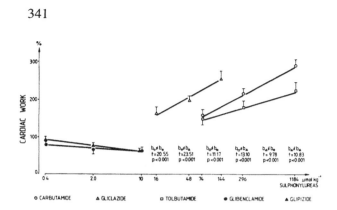

Figure 8. Effects of hypoglycaemic sulphonylureas on cardiac work in dogs. The figure shows that the dose-response curves on alterations in cardiac work are influenced differently by the first and second generation sulphonylureas. The first generation sulphonylureas increase, while second generation sulphonylureas do not influence or decrease cardiac work.

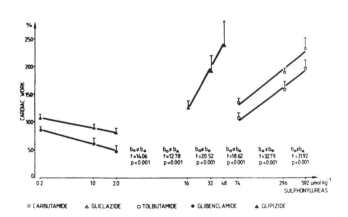

Figure 9. Effects of hypoglycaemic sulphonylureas on cardiac work in rabbits. The figure shows that the dose-response curves on alterations in cardiac work are influenced differently by the first and second generation sulphonylureas. The first generation sulphonylureas increase, while second generation sulphonylureas did not influence or decrease the cardiac work.

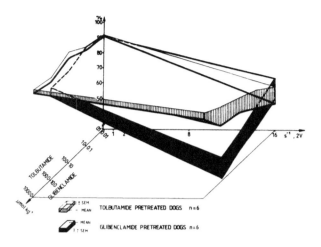

Figure 10. Effects of glibenclamide and tolbutamide on alterations in heart rate induced by electrical stimulation of vagus nerve in dogs.
The space-diagram of dose-response curves demonstrates that the second generation compound glibenclamide increases, while the first generation compound tolbutamide diminishes the effect of electrical stimulation of vagus nerve on heart rate.

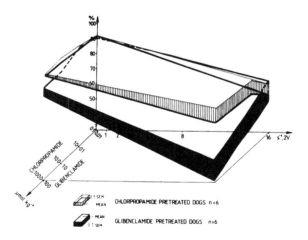

Figure 11. Effects of glibenclamide and chlorpropamide on alterations in heart rate induced by electrical stimulation of vagus nerve in dogs.
The space-diagram of dose-response curves demonstrates that the second generation compound glibenclamide increases, while the first generation compound chlorpropamide diminishes the effect of electrical stimulation of vagus nerve on heart rate.

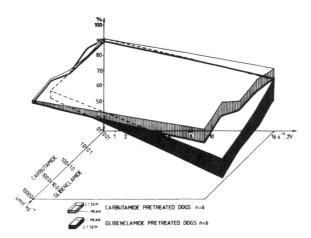

Figure 12. Effects of glibenclamide and carbutamide on alterations in heart rate induced by electrical stimulation of vagus nerve in dogs.
The space-diagram of dose-response curves demonstrates that the second generation compound glibenclamide increases, while the first generation compound carbutamide diminishes the effect of electrical stimulation of vagus nerve on heart rate.

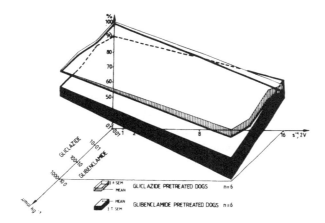

Figure 13. Effects of glibenclamide and gliclazide on alterations in heart rate induced by electrical stimulation of vagus nerve in dogs.
The space-diagram of dose-response curves demonstrates that the second generation compound glibenclamide increases, while the first generation compound gliclazide diminishes the effect of electrical stimulation of vagus nerve on heart rate.

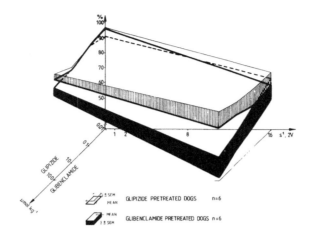

Figure 14. Effects of glibenclamide and glipizide on alterations in heart rate induced by electrical stimulation of vagus nerve in dogs.
The space-diagram of dose-response curves demonstrates that the second generation compound glibenclamide increases, while the first generation compound glipizide diminishes the effect of electrical stimulation of vagus nerve on heart rate.

for their different effects on blood pressure taking its origin from the different chemical structure of the first and second generations of these drugs (5). The present work contributes further support of this statement.

On the other hand, the higher mortality of diabetic patients with acute myocardial infarction in coronary care units are attributed to the more frequent onset of cardiogenic shock and that of lethal arrhythmias compared with a metabolically healthy population (21). The present work is enabling another possible explanation. The arrhythmogenic effect (22,5,10) of first generation hypoglycaemic sulphonylureas is namely supposed to be responsible for higher mortality rate in coronary heart disease, since with the exception of the higher systolic blood pressure, no difference could be detected relating the metabolic variables or risk factors among the investigated groups.

Furthermore, the results on rabbits suggest that the first generation sulphonylureas increases the cardiotoxicity of cardiac glycosides, while glibenclamide and glipizide diminish it (Fig. 6). Accordingly, the conclusion could be drawn that in spite of first generation sulphonylureas, the second generation compounds increase the stability of heart rhythm. Taking into consideration the fact that the long term existence of diabetes contributes to developing of diabetic cardiac and vascular alterations which could effect the administration of cardiac glycosides. Therefore, great caution must be exercised in the simultaneous administration of cardiac glycosides and hypoglycaemic sulphonylureas, since the interaction between cardiac glycosides and first generation sulphonylureas may enhance the incidence of drug-induced ventricular ectopic beats or sudden death.

The clinical results suggests further that glibenclamide has an antiarrhythmic effect, whereas the first generation sulphonylureas are arrhythmogenic. The investigation of ischaemic rat hearts shows that second generation sulphonylureas are minimalizing the incidence of ventricular ectopic beats and ventricular fibrillation, while tolbutamide, carbutamide and gliclazide are increasing the appearance of this unfavorable phenomenon (Fig. 7). These results support further the fact that the first generation sulphonylureas contribute to the high incidence of cardiovascular mortality of diabetics.

Moreover, the investigation of the hemodynamic effects of hypoglycaemic sulphonylureas on dogs and rabbits shows that glibenclamide and glipizide does not influence the heart work, while tolbutamide, gliclazide and carbutamide increases it (Figs. 8 and 9). This pressed exercise evokes an increase in myocardial oxygen demand and contributes to cardiac alterations in the ischaemic heart.

Finally, information would be obtained whether the neuroregulation of the heart is also influenced by the hypoglycaemic sulphonylureas (Figs. 10, 11, 12, 13 and 14). It could be seen that the effect of the electrical stimulation of the vagus nerve on the heart rate is increased only by glibenclamide. Tolbutamide and carbutamide decreased while gliclazide and glipizide practically did not influence this effect. These experiments show that there are some differences between the effects of glibenclamide and glipizide. This fact could be a critical point at developing the new compounds of hypoglycaemic sulphonylureas.

The clinical importance of these results enables the conclusion to be drawn, that in the therapy of diabetic patients, glibenclamide must be preferred instead of the first generation sulphonylurea compounds, especially in the case of manifest coronary heart disease, or if a risk for it is existing.

Summary

The authors investigated the cardiovascular effects of different hypoglycaemic sulphonylureas. It could be demonstrated that the investigated first generation sulphonylureas increase the cardiotoxicity of cardiac glycosides, enhance the arrhythmogenicity of the ischaemic myocardium and reduce the survival of patients suffering from coronary heart disease. On the contrary, glibenclamide and glipizide decreased the cardiotoxicity of cardiac glycosides, diminished the arrhythmogenicity of the ischaemic myocardium and glibenclamide did not influence the survival of patients suffering from coronary heart disease. Glibenclamide enhanced further, in contrary to the other investigated sulphonylureas, the effect of electrical stimulation of vagus nerve on heart rate. Therefore, it could be concluded that in the therapy of diabetic patients, glibenclamide must be preferred instead of first generation sulphonylurea compounds, especially in the case of coronary heart disease or digitalization.

References

1. University Group Diabetes Program. A study of the effects of agents on vascular complications in patients with adult onset diabetes. 11 Mortality results. Diabetes 1970;19(Suppl. 2):789-830.
2. Williams GH, Braunwald E. Endocrine and nutritional disorders and heart disease: Diabetes mellitus. In: Braunwald E/ed./: Heart disease. A textbook of cardiovascular medicine. WB Saunders Compnay, Philadelphia, London, Toronto, Mexico City, Rio de Janeiro, Sydney, Tokyo 1984, pp. 1722-1747.
3. Pogátsa G, Németh M. Electrophysiological effects of hypoglycaemic sulphonylureas on rabbit heart. Eur J Pharmacol 67, 333-338, 1980.
4. Levey GS, Lasseter KC, Palmer RF. Sulphonylureas and the heart. Ann Rev Med 1974;25:69-74.
5. Pogátsa G, Dubecz E. The direct effect of hypoglycaemic sulphonylureas on myocardial contractile force and arterial blood pressure. Diabetologia 1977;13:515-519.
6. Ballagi-Pordány G, Köszeghy A, Koltai MZs and Pogátsa G. Effect of tolbutamide, gliclazide and glipizide on the ventricular ectopic beats and fibrillation caused by coronary occlusion in rats. Diabetologia 1987;30:496A.

7. Ballagi-Pordány G, Köszeghy A, Koltai MZs, Pogátsa G. Effect of first and second generation sulphonylureas on the cardiotoxicity of strophanthidine in rabbits. Diabetologia 1988;31:467A.
8. Lasseter KC, Levey GS, Palmer RF, McCarthy JS. The effect of sulphonylurea drugs on rabbit myocardial contractility, canine Purkinje fiber automaticity, and adenyl cyclase activity from rabbit and human hearts. J Clin Invest 1972;51:2429-2434.
9. Crass MF, Spanheimer RG, Stone DB, Brown RJ. Tolbutamide induced inotropic responses in the perfused working heart: effects of albumin. Proc Soc Exp Biol Med 1973;142:861-866.
10. Pogátsa G, Koltai Mzs, Balkány I, Dévai J, Kiss V. Effects of various hypoglycaemic sulphonylureas on the cardiotoxicity of glycosides. Eur J Clin Pharmacol 1985;28:367-370.
11. Koltai MZ, Kammerer L, Jermendy G, Pogátsa G. Ober die Inzidenz des Myokardinfarktes bei Zuckerkranken. Wien Med Wschr 1985;185(Suppl 71):10.
12. Balant L. Clinical pharmacokinetics of sulphonylurea hypoglycaemic drugs. Clinical Pharmacokinetics 1981;6:215-241.
13. Ballagi-Pordány G, Köszeghy A, Koltai MZ, Pogátsa G. Az elsö és második generációs, vércukorszintet csökkentö sulphonylureák eltérö hatása a strophantin toxicitására nyulakon. Kisérletes Orvostudomány 1988;40:305-310.
14. Lepran I, Koltai M, Werner S, Szekeres L. Coronary artery ligation in early arrhythmias and determination of the ischemic area in conscious rat. J Pharmacol Methods 1983;9:219-230.
15. Ballagi-Pordány G, Köszeghy A, Koltai M, Pogátsa G. A szulfonilureák eltérö hatása a ritmuszavarokra ischaemiás patkánysziven. Kisérletes Orvostudomány 1988;40:300-304.
16. Ballagi-Pordány G, Köszeghy A, Koltai MZ, Aranyi Z, Pogátsa G. A vércukorszintet csökkentö szulfonilureák hatása a hemodinamikai paraméterekre kutyán. Kisérletes Orvostudomány 1989;41:330-335.
17. Ballagi-Pordány G, Köszeghy A, Koltai MZ, Aranyi Z, Pogátsa G. A vércukorszintet csökkentö szulfonilureák közvetlen hátasa a sziv- és érrendszerre nyulon. Kisérletes Orvostudomány 1989;41:401-406.
18. Laube H, Krausch H. Einfluss unterschiedlicher Behandlungsformen auf den Fettstoffwechsel beim Diabetes mellitus. Med Welt 1988;39:358.

19. Christlieb AR. Diabetes and hypertensive vascular disease, mechanisms and treatment. Am J Cardiol 1973;32:592-606.
20. Wales JK, Grant AM, Wolf EW. The effect of tolbutamide on blood pressure. J Pharmacol Exp Ther 1971;178:130-140.
21. Kereiakes DJ, Naughton JL. The heart in diabetes. West J Med 1983;140:583-593.
22. Ballagi-Pordány G, Koltai MZ, Köszeghy A, Pogátsa G. Effect of tolbutamide, gliclazide and glipizide on the ventricular ectopic beats and fibrillation by coronary occlusion in rats. Diabetologia Croatica 1988;30:496-503.

Reversibility of Diabetic Cardiomyopathy by Therapeutic Interventions in Mild Diabetes

D. Stroedter, M. Schmitt, T. Broetz, K. Federlin, W. Schaper*

3rd Medical Clinic and Policlinic, Univ. of Giessen, Rodthohl 6, 6300 Giessen, Germany, and Max-Planck-Institute*, 6350 Bad Nauheim, Germany

Introduction

Severe experimental diabetes, induced by streptozotocin in a dose of 65 mg/kg body weight, resulting in blood glucose levels of 500 mg/dl, leads to a cardiomyopathy, characterized by reduced cardiac output, due to reduced stroke volume and reduced heart rate. Investigating these hearts in the isolated working rat heart model, the development of a cardiomyopathy can be seen after 1 week of diabetes as well as after 2 weeks, 8 weeks, 16 and 24 weeks (1,2,3).

The different duration of severe diabetes leads to some differences in the extent of cardiac failure. In contrast to short-term diabetes, 4 months and 6 months diabetes leads to progressive premature heart failure, allowing an investigation in the working heart model for about 30 min only. Moreover the addition of insulin (20 mU/ml) to the perfusion medium, leading to a normalization of cardiac output in short-term diabetes, does not result in a complete normalization in 4 months diabetic hearts. These data are in agreement with results of Tahiliani et al (4,5) in 5 months diabetic hearts and an insulin therapy about 4 weeks. Otherwise insulin enables these hearts to perform longer cardiac work, but at a lower cardiac output level, than without insulin in the perfusion medium, e.g. insulin prevents premature cardiac failure in diabetic hearts. The question is: Are these results only seen in severe diabetes or is mild diabetes, more often seen in clinic, also able to induce a cardiomyopathy? Therefore the goals of the presented study are:
1. To clarify cardiac performance and metabolism in mild diabetes lasting for 2 and 4 months.
2. To compare the effect of 2 forms of therapy, islet transplantation and insulin therapy (s.c.) lasting for 2 months in regard to the

reversibility of cardiomyopathy and cardiac metabolic alterations. Although islet transplantation is more difficult than insulin therapy (s.c.) and still in experimental status in diabetes therapy, we have chosen this way of therapy because of its more physiological release of insulin, possibly resulting in better effects in regard to diabetic complications.

Material and Methods

For this study male Lewis rats were employed. The diabetes was induced by streptozotocin in a dose of 40 mg/kg body weight. The blood glucose levels are plotted in Fig. 1. A 2 or 4 months diabetic period was followed by a 2 months therapeutic phase. The insulin therapy (s.c.) as well as the islet transplantation results in a fairly complete normalization of the blood glucose levels. The fasting blood glucose levels are under the therapy in the normal range.

As there is no difference in metabolism and hemodynamics after 2 and 4 months of diabetes and the same results are seen after 2 months of therapy without any significant difference, too, the results of the 4 months diabetes study are only shown.

The experiments were done in the isolated working rat heart model, described earlier (1), a modification of that described by Neely et al (6) and Taegtmeyer et al (7). The hearts were paced with a frequency of 300/min. After a 10 min Langendorff-washout perfusion from a reservoir 100 cm above the heart, containing Krebs-Henseleit-buffer (37°C) and 5.5 mmol/l glucose, gassed by 95% O_2 and 5% CO_2, the hearts were perfused in the working heart model about 60 min at a physiological workload, e.g. a preload of 15 cm H_2O and an afterload of 110 cm H_2O, using a recirculating system. Perfusion medium was a Krebs-Henseleit-buffer, containing 5.5 mmol/l glucose as substrate, too, and gassed by 95% O_2 and 5% CO_2. Samples of the perfusion medium were taken every 15 min for analysis. At the end of the perfusion the hearts were freeze-clamped in aluminum tongs chilled in liquid N_2.

Statistics: Analysis variance, n=6 in every group, * = 0.05, ** = 0.001. Data are presented as means and the standard error of the means.

Results

I. Hemodynamics
1. Diabetic hearts had significantly lower cardiac output when compared to normal healthy controls (Fig. 2).

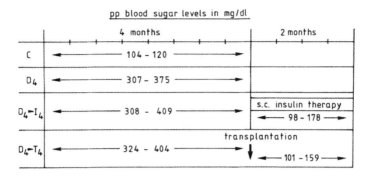

Figure 1. Postprandial blood glucose levels during 4 months of diabetes and during 2 months of therapy. C = control, D_4 = diabetic hearts, I_4 = hearts after insulin therapy (s.c.), T_4 = hearts resp. animals after islet transplantation.

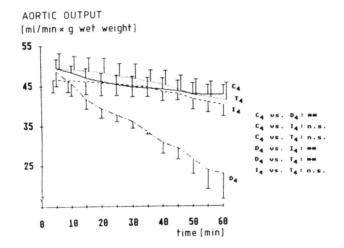

Figure 2. Aortic output during 60 min of perfusion in control and diabetic hearts and after 2 months of insulin therapy (s.c.) (I_4) or islet transplantation (T_4).

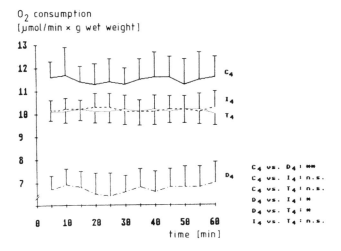

Figure 3. O_2-consumption of normal and diabetic hearts and after therapy.

2. A normalization of cardiac performance was achieved with both therapies, which do not differ in the extent of amelioration.
3. Similar results were observed with regard to oxygen consumption (Fig. 3); diabetic hearts were 41% lower when compared to control hearts or therapeutically adjusted hearts.

II. Metabolism

1. The glucose uptake (Fig. 4) of the diabetic heart was only half that of a normal heart. A normalization of the glucose uptake was achieved through both forms of therapy. The lactate and pyruvate production of the diabetic heart was twice as high as that of normal healthy hearts. Lactate and pyruvate production were also normalized through both therapies.
2. After a 10 min Langendorff-perfusion (Fig. 5) the hearts were examined for the metabolic balance. Characteristic for diabetic hearts were increased glycogen and triglyceride stores as well as decreased ATP and CP levels. After therapy the ATP levels were in the normal range again.
3. Also after 1 hour of work (Fig. 6) the ATP and CP levels were lower in diabetic hearts, whereas in the therapeutic series there were normal or significantly higher levels.

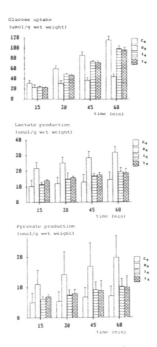

Figure 4. The cumulative glucose uptake, the cumulative lactate and pyruvate production during 60 min of work of normal and diabetic hearts and after therapy.

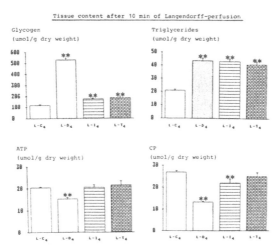

Figure 5. Tissue content of glycogen, triglycerides, ATP and CP after 10 min of Langendorff-washout-perfusion in normal and diabetic hearts and after therapy in comparison to normal hearts.

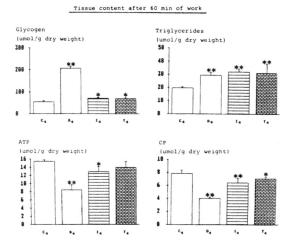

Figure 6. Tissue content of glycogen, triglycerides, ATP and CP after 60 min of work in comparison to normal hearts (C_4).

III. Energy balance
1. In this model the glucose utilization (Table 1) was calculated from exogenous glucose uptake plus glycogen breakdown minus (lactate plus pyruvate production)/2. The results show that healthy normal hearts acquire 10% of their energy needs from endogenous reserves, whereas diabetic hearts acquire 50%. The glucose utilization in diabetic hearts was 42% less than in the healthy normal hearts.
2. The myocardial ATP and CP levels (Table 2) characterize the energy status of the heart. A closer examination of these values is necessary. The sum of the ATP and CP levels was 44% lower in diabetic hearts; this percentile correlates well with the reduced glucose utilization of 42% and the reduced oxygen uptake of 41%.

    A reduced level of high energy phosphates does not explain the reduced hemodynamics, because a compensated increase in ATP turnover would be able to compensate for this reduction. As the turnover calculations show, the ATP turnover in diabetic hearts as sign for a reduced oxidative phosphorylation was not increased.

IV. What can we conclude from the relationship between measured and calculated O_2-uptake?

    In the comparison of the measured O_2-uptake with the O_2-consumption

Table 1. Glucose utilization, calculated from glucose uptake plus glycogen breakdown minus (lactate plus pyruvate production)/2.

Balance of energy

	Glucose uptake	Glycogen breakdown	Lactate+ Pyruvate prod./2	Glucose utilization
C_4	115.98	9.65	10.70	114.93
D_4	44.76	48.53	25.80	67.49
I_4	100.17	15.88	15.05	101.00
T_4	96.89	17.41	14.31	99.99

in umol/h x g wet weight
** $p < 0.001$

Table 2. ATP turnover. From glucose utilization the ATP production per min and per beat is calculated; 1 mole glucose yields 36 moles ATP. According to the premise that ATP, which is produced, is used, the ATP turnover per beat can be calculated. Basis of the calculation is: 1 mole glucose yields 36 moles ATP and needs 6 moles O_2 for oxidation, 1 mole palmitic acid yields 129 moles ATP and needs 23 moles O_2 for oxidation.

ATP - turnover

	C_4	D_4	I_4	T_4
$\sum$ ATP + CP (umol/g wet weight)	3.47	1.93	2.89	3.15
ATP-production (umol/min x g wet w.)	68.96	40.49	60.60	59.99
ATP-prod./beat (umol/beat x g wet w.)	0.230	0.135	0.202	0.200
ATP-turnover/beat = % of tissue level/beat	6.63	6.99	6.99	6.35

Table 3. Relation of measured and calculated O_2-consumption.

Relation of measured and calculated O_2-consumption

	C_4	D_4	I_4	T_4
O_2-consumption (umol/min x g wet w.) calculated for				
a. Glucose	11.49	6.75	10.10	10.00
b. Triglycerides	0.19	2.38	1.88	1.22
c. Sum of a. + b.	11.68	9.13	11.98	11.22
O_2-consumption (umol/min x g wet w.) measured	11.47	6.72	10.26	10.11

(Table 3), calculated from glucose utilization, we can see that these values are identical - the difference is only 0.5 to 1.5%. This indicates that in the model used here the normal as well as the diabetic heart cover their energy requirements completely by carbohydrates. A lipolysis is seen, but without any indication of a beta-oxidation.

This conclusion is underlined by other observations (1), namely: Perfusing with substrate-free medium diabetic hearts perform longer cardiac work with a higher output than normal hearts, due to the increased glycogen stores, but not so long as it could be expected by a contribution of triglycerides as fuel for energy production. Secondly, the addition of iodoacetate, an inhibitor of glycolysis, leads in normal as well as in diabetic hearts to an acute heart failure (aortic output decreases within 2 min to 0 ml/min). Only after addition of octanoate to the perfusion medium, containing 5.5 mmol/l glucose, a normalization of cardiac output is seen (unpublished results).

Conclusions
1. Mild diabetes of 4 months duration leads to cardiomyopathy. The

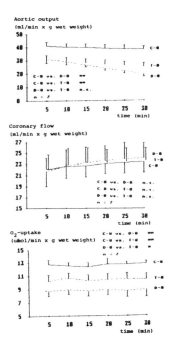

Figure 7. Aortic output, coronary flow and O_2-uptake of normal hearts and after 8 months of mild diabetes resp. 2 months of diabetes therapy by islet transplantation.

reduction in cardiac performance was the same as after 2 months of mild diabetes.

2. The diabetic cardiomyopathy is due to reduced glucose utilization (42%), leading to reduced oxidative phosphorylation, indicated by reduced O_2-uptake (41%) and reduced myocardial levels of high energy phosphates (44%).

3. Both islet transplantation and insulin therapy (s.c.) are able to normalize cardiac performance as well as cardiac metabolism after 2 months of diabetes as well as after 4 months of diabetes, indicating that this diabetic cardiomyopathy is a reversible damage due to insulin deficiency.

4. Both therapeutic interventions do not differ in the quality of reversibility.

In the meantime we have investigated hearts after 8 months of mild diabetes and after an additional therapeutic phase of 2 months by islet transplantation. After 8 months of diabetes this therapy does not lead to a normalization of cardiac output in the working heart model, e.g. between 4 and 8 months of mild diabetes a point of no return is achieved, indicating that here other mechanisms than reduced glucose utilization must be discussed (Fig. 7).

In contrast to these results in vitro after 8 months of mild diabetes a normalization of cardiac performance in vivo is seen using the measurement of dp/dt via a catheter in the left ventricle (Results in co-operation with Prof. Dr. P. Rösen, Düsseldorf, FRG.).

Summary

The aim of this study was to clarify cardiac performance and metabolism in mild diabetes of 4 months duration (blood sugar levels 16.5 - 22 mmol/l, normal fasting blood glucose) using the working rat heart model at physiological workload, and to compare the effect of 2 forms of diabetes therapy, islet transplantation and insulin therapy (s.c.) about 2 months. Diabetes resulted in a significant reduction of cardiac output, accompanied not only by a 41% reduction of oxygen uptake, but of a 42% reduction of glucose utilization/h, too. Myocardial ATP and CP levels were decreased by 44%. The two therapeutic interventions produced a complete reversibility of both hemodynamic and metabolic alterations. In this experimental model mild diabetes leads to a cardiomyopathy, caused by reduced utilization of carbohydrates, leading to a reduced energy production with reduced oxygen uptake and reduced high energy phosphate levels. All these parameters were reduced to the same extent. The results show that diabetic cardiomyopathy in mild diabetes is due to insulin deficiency, and that both therapeutic interventions do not differ in the quality of reversibility.

Acknowledgements

This research was supported by DFG Str 289/1-1 - Deutsche Forschungsgemeinschaft.

References

1. Stroedter D, Willmann P, Willmann J, Federlin K, and Schaper W. Results of a balance of energy in the diabetic heart. In: The Diabetic Heart, eds. Nagano M and Dhalla NS, Raven Press, New York, pp 383-393, 1991.

2. Stroedter D, Schuster KR, Mogk M, Bretzel RG, and Federlin K. Reversibility of diabetic cardiomyopathy with islet transplantation in rats. Diabetes 1989;38 Suppl 1:319-320.
3. Stroedter D. Diabetische Kardiomyopathie - Tatsache oder Fiktion? Habilitationsschrift, Univ. Giessen, FRG, 1987, pp 1-334.
4. Tahiliani AG, Lopaschuk GD and McNeill JH. Effect of insulin treatment on long-term diabetes-induced alteration of myocardial function. Gen Pharmacol 1984;15:545-547.
5. Tahiliani AG and McNeill JH. Diabetes-induced abnormalities in the myocardium. Life Sci 1986;38:959-974.
6. Neely JR, Liebermeister H, Battersby EJ and Morgan HE. Effect of pressure development on oxygen consumption by isolated rat heart. Am J Physiol 1967;212:804-812.
7. Taegtmeyer H, Hems R and Krebs HA. Utilization of energy-providing substrates in the isolated working rat heart. Biochem J 1980;186:701-711.

Improvement of Myocardial Function and Metabolism in Diabetic Rats By the Carnitine Palmitoyltransferase Inhibitor Etomoxir

P. Rösen, F.J. Schmitz, H. Reinauer

Dept. of Clinical Biochemistry, Diabetes-Forschungsinstitut, D-4000 Düsseldorf, Germany

Introduction

The cardiac risk of diabetic patients is increased and the outcome from myocardial infarction impaired in diabetes (1). Additionally, in clinical and experimental studies, evidence has been presented that the ventricular function can be disturbed very early in diabetes, even in the absence of atherosclerotic coronary disease (2-8). These findings led to the hypothesis of a specific "diabetic cardiomyopathy" causing impairment of heart performance and thereby an increased cardiac risk of diabetics (2-4). Besides changes in regulation of coronary perfusion (9) and in the myocardial conducting system (10), metabolic alterations might contribute to impairment of cardiac function in diabetes (2,7,8,11). A reduced rate of glycolysis and enhanced reliance of the diabetic heart on fatty acids as the major energy substrate might cause a diminished generation of glycolytic ATP and limit the energy production of the heart especially if the coronary perfusion is impaired. In agreement with this hypothesis myocardial creatine-phosphate and ATP has been described to be reduced in hearts of chemically induced and spontaneously diabetic rats (8,12,13). Furthermore, accumulation of acylcarnitines and other intermediates of fatty acid metabolism has been directly implicated in the development of insulin resistance, the reduced uptake and conversion of glucose as well as in disturbances of calcium homeostasis (11, 14-17).

Accordingly, an inhibition of fatty acid metabolism and a shift of myocardial metabolism to glucose as the major energy substrate might be desirable and protective for the heart in diabetes. Such a metabolic shift has been suggested to be achieved by pharmacological inhibition of carnitine palmitoyltransferase I (18-21). Thus, it has been already shown that

Nagano, M., Mochizuki, S., Dhalla, N.S. (eds.), CARDIOVASCULAR DISEASE IN DIABETES. Copyright © 1992. Kluwer Academic Publishers, Boston. All rights reserved.

inhibitors of carnitine palmitoyltransferase I (CPT-I) effectively inhibit fatty acid oxidation (21) and stimulate the oxidation of glucose and lactate several-fold in isolated perfused hearts of control and diabetic rats (19,20). These acute metabolic effects of CPT inhibition are discussed to cause the increased insulin sensitivity and the protection of the diabetic heart against ischemic damage if perfused with CPT inhibitors (19, 20, 22).

To evaluate the therapeutical potential of these pharmacologically active compounds, it is important to study not only the acute effects of such CPT I inhibitors in an isolated heart preparation, but also the influence of a long lasting treatment on the performance and the metabolism of the diabetic heart in vivo. Chronically diabetic rats were therefore treated with etomoxir, a recently developed inhibitor of CPT-I (2-(6-(4-chlorophenoxy)-hexyl)-oxirane-2-carboxylate), for 8 days in a non-toxic dosage and the effect of etomoxir on heart function, on serum and myocardial lipids as well as on carnitine content in heart and liver was investigated.

Methods

Diabetes was induced by streptozotocin (60 mg/kg body weight) in male Wistar rats (250-300 g) as already described in detail (9, 19, 20).

Heart function; heart rate, maximal left ventricular systolic pressure (LVSP) and the increment in pressure development and relaxation (+dp/dt max, -dp/dt max) were measured by a Millar tip catheter (PR 249) inserted into the left ventricle as described (8). The electrocardiogram (ECG) was determined in the three standard leads after anaesthetizing the rats by injection of nembutal (30 mg/kg body weight).

Biochemical analysis; analysis of serum lipids, blood glucose ß-hydroxybutyrate, hemoglobin A_1 were performed by standard techniques (8, 19, 20). Triglycerides, phospholipids and fatty acids were extracted by chloroform-methanol and separated by thin layer chromatography, and the fatty acid composition was determined by gas chromatography (23).

Carnitine and its derivatives were extracted and determined using a radioenzymatic procedure (24).

Treatment of rats with etomoxir; control and diabetic rats were treated with etomoxir (Byk-Gulden Konstanz, FRG) dissolved in saline. The daily dosage was 18 mg/kg body weight, which was applied for 8 days by i.p. injection. The treatment was started 5 weeks after induction of diabetes by streptozotocin and verification of the diabetic state.

Results

As already described (8) myocardial performance was impaired after induction of diabetes (Table 1). Maximal impairment was achieved after a diabetes duration of 4-6 weeks. In parallel to the reduction of heart rate, the velocities of contraction and relaxation disturbances in the ECG became evident as indicated by the broadening of the QRS complex. A more detailed analysis of myocardial conduction using an isolated perfused heart, to the surface of which a multi-electrode matrix was attached has recently been reported (10).

Treatment of healthy rats with etomoxir for eight days did not influence heart performance in vivo at all. In diabetes, however, treatment with etomoxir led to an increase of maximal left ventricular systolic pressure and a significant acceleration of the velocities of contraction and relaxation (Table 1). Additionally, the QRS- and QT-times prolonged in diabetes became shortened by the treatment with etomoxir from 0.06 and 0.096 to 0.054 and 0.089 respectively ($p<0.05$), whereas heart rate was not affected. Thus, the impairment of cardiac function developed during diabetes for 4 to 6 weeks can be partially normalized or significantly improved by treatment of diabetic rats with etomoxir within 8 days (Table 1).

Treatment of diabetic rats with etomoxir resulted in only a small decrease in blood sugar level and did not reduce the percentage of glycated hemoglobins. Thus, etomoxir has only a mild hypoglycemic potency in the applied dosage (Table 2).

Ketogenesis and lipid metabolism were, however, strongly affected by treatment of control and diabetic rats with etomoxir as indicated by the remarkable reduction of ß-hydroxybutyrate, glycerol, cholesterol, and triglycerides in serum (Table 2). Only the concentration of free fatty acids in serum became elevated by about 30-40% as compared to untreated diabetic rats.

In contrast to serum, lipids in myocardium and liver including free fatty acids, triglycerides, phospholipids, and cardiolipin were generally elevated in both healthy and diabetic rats treated with etomoxir. Histologically small, but not yet pathological, lipid deposits were detected in liver and heart already one week after treatment of rats with etomoxir (Table 3).

Table 1. Influence of etomoxir and myocardial performance of diabetic rats.

	Control		Diabetes	
Etomoxir	−	+	−	+
Heart rate (min^{-1})	416 ± 8	390 ± 10	312 ± 10*	313 ± 11
LVSP (mmHg)	149 ± 6	152 ± 3	100 ± 5*	129 ± 8**
+ dp/dt (mmHg/s)^{max}	9161 ± 552	8970 ± 311	5434 ± 426*	7183 ± 215**
− dp/dt (mmHg/s)^{max}	7954 ± 253	7211 ± 484	3432 ± 36*	5666 ± 196**

Values are means ± SEM of 6 to 8 experiments. Diabetes was induced by streptozotocin. After a diabetes duration of 6 weeks heart function was measured by a Millar tip catheter inserted into the left ventricle. A part of the animals were treated with etomoxir for 8 days (18 mg/kg body weight).
LVSP = maximal left ventricular systolic pressure
* $p < 0.05$ diabetes vs control.
** $p < 0.05$ untreated vs etomoxir treated animals.

Whereas the fraction of acylcarnitines was only slightly influenced by the induction of diabetes, diabetes led to a large reduction in the amount of total and free myocardial carnitine as previously reported (25). This loss of carnitines could totally be prevented by etomoxir so that the amounts of total and free myocardial carnitine in treated diabetic rats were no longer different from those in healthy rats (Table 4). In contrast to heart, in liver diabetes did not cause a decrease in free and total carnitine. Nevertheless, treatment of the animals with etomoxir caused a remarkable increase in both free and total carnitine. Thus, treatment of the animals with etomoxir led to an increased intracellular concentration of carnitine, but did not cause an accumulation of acylcarnitines in heart and liver.

Discussion

Fatty acids and ketone bodies are the main substrates for energy generation in the diabetic heart (11) and the accelerated oxidation of these substrates leads to an inhibition of glucose and lactate oxidation and insulin

Table 2. Influence of the carnitine palmitoyltransferase inhibitor etomoxir on blood glucose, ß-hydroxybutyrate, cholesterol and triglycerides.

	Control		Diabetes	
+ Etomoxir	−	+	−	+
Glucose (mg/dl)	162 ± 7	120 ± 9**	452 ± 37*	380 ± 33**
HbA$_1$ (%)	4.3 ± 0.1	4.6 ± 0.2	10.9 ± 0.3*	12.5 ± 0.5
ß-OHB (nmol/ml)	140 ± 28	172 ± 15	1134 ± 214*	401 ± 46**
Glycerides (mg/dl)	77 ± 8	50 ± 7**	323 ± 62*	218 ± 33**
cholesterol (mg/dl)	60 ± 4	57 ± 6	80 ± 5*	69 ± 4**

Means ± of 5 to 9 animals are given. Diabetes was induced by streptozotocin and lasted for 6 weeks. A part of the animals were treated with etomoxir for 8 days (18 mg/kg body weight). Blood and serum was analysed as described in methods.
* $p < 0.05$ diabetes vs controls
** $p < 0.05$ untreated vs etomoxir treated animals
ß-OHB = ß-hydroxybutyrate

Table 3. Influence of etomoxir on lipids in myocardium

	Control		Diabetes	
Etomoxir	−	+	−	+
FFA (nmol/ g w.w.)	152 ± 52	193 ± 35	264 ± 64*	315 ± 102
Pls (umol/g w.w)	48.4 ± 3.5	66.8 ± 4.0**	51.8 ± 3.7	72.5 ± 4.2**
Cl (umol/g w.w)	8.9 ± 0.5	13.6 ± 0.7**	8.3 ± 0.3	10.5 ± 0.6**

Means ± SEM of 6 to 7 experiments are given. Methodological details are given in legend to Table 1. Pls = phospholipids   Cl = cardiolipin
* $p < 0.05$ control vs diabetes
** $p < 0.05$ etomoxir treated vs untreated animals

Table 4. Influence of etomoxir on carnitines in heart and liver

	Control		Diabetes	
Etomoxir	−	+	−	+
In Heart:				
free	919 ± 41	1281 ± 103**	287 ± 28*	1006 ± 27**
short chain	105 ± 23	345 ± 59**	290 ± 18*	261 ± 33**
long chain	32 ± 2	37 ± 2	24 ± 1	32 ± 2**
total	1056 ± 158	1664 ± 225**	600 ± 115*	1299 ± 179**
total/free	1.1	1.3	2.1	1.3
In Liver:				
free	150 ± 9	323 ± 32**	183 ± 14	350 ± 44**
total	346 ± 27	621 ± 33**	490 ± 44	674 ± 46**
total/free	2.3	1.9	2.7	1.9

Means ± SEM of 6 to 8 experiments are given. The carnitine derivatives are given in nmol/g w.w. and were determined by a radio-enzymatic method (24).
* $p < 0.05$ control vs diabetes
** $p < 0.05$ etomoxir treated vs untreated rats

resistance (14,19,20). It has been speculated that the increased reliance of the heart on lipid oxidation leads to an increased production of acylcarnitines and to various deleterious effects of these compounds on myocardial mitochondria, sarcoplasmic reticulum and sarcolemma resulting in an impairment of myocardial function (15-17). Since inhibitors of CPT-I have been shown to have no direct, immediate effect on myocardial performance, but to effectively inhibit ketogenesis and ß-oxidation (18) it has been further assumed that by inhibition of CPT-I myocardial metabolism can be shifted from lipids to glucose as the main energy substrate and that such a metabolic shift could be protective for the heart. In line with this hypothesis, cardiac performance of diabetic rats became improved by treatment of the animals for only 8 days with etomoxir. The velocities of contraction and relaxation as well as the conduction were improved by this treatment, whereas the innervation of the heart was not influenced by etomoxir. This interpretation that the improvement of cardiac function results from the metabolic shift from lipid to glucose oxidation is not only supported by previously published findings such as inhibition of ß-oxidation and ketogenesis (18,21), acceleration of oxidation of glucose and lactate, activation of pyruvate dehydrogenase (19,20), but also by the metabolic data reported here: the concentration of ß-hydroxybutyrate is strongly reduced, fatty acids are preferentially incorporated into complex lipids resulting in a slight accumulation of lipids in heart and liver. Furthermore, we did not observe any direct immediate effect of etomoxir or a very similar inhibitor of CPT-I (POCA) on myocardial function. The compensatory stimulation of glucose metabolism might result in an improved energy provision and especially of glycolytic ATP which has been show to play a specific role for the maintenance of various ATPase activities in the heart (26). Additionally, such a metabolic shift might also be followed by changes in the isomyosin pattern. There are several lines of evidence that in the diabetic state the isomyosins change from V_1 to V_3 (27,28), but also that a forced metabolism of glucose can reverse this alteration (29) resulting in an improved contractility and relaxation of the heart.

In line with this interpretation Lee et al. (30) could demonstrate that all affects of CPT inhibition could be abrogated by octanoate, a short fatty acid, which can be metabolized without the CPT shuttle. Thus, all actions are mediated via inhibition of long chain fatty acid oxidation. Furthermore, treatment of diabetic animals with L-carnitine similarly prevented the loss of myocardial carnitine and the depression of myocardial performance (31). It is interesting to note that there is a loss of carnitines from heart also in other forms of cardiopathy as in Syrian hamsters, whereas carnitines in skeletal muscle and liver are not affected (32). All these findings suggest a direct link between myocardial carnitines, lipid oxidation and the development of cardiac dysfunction.

It is interesting to note that heart rate was not influenced by etomoxir indicating that the observed changes in contractility and relaxation are independent from changes in heart rate. It remains to be proven whether stimulation of sympathetic innervation and treatment with etomoxir together completely normalize the impaired function of the diabetic heart. Our results also suggest that different pathophysiological mechanisms contribute to impairment of cardiac function in diabetes: one mechanism may concern the decreased glucose metabolism and thus affect the glycolytic ATP and the energy state, the isomyosin pattern and thereby the calcium homeostasis of the heart. Another mechanism seems to be independent from glucose metabolism and contribute to disturbances of myocardial innervation.

In spite of the accelerated conversion of glucose by the heart we only observed a very weak hypoglycemic affect of etomoxir. This finding might indicate either that mainly myocardial metabolism is altered with respect to glucose oxidation, whereas no changes occur in skeletal muscle, the major consumer of glucose. Alternatively, the in vivo applied dosage of etomoxir was not sufficient to effectively inhibit gluconeogenesis in liver. Both explanations would limit the hypoglycemic activity of this CPT-I inhibitor.

One most striking finding of this study is that the loss of total and free carnitines in heart of diabetic rats (25) could be totally prevented by etomoxir. Since the uptake of carnitine by the heart is not hampered in diabetes, however, a marked reduction in serum carnitine and an increased urinary excretion rate have been observed (33), it is obvious that the carnitine concentration in the heart reflects the diminished concentration in serum. The restoration of myocardial carnitine by etomoxir is therefore indicative for a non-cardiac effect of etomoxir presumably an inhibition of the accelerated urinary excretion. Since the acylcarnitines in the non-ketotic diabetic rat heart are only slightly elevated in spite of the hyperlipidemic conditions and the reduced oxidative capacity of the heart in diabetes (8,22), it is intriguing to assume that some carnitine is also lost from the heart by an efflux of acylcarnitines. It is conceivable that this efflux of carnitines is reduced by etomoxir and myocardial carnitine is thereby conserved, since the formation of acylcarnitines from CoA-derivatives is inhibited and less acylcarnitines are available. As a consequence of inhibition of CPT-I a preferential formation of complex lipids has to be expected in line with the biochemical and histological findings.

It has been shown that inhibition of CPT-I might be useful for breaking the insulin resistance observed very often in Type II diabetics, and also in Type I diabetes (19,20). It also improves the depressed cardiac function and protects the diabetic heart against ischemic damage (22). Thus, inhibition of CPT-I might be therapeutically useful if the accumulation of lipids demonstrated in this study remains moderate and results from metabolic adaptation processes after start of the treatment with etomoxir.

Summary

Inhibitors of carnitine palmitoyltransferase (CPT) have been shown to effectively inhibit fatty acid oxidation, to stimulate glucose consumption, and to break insulin resistance (19,20). These metanolic effects might be desirable and protective for the diabetic heart, the cardiac performance of which is strongly reduced (8,19). Therefore the influence of the newly developed CPT-I inhibitor etomoxir on heart function and metabolism was studied to evaluate the therapeutic potential of this compound. Treatment of diabetic rats (streptozotocin, 60 mg/kg body weight) with etomoxir (18 mg/kg body weight/day) for eight days led to an improvement of heart function of diabetic rats. Maximal left ventricular systolic pressure, and the velocities of contraction and relaxation were accelerated whereas heart rate was not affected. In the ECG, the QRS- and QT-complexes broadened in diabetes became shortened. Etomoxir had only a mild hypoglycemic potency, but strongly inhibited ketogenesis. Whereas serum lipids were reduced, the amounts of various lipids in myocardium and liver of healthy and diabetic rats were elevated by etomoxir, and histologically definite, but not yet pathological lipid deposits were detected. Etomoxir totally prevented the loss of carnitine generally associated with diabetes. The demonstrated improvement of cardiac performance in diabetes is suggested to be caused by a shift of myocadial metabolism from fatty acid oxidation to an accelerated glucose consumption and mainly by the preservation of myocardial carnitine. In summary, the highly specific inhibitor of CPT-I etomoxir might be therapeutically useful to protect the heart in diabetes, if the accumulation of lipids in liver and heart remains tolerable.

References

1. Jarrett RJ. The epidemiology of coronary heart disease and related factors in the context of diabetes mellitus and impaired glucose tolerance. In: Diabetes and heart disease, Jarrett RJ (ed), Elsevier, Amsterdam, pp. 1-24, 1984.
2. Ledet T, Gotzsche O, Heickendorff L. The pathology of diabetic cardiopathy. In: Diabetes and heart disease, Jarrett RJ (ed), Elsevier, Amsterdam pp. 25-46, 1984.
3. Regan T, Lyons MM, Ahmed SS, Levinson GE, Oldewurtl HA, Ahmed MR, Haider B. Evidence for cardiomyopathy. J Clin Invest 1977;60:885-899.

4. Shapiro LM. Specific heart disease in diabetes mellitus. Br J Med 1982;284:140-141.
5. Regan TJ, Ettinger PO, Khan MI, Jesrani MI, Lyons MM, Oldewurtl HA, Weber M. Altered myocardial function and metabolism in chronic diabetes mellitus without ischemia in dogs. Circ Res 1974;35:222-237.
6. Fein FS, Kornstein LB, Strobeck JE, Capasso JM, Sonnenblick EH. Reversibility of diabetic cardiomyopathy with insulin in rats. Circ Res 1980;47:922-933.
7. Penpargkul S, Schaible T, Yiptinsoi T, Scheuer J. The effect of diabetes on performance and metabolism of rat hearts. Circ Res 1980;47:911-921.
8. Rösen P, Windeck P, Zimmer HG, Reinauer H. Myocardial hearts. Basic Res Cardiol 1986;81:620-635.
9. Rösen P, Rösen R, Hohl C, Klaus W, Reinauer H. Reduced transcoronary exchange and prostaglandin synthesis in diabetic rat heart. Am J Physiol 1984;247:H563-H569.
10. Dhein S, Tschöpe D, Rösen P, Rösen R. Defect in the myocardial conducting system of streptozotocin-diabetic rats. In: Diabetic Neuropathy Proceedings, Ward JD (ed), J. Wiley & Sons, Baffins Lane, in press.
11. Neely JR, Morgan HE. Relationship between carbohydrates and lipid metabolism and energy balance of heart muscle. Ann Rev Physiol 1974;36:413-459.
12. Atkinson DE. Reduced high energy phosphate levels in rat hearts. Effect of alloxan diabetes. Am J Physiol 1976;230:1744-1750.
13. Jenkins RL, McDaniel HG, Digerness S, Parrish SW, Ong RL. Adenine nucleotide metabolism in hearts of diabetic rats. Diabetes 1988;37:629-636.
14. Randle PJ, Garland PB, Hales CN, Newsholme EA. The glucose fatty acid cycle. Its role in insulin sensitivity and the metabolic disorders of diabetes mellitus. Lancet 1963;785-789.
15. Lamers JMJ, Dejonge-Stinis JT, Verdouw PD, Hülsmann WC. On the possible role of long chain fatty acid acylcarnitine accumulation in producing junctional and calcium permeability changes in membranes during myocardial ischemia. Cardiovas Res 1987;21:313-322.
16. Ganguly PK, Pierce GN, Dhalla KS, Dhalla NS. Defective sarcoplasmic

reticular calcium transport in diabetic cardiopathy. Am J Physiol 1983;244:E528-E535.
17. Baydoun AR, Markham A, Morgan RM, Sweetman AJ. Palmitoyl carnitine: An endogenous promoter of calcium efflux from rat heart mitochondria. Biochem Pharmacol 1988;37:3103-3107.
18. Bressler R, Corredor C, Brendel K. Hypoglycin and hypoglycin-like compounds. Pharmacol Rev 1969;21:105-130.
19. Rösen P, Reinauer H. Inhibition of carnitine palmitoyl-transferase 1 by phenylalkyloxiranecarboxylic acid and its influence on lipolysis and glucose metabolism in isolated perfused hearts of streptozotocin-diabetic rats. Metabolism 1984;23:177-185.
20. Rösen P, Herberg L, Reinauer H. Different types of post-insulin receptor defects contribute to insulin resistance in hearts of obese Zucker rats. Endocrinol 1986;119:1285-1291.
21. Sherratt HS, Gathey SJ, DeGrado TR, Ng CK, Holden JE. Effects of 2-(5(4-chlorophenyl)pentyl)oxirane-2-carboxylate on fatty acid and glucose metabolism in isolated perfused rat hearts determined using iodine-125-hexadecanoate. Biochem Biophys Res Commun 1983;117:653-657.
22. Lopaschuck GD, Wall SR, Olley PM, Davies NJ. Etomoxir, a carnitine palmitoyltransferase I inhibitor, protects hearts from fatty acid-induced ischemic injury independent of changes in long chain acylcarnitine. Circ Res 1988;63:1036-1043.
23. Rösen P, Senger W, Feuerstein J, Grote H, Reinauer, H. Influence of streptozotocin diabetes on myocardial lipids and prostaglandin release by the rat heart. Biomed Med 1983;30:19-33.
24. Pande SV, Caramancion MN. A simple radioisotopic assay of acetylcarnitine and acetyl-CoA at picomolar levels. Anal Biochem 1981;112:30-38.
25. Vary TC, Neely JR. A mechanism for reduced myocardial carnitine levels in diabetic animals. Am J Physiol 1982;243:H154-H158.
26. Bricknell OL, Daries PS, Opie LH. A relationship between ATP, glycolysis and ischemic contracture in the isolated rat heart. J Mol Cell Cardiol 1981;13:941-945.
27. Dillmann WH. Diabetes mellitus-induced changes in the concentration of specific mRNAs and proteins. Diabetes/Metabolism Rev 1988;4:789-797.
28. Malhotra A, Mordes JP, McDermott L, Schaible TF. Abnormal cardiac

biochemistry in spontaneously diabetic Bio-Breeding/Worcester rat. Am J Physiol 1985;249:H1051-H1055.
29. Dillmann WH. Diabetes and thyroid-hormone induced changes in cardiac function and their metabolic basis. Ann Rev Med 1989;40:373-394.
30. Lee SM, Bahl JJ, Bressler R. Prevention of the metabolic effects of 2-tetradecylglycidate by octanoid acid in the genetically diabetic mouse (db/db). Biochem Med 1985;33:104-109.
31. Rodrigues B, Xiang H, McNeill JH. Effect of L-carnitine treatment on lipid metabolism and cardiac performance in chronically diabetic rats. Diabetes 1988;37:1358-1364.
32. Yamashita T, Hayashi H, Kaneko M, Kamikawa T, Kobayashi A, Yamazaki N, Miura K, Shirasawa H, Nishimura M. Carnitine derivatives in hereditary cardiomyopathic animals. Jpn Heart J 1985;26:833-844.
33. Brooks SD, Bahl JJ, Bressler R. Carnitine in the streptozotocin-diabetic rat. J Nutr 1985;115:1267-1273.

Abnormal Mitochondrial Oxidative Phosphorylation of Ischaemic and Reperfused Myocardium Reversed by L-Propionyl-Carnitine

R. Ferrari, E. Pasini, A. Cargnoni, E. Condorelli,
F. De Giuli, A. Albertini

*Departments of Cardiology and Chemistry, University of Brescia,
Brescia, ITALY*

Introduction

In the experimental animal, L-propionyl-carnitine, one of the most potent analogues of carnitine (1,2,3) exert a cardioprotective action on ischaemic and reperfused myocardium (4,5,6,7). Despite considerable efforts to find explanation for these beneficial effects, a commonly accepted basic mechanism is still lacking. Recently it has been suggested that L-propionyl-carnitine protects the ischaemic myocardium by improving mitochondrial function (7,8,9). We now describe the effect of L-propionyl-carnitine on the deterioration on mitochondrial function caused by ischaemia and reperfusion in the isolated rabbit hearts. L-propionyl-carnitine was used at the concentration of 10^{-7} M, as it has been shown to be an optimal dose for cardioprotection (9). Some of the present data have been published (6,9).

Materials and Methods

Perfusion of the hearts

Adult New Zealand white rabbits (2.5 to 3.0 kg) were stunned by a blow on the head. The hearts were rapidly excised and perfused with a modified Krebs-Henseleit (10) buffer solution by the non-recirculating Langendorff technique as previously described (11). The buffer solution was delivered to the aortic cannula at 37°C and at a perfusion pressure of 60 to 80 mmHg, maintained with a Watson Marlow rotary pump (MHRE MK3). The perfusion pressure was monitored at the head of the aortic inflow cannula with a Statham P 23 transducer. This provided a constant flow of 25 ± 1.7 ml/min. The hearts were paced at 180 beats/min using suprathreshold rectangular pulses of

*Nagano, M., Mochizuki, S., Dhalla, N.S. (eds.), CARDIOVASCULAR
DISEASE IN DIABETES. Copyright © 1992. Kluwer Academic Publishers,
Boston. All rights reserved.*

1.0 ms duration. A period of 30 min equilibration was allowed before any experimental intervention. Then a perfusion containing L-propionyl-carnitine dissolved at 10^{-7} M was started and maintained until the end of the experiment. Thirty minutes later, either the control or the treated hearts were divided into three groups. Those in one group were further perfused under aerobic conditions (coronary flow 25 ± 1.7 ml/min) for 90 min. The hearts of the second group were made ischaemic by reducing coronary flow from 25 to 1 ml/min for 60 min and those of the third group were made ischaemic for 60 min and then reperfused. Reperfusion was for 30 min at the aerobic pre-ischaemic coronary flow. Left ventricular wall temperature was maintained at 36°C to 37°C, irrespective of coronary flow.

Left ventricular pressure measurements

To obtain an isovolumetrically beating preparation, a fluid-filled balloon was inserted into the left ventricular cavity via the atrium. The intraventricular balloon was then connected by a fluid-filled polyethylene catheter to a Statham pressure transducer (P 23 D6) for the determination of left ventricular pressure, as previously described (11).

Mitochondrial studies

1 - Isolation of the mitochondria:

Mitochondria were isolated at the end of each perfusion by differential centrifugation as previously described (11,12,13). Two different isolation media were used. The mitochondria required for oxygen consumption studies were isolated in the medium described by Sordhal et al (14) (180 mM KCl, 10 mM EDTA, 0.5% BSA). The mitochondria used for the determination of endogenous calcium and of ATP production were extracted in a medium containing sucrose (250 mM) and ruthenium red (5 uM) (13,15).

2 - Oxygen consumption measurements:

Rates of oxygen consumption were monitored polarographically at 25°C using a Clark type electrode. The reaction medium consisted of 250 mM sucrose, 3 mM KH_2PO_4, 0.5 mM EDTA and 3 mM K glutamate, pH 7.4 adjusted with Tris buffer. Mitochondria (to provide a final concentration of 1.25 mg mitochondrial protein/ml reaction medium) were added to the reaction chamber and allowed to equilibrate for 1 min. State 3 respiration was initiated by adding 0.5 mM ADP, pH 7.4. Mitochondrial function was assessed in terms of RCR, QO_2 and ADP/O here RCR (respiratory control ratio) is the ratio of oxygen used in the presence of ADP to that used in the absence of ADP. QO_2 are n atoms of oxygen used per mg of mitochondrial protein per min in response to the addition of ADP. ADP/O ratio is the manomoles ADP used per n atoms of oxygen consumed.

3 - Protein determination:

Mitochondrial protein concentration was determined by the method of Bradford (16) using BSA as standard.

4 - Mitochondrial ATP production:

ATP synthesis was determined in the medium used for oxygen consumption. Synthesis was initiated by adding ADP (0.5 mM). Two hundred ul samples were taken before and at 6, 15, 30, 45, 60, 100 and 120 seconds after adding ADP. They were then mixed with 50 ul of 10% perchloric acid on ice. Precipitated protein was separated by centrifugation and the ATP content of the supernatant was determined enzymatically using the method of Lamprecht and Trautschold (17). The total amount of ATP produced was calculated as the ATP present in the reaction chamber 15 seconds after the transition from state 3 to state 4 respiration.

5 - Mitochondrial calcium content:

Calcium content was determined by atomic absorption spectrometry. Mitochondrial pellets were digested overnight in 500 ul HNO_3. Lanthanum chloride was added to provide a final concentration of 0.1%; $CaCO_3$ was used as standard.

Tissue ATP and CP determination

The perfusion of the hearts in which ATP and CP levels were to be determined, was terminated by freeze-clamping the left ventricular apex with aluminum tongs pre-cooled in liquid nitrogen. The frozen muscle was then pulverized, homogenized and assayed for ATP and CP following the method of Lamprecht and Trautschold (17).

Experimental compounds and statistical evaluation

The reagents were analytical reagent grade quality. All enzyme used for the biochemical determinations were obtained from the Sigma Company (USA). L-propionyl-carnitine was kindly supplied by Sigma-Tau, Rome (Italy). The data are expressed as mean ± S.E. of n experiments, where each experiment is an individual perfusion. Statistical significance was calculated by Student's t-test, taking P = 0.05 as the limit of significance.

Results

Contractile activity

From Figure 1 it appears that infusion of L-propionyl-carnitine did not cause significant changes in cardiac performance during the 30 minutes of aerobic perfusion. Ischaemia resulted in a rapid decline of developed pressure to almost zero. The period of still detectable contractile activity during the first minutes after ischaemia was equal for control and L-propionyl-carnitine treated hearts (2.5 to 3.5 min). In control hearts diastolic pressure began to rise progressively 20 min after the onset of ischaemia and by the end of 60 min it had increased to 31 ± 2.1 (S.E.) mmHg. Readmission of flow to these hearts resulted in a rapid, further increase of coronary perfusion pressure and diastolic pressure, with only a small recovery of developed pressure. Administration of L-propionyl-carnitine (10^{-7}M) significantly delayed and reduced the rise in diastolic pressure that occurs during ischaemia. In addition, L-propionyl-carnitine, attenuated the reperfusion-induced increase in diastolic pressure and significantly improved the recovery of developed pressure.

Isolated mitochondrial function

Table 1 summarizes the data obtained from mitochondria isolated by using the two extraction media described in the methods section. Initial rate, total amount of mitochondrial ATP produced and calcium content are shown in Figure 2.

The data reported in Table 1 as series I refer to mitochondria isolated in a medium containing KCl, EDTA and albumin, whilst those reported as series II refer to mitochondria isolated in the EDTA-free medium containing sucrose and ruthenium red. Preliminary experiments indicated that there is no significant difference between RCR, QO_2, ADP/O, yield and calcium content values of mitochondria isolated from hearts after 30 or 120 minutes of aerobic perfusion and those obtained for mitochondria from freshly excised, non-

Table 1. Effect of L-propionyl-carnitine (L-P-C) on the ischaemic and reperfusion induced alterations in isolated mitochondrial function.

Experiments	RCR		QO_2		ADP/O		Yield	
Series	I	II	I	II	I	II	I	II
150 min aeorbic perfusion								
Control	17.8 ± 1.7	7.6 ± 1.7 $P_1 < 0.001$	247 ± 17.1	196 ± 11.0 $P_1 < 0.05$	2.8 ± 0.1	2.2 ± 0.5 $P_1 < 0.05$	12.4 ± 2.3	7.0 ± 0.9 $P_1 < 0.05$
+ L-P-C 10^{-7} M	16.9 ± 2.3	7.4 ± 0.9 $P_1 < 0.001$	240 ± 18.1	171 ± 9.3 $P_1 < 0.05$	2.7 ± 0.1	2.2 ± 0.7 $P_1 < 0.05$	12.6 ± 2.7	8.3 ± 1.6 $P_1 < 0.05$
60 min ischaemic perfusion								
Control	7.3 ± 1.6	3.4 ± 2.0 $P_1 < 0.001$	159 ± 9.8	104 ± 3.9 $P_1 < 0.05$	2.5 ± 0.5	1.8 ± 0.7 $P_1 < 0.05$	7.9 ± 2.6	3.0 ± 0.6 $P_1 < 0.05$
+ L-P-C 10^{-7} M	12.1 ± 1.9*	6.7 ± 1.4** $P_1 < 0.001$	214 ± 7.1*	181 ± 2.7** $P_1 < 0.05$	2.7 ± 0.3*	2.2 ± 0.2* $P_1 < 0.05$	1.0 ± 1.3*	7.0 ± 1.1** $P_1 < 0.05$
Ischaemia + 30 min reperfusion								
Control	7.1 ± 1.9	2.1 ± 0.6 $P_1 < 0.001$	111 ± 12.1	60.5 ± 4.0 $P_1 < 0.05$	2.3 ± 0.3	1.5 ± 0.6 $P_1 < 0.05$	6.3 ± 1.9	2.8 ± 1.0 $P_1 < 0.05$
+ L-P-C 10^{-7} M	14.1 ± 1.2**	7.1 ± 1.1** $P_1 < 0.001$	199 ± 12.1	151 ± 2.9** $P_1 < 0.05$	2.7 ± 0.1*	2.1 ± 0.3** $P_1 < 0.05$	11.3 ± 1.1**	6.9 ± 0.5** $P_1 < 0.05$

The data are expressed as mean ± S.E. Series I refers to the results obtained for KCl, EDTA and albumine containing media; series II to those obtained using sucrose-ruthenium red containing media. P_1 relates to the significance of the difference between the value obtained using medium I and II in each experimental condition. *P_2 < 0.05; *P_2 < 0.01, where P relates to the significance of the difference between the control and the relative L-propionyl-carnitine treated group. QO_2 is expressed as nmoles O_2/mg prot and yield as mg prot/g wt weight.

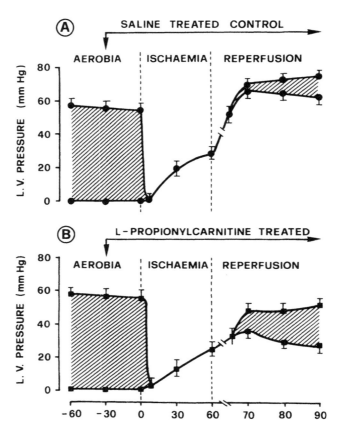

Fig. 1. Effect of L-propionyl-carnitine on the ischaemic and reperfusion induced alterations of left ventricular developed and diastolic pressure. Under aerobic and reperfusion conditions the hearts were perfused at a mean coronary flow of 25 ml/min. Ischaemia was induced (at time 0) by reducing coronary flow to 1 ml/min. L-propionyl-carnitine administration was started 30 min before the onset of ischaemia. Each point is the mean of six separate experiments and results are expressed as mean ± S.E. P relates to the significance of the difference between the controls, and the relative L-propionyl-carnitine treated group.

perfused hearts.

Table 1 shows that The RCR, QO_2, and ADP/O values obtained for mitochondria isolated in medium I, were always significantly higher than those obtained for mitochondria extracted after the same experimental conditions but using medium II. The yield of mitochondria extracted in medium I was also higher than that obtained in medium II, indicating that fewer mitochondria can be isolated using this medium. As expected, the calcium content of mitochondria from series I was, in each condition, significantly lower than that of mitochondria isolated in the presence of ruthenium red and absence of EDTA.

From Table I it appears that in control hearts 60 minutes of ischaemia, induced a reduction of mitochondrial RCR and QO_2 independently from the medium used, whilst ADP/O ratio was reduced only for ischaemic mitochondria isolated in medium II. This suggests that the composition of medium I was able to maintain the phosphorylating capacity (ADP/O) of the ischaemic mitochondria despite the reduction in the respiration rate (QO_2 and RCR). This is also evident from the data reported in Figure 2, showing that ischaemia induced a reduction in the rate of ATP production but no changes in the total amount of ATP produced.

The RCR, QO_2, ADP/O of reperfused mitochondria were also significantly reduced, irrespective of the medium used. The calcium content of mitochondria isolated in medium II from ischaemic and, particularly, from reperfused myocardium was significantly increased. In contrast, calcium content of the mitochondria from the same ischaemic and reperfused hearts, but isolated in medium I, was unchanged from that of the aerobic mitochondria, indicating that the EDTA content of medium I was able to buffer all the calcium during the extraction procedure.

Administration of L-propionyl-carnitine made no difference to the oxidative phosphorylating activity or to the calcium content of mitochondria isolated after aerobic perfusion. The yield was also unchanged. The deterioration of mitochondrial respiration and the increase in calcium content induced by ischaemia and reperfusion can be prevented by L-propionyl-carnitine administration at 10^{-7} M, irrespective of which extraction medium was used. Nevertheless, the differences in RCR, QO_2, and ADP/O values between mitochondria from hearts treated with L-propionyl-carnitine and those from control hearts were always higher when the extraction was carried out with medium II.

Figure 2 shows the pattern of ATP production from mitochondria harvested after the different experimental condition. In the control, aerobic mitochondria about 1 minute after the addition of ADP, 390 n moles of ATP/mg protein were produced and 144 n atoms of oxygen/mg of protein were consumed, yielding an ATP/O ratio of 2.70. Figure 2 shows that ischaemia induced a

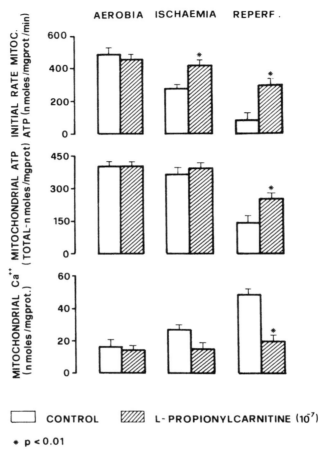

Fig. 2. Effect of L-propionyl-carnitine on initial rate, total ATP production and calcium content of mitochondria isolated after 150 min of aerobic perfusion, or after 60 min of ischaemic perfusion or after ischaemia followed by reperfusion. Each point is the mean of at least six separate experiments and results are expressed as mean ± S.E.

decline of the rate of mitochondrial ATP production, although the total production of ATP was maintained. Reperfusion further reduced the rate and the net ATP production, yielding an ATP/O value of only 0.33 ± 1.5. Treatment with L-propionyl-carnitine had no effect on the total amount or on the initial rate of ATP production from mitochondria isolated from aerobic perfused hearts. L-propionyl-carnitine at 10^{-7} M increased the initial rate of ATP production of the ischaemic mitochondria. Furthermore, L-propionyl-

Table II. Effect of direct administration of L-propionyl-carnitine (L-P-C) to the isolated mitochondria after 120 minutes aerobic perfusion, 60 minutes ischaemia and 60 minutes ischaemia + 30 minutes reperfusion.

Experiments	RCR		QO_2		ADP/O	
Series	I	II	I	II	I	II
150 min aerobic perfusion						
Control	16.0	5.6	251	194	2.78	2.33
L-P-C (5 uM)	15.9	5.2	248	190	2.77	2.31
L-P-C (15 uM)	15.9	5.2	250	192	2.77	2.33
60 min ischaemic perfusion						
Control	10.7	3.4	187	124	2.52	1.91
L-P-C (5 uM)	10.4	3.2	187	120	2.53	1.78
L-P-C (15 uM)	10.1	3.1	188	121	2.45	1.90
60 min ischaemia + 30 min reperfusion						
Control	5.8	1.1	121	62	2.25	1.55
L-P-C (5 uM)	5.6	1.0	122	62	2.24	1.53
L-P-C (15 uM)	5.5	1.2	120	62	2.22	1.45

The data represent the mean of at least 5 experiments. Series I refers to results obtained with KCl, EDTA, albumin containing media, Series II to mitochondria extracted using sucrose-ruthenium red media. L-propionyl-carnitine (L-P-C) was added to the incubation media to provide a final conc. of 5 or 15 uM. Because there was no difference after the addition L-propionyl-carnitine, standard errors and statistical analysis are not reported. QO_2 is expressed as nmoles O_2/mg prot.

carnitine significantly increased total and initial rate of ATP production of the mitochondria isolated after reperfusion.

Finally, Table II shows that when L-propionyl-carnitine was added directly to the isolated mitochondria in the reaction medium to provide a final concentration of 5 uM and 15 uM there was no significant change in their oxidative phosphorylating capacities.

ATP and CP reserves

The results are summarized in Figure 3. As expected, in control heart ischaemia resulted in a decline of endogenous stores of ATP and CP and reperfusion failed to restore tissue content of these nucleotides.

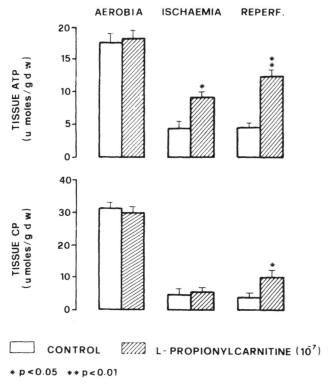

Fig. 3. Effect of L-propionyl-carnitine treatment on the ischaemic and reperfusion induced deterioration of tissue ATP and CP content. Results are expressed as mean ± S.E. of six individual experiments. Tests of significance calculated with respect to the difference between the control and the relative treated groups.

Administration of L-propionyl-carnitine had no effect on the ATP and CP content of the aerobically perfused heart. Administration of L-propionyl-carnitine reduced the ischaemic induced depauperation of ATP but failed to maintain CP stores. In addition, L-propionyl-carnitine significantly improved the recovery of tissue ATP and CP after reperfusion, but no complete restoration of energy stores was found.

Discussion

The results in this study indicate that administration of L-propionyl-carnitine was able to reduce some of the damage caused by ischaemia and subsequent reperfusion in the isolated and perfused rabbit hearts. There are four confirmatory groups of evidence in support of the general conclusion that L-propionyl-carnitine has a protective effect: -1) the rise of diastolic pressure during ischaemia and reperfusion was diminished with a greater percentage of recovery of developed pressure; -2) the oxygen consumption and ATP generating capacity of mitochondria were well maintained despite the prolonged period of ischaemia and subsequent reperfusion -3) mitochondrial calcium overload was reduced; -4) there was preservation of endogenous ATP and CP stores. This protective effect is specific for L-propionyl-carnitine as we have previously shown that, in the same experimental model, L-carnitine (7,18) and propionic acid (7,9) were not active.

In the experiments reported here, total coronary flow was controlled by a constant flow pump. During readmission of flow, coronary perfusion pressure, which in the presence of constant flow is an indirect measurement of coronary resistances, did not differ between the control and the treated hearts. It seems, therefore, that coronary vasodilation or enhancement of tissue perfusion are not important factors in the cardioprotective effect of L-propionyl-carnitine which we have observed. A lowered myocardial oxygen demand prior or at the time of ischaemia is also an unlikely factor as L-propionyl-carnitine did not modify peak of developed pressure before ischaemia or the onset of quiescience during ischaemia. Heart rate was also kept constant by atrial stimulation in all groups. However, it should be recalled here that in the hearts receiving L-propionyl-carnitine, tissue levels of ATP after ischaemia were significantly better maintained. These findings are in agreement with the data reported by Paulson et al. (4) showing that L-propionyl-carnitine increased the concentration of ATP and CP of isolated rat hearts subjected to 90 min of ischaemia.

It is likely that L-propionyl-carnitine improved the residual oxidative metabolism of the ischaemic myocytes by enhancing palmitate oxidation (7). Amelioration of oxidative metabolism under the severe condition of ischaemia which we used is limited by the drastic reduction of coronary flow and, therefore, of oxygen availability. However, it should be taken into consideration that maintenance of active contraction utilizes as much as the 75 - 80% of total cellular ATP production. Therefore, the ischaemic-induced cessation of contraction already removes an enormous energy drain on the cell. Under these conditions, even a small improvement of residual oxidative metabolism is likely to yield the enhanced tissue ATP content reported in this study, which in turn, may be important for assuring normal ion homeostasis and membrane integrity (11,13). In accordance to this hypothesis is the finding that L-propionyl-carnitine protected the function of mitochondria isolated after ischaemia and reperfusion.

In this study several precautions have been taken to determine isolated mitochondria function. Two different isolation media have been used and the data shown in Table 1 indicate that conditions of isolation are important in the interpretation of the results. Interestingly the effects of L-propionyl-carnitine were always more evident for the mitochondria isolated in medium II than for those in medium I. Amelioration of the ischaemic induced-mitochondrial dysfunction by L-propionyl-carnitine has been reported before in dogs (19) and in rats (7) and it has been suggested to be dependent upon a reduction in long-chain acyl CoA accumulation (7,19), although Paulson et al. (4) reported that L-propionyl-carnitine does not significantly affect the amount of long-chain acyl CoA in the ischaemic myocardium. Since L-propionyl-carnitine is supposed to have no direct effect on mitochondrial calcium transport (7), and when administered directly to the isolated mitochondria failed to improve their function, it must be assumed that its beneficial action depends on an "in vivo" effect. Two possibilities should be considered in this regard. Firstly, administration of L-propionyl-carnitine might preserve mitochondria function by promoting the formation in the myocardium of both propionyl CoA and carnitine. L-propionyl-carnitine is easily transported in the myocytes and within the cell into mitochondria via the carnitine-dependent translocase system. Once in the mitochondria it is converted into propionyl-CoA and carnitine (20). Propionyl-CoA is then converted into succinyl-CoA (21) increasing the flux through the Krebs cycle and the utilization of acetyl-CoA. Carnitine, on the other hand, removes long-chain-acyl-CoA accumulated in the ischaemic conditions, thus again increasing the flux in the Krebs cycle.

In addition, L-propionyl-carnitine could preserve cellular and mitochondrial membrane integrity during the ischaemic period. We have previously demonstrated (22) that L-propionyl-carnitine is able to protect isolated heart mitochondria against the ferrous ions-induced lipid peroxidation damage. This protective effect of L-propionyl-carnitine could not be explained in terms of a reduction of lipid peroxidation, as malondialdehyde formation was not modified (22). We concluded that the most likely explanation was an interaction of the compound with the lipid bilayer, leading to a stabilizing effect. It is possible that the length of the esterified acid with L-carnitine regulates this interaction. This would explain the ineffectiveness of L-carnitine to protect mitochondrial function (18,22) and the reported higher efficiency of long-chain acyl-carnitine in protecting the myocardium from enzyme release (23).

In summary, we have provided specific evidence that L-propionyl-carnitine exerts a dose dependent cardioprotection against ischaemia and reperfusion in the isolated and perfused rabbit hearts. The beneficial effect is extended to mitochondrial function characterized by maintenance of oxidative-phosphorylating capacity, ATP production and prevention of calcium overload. This, in turn, is likely to depend on the metabolic and membranes stabilizing properties of L-propionyl-carnitine.

Summary

The aim of the present study was to investigate if treatment with L-propionyl-carnitine is able to reduce some of the deleterious effects caused by ischaemia and reperfusion in the isolated Langendorff perfused rabbit hearts. L-propionyl-carnitine (10^{-7}M) delivered in the perfusate 30 min before ischaemia-reduced the ischaemic-induced deterioration of mitochondrial function and the depauperation of tissue stores of ATP. On reperfusion, hearts treated with L-propionyl-carnitine recovered better than the untreated hearts with respect to left ventricular performance, replenishment of ATP and CP stores and mitochondrial function. The reperfusion-induced mitochondrial calcium overload was also reduced. It is concluded that L-propionyl-carnitine protects the myocardium against some of the deleterious effects of ischaemia and reperfusion and, in particular, prevents mitochondrial calcium overload and maintains mitochondrial function. Because this protection occurred in absence of negative inotropic effect during normoxia or of a coronary dilatatory effect during ischaemia, it cannot be attributed to an energy sparing effect or to improvement of oxygen delivery. Therefore, alternatively, mechanisms of action are to be considered.

Acknowledgements

This work was supported by the Italian C.N.R. grant 087432. We thank Miss Roberta Bonetti for secretarial assistance in preparing the manuscript and Miss Michela Palmieri for her technical assistance. We wish to thank Sigma-Tau, Rome, for kindly providing L-propionyl-carnitine.

References

1. Shug AJ, Thomsen JH, Folts JD, Bittar N, Klein MI, Koke JR, Huth PJ. Changes in tissue levels of carnitine and other metabolites during myocardial ischaemia and anoxia. Arch Biochem Biophys 1978;187:25-33.
2. Suzuki Y, Kamikawa T, Kobayashi A, Masumura Y, Yamazachi N. Effects of L-carnitine on tissue levels of acyl carnitine, acyl coenzyme A and high energy phosphate in ischemic dog hearts. Jap Circ J 1981;45:687-694.
3. Folts JD, Shug AL, Koke JR, Bittar N. Protection of the ischemic dog myocardium with carnitine. Am J Cardiol 1978;41:209-214.
4. Paulson DJ, Traxler J, Schmidt M, Noonan J, Shug AL. Protection of the ischemic myocardium by L-propionyl-carnitine: Effects on the recovery of cardiac output after ischaemia and reperfusion, carnitine transport, and fatty acid oxidation. Cardiovasc Res 1986;20:536-541.
5. Liedtke AJ, Demaison L, Nellis S. Effects of L-propionyl-carnitine on mechanical recovery during reflow in intact hearts. Am J Physiol 1988;255:H169-H176.
6. Ferrari R, Curello S, Ceconi C, Guarnieri C, Albertini A, Visioli O. Alteration of glutathione metabolism and of GDP activity during myocardial ischaemia and reperfusion. J Mol Cell Cardiol 1984;16:18.
7. Siliprandi N, Di Lisa F, Pivetta A, Miotto G, Siliprandi D. Transport and function of L-carnitine and L-propionyl-carnitine: relevance to some cardiomyopathies and cardiac ischaemia. Z Kardiol 1987;76(Suppl. 5):34-40.
8. Ferrari R, Ceconi C, Curello S, Pasini E, Visioli O. Protective effect of propionyl-l-carnitine against ischaemia and reperfusion-damage. Mol Cell Biochem 1989;88:161-168.
9. Ferrari R, Cargnoni A, Pasini E, Boffa GM, Ceconi C, Curello S. The effects of L-propionyl-carnitine on the ischaemic and reperfused myocardium. Cardiovasc Drugs Ther. In press, 1991.
10. Krebs HA, Henseleit K. Untersuchungen uber die Harnstoffbildung im Tierkorper. Hoppe-Seyler's Physiol Chem 1932;210:33-66.
11. Ferrari R, Albertini A, Curello S, Ceconi C, Di Lisa F, Raddino R, Visioli O. Myocardial recovery during post-ischaemic reperfusion. Effect of nifedipine, calcium and magnesium. J Mol Cell Cardiol 1986;18:487-498.

12. Ferrari R, Williams AJ, Di Lisa F. The role of mitochondrial function in the ischaemic and reperfused myocardium. In: Advances in Studies on Heart Metabolism, (edited by CM Caldarera, P Harris). Clueb Publications, Bologna, Italy, 1982, pp. 245-255.
13. Ferrari R, Williams AJ. The role of mitochondria in myocardial damage occurring on post-ischaemic reperfusion. J Appl Cardiol 1986;1:501-519.
14. Sordhal LA, McCollum WB, Wood WG, Schwartz A. Mitochondria and sarcoplasmic reticulum function in cardiac hypertrophy and failure. Am J Physiol 1973;244:497-502.
15. Peng GF, Rane JJ, Murphy ML, Straub KD. Abnormal mitochondrial oxidative phosphorylation of ischaemic myocardium reversed by calcium diluting agents. J Mol Cell Cardiol 1977;9:897-908.
16. Bradford MM. A rapid and sensitive method for the qualification of microgram quantities of protein utilizing the principle for protein binding. Anal Biochem 1978;72:248-254.
17. Lamprecht W, Trautschold E. Adenosine-5'-triphosphate determination with hexokinase and glucose-6-phosphate dehydrogenase. In: Method of Enzymatic Analysis, (edited by HU Bergmeyer). Academic Press Inc, New York, 1974, pp. 2101-2105.
18. Di Lisa F, Raddino R, Ferrari R. Modificazioni metaboliche e contrattili indotte da diversi substrati in corso di ischemia sperimentale e successiva riperfusione. G Clin Fisiopatol Cardiovasc 1982;1:65-75.
19. Kotaka K, Miyazaki Y, Ogawa K, Satake T, Kitazawa M, Sugitama S, Ozawa T. Protective effects of carnitine and its derivatives against free fatty acid-induced myocardial dysfunction. J Appl Biochem 1981;3:328-336.
20. Clarke PRH, Bieber LL. Effect of micelles on the kinetics of purified beef heart mitochondrial carnitine Palmitoyltransferase. J Biol Chem 1981;256:9869-9873.
21. Davis EJ, Spydevold O, Bremer J. Pyruvate carboxylase and propionyl-CoA carboxylase as anaplerotic enzymes in skeletal muscle mitochondria. Eur J Biochem 1980;110:255-262.
22. Ferrari R, Ciampalini G, Agnoletti G, Cargnoni A, Ceconi C, Visioli O. Effect of L-carnitine derivatives on heart mitochondrial damage induced by lipid peroxidation. Pharmacol Res Comm 1988;20:125-132.

23. Hülsmann WC, Dubelaar ML, Lamers JMJ, Maccari F. Protection by acylcarnitines and phenylmethylsulfonyl fludride of rat heart subjected to ischemia and reperfusion. Biochimica et Biocpysica Acta 1985;847:62-66.

CPSIA information can be obtained at www.ICGtesting.com
Printed in the USA
LVOW011748210413

330169LV00003B/73/P

9 781461 365587